a LANGE medical book

CURRENT
Diagnosis &
Treatment of Sexually
Transmitted Diseases

Edited by

Jeffrey D. Klausner, MD, MPH
Director, STD Prevention and Control Services
San Francisco Department of Public Health
Associate Clinical Professor of Medicine
Department of Medicine, Divisions of AIDS
  and Infectious Diseases
University of California, San Francisco

Edward W. Hook III, MD
Professor of Medicine, Microbiology, and Epidemiology
University of Alabama at Birmingham
Director, STD Control Program
Jefferson County Department of Public Health
Birmingham, Alabama

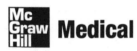 **Medical**

New York   Chicago   San Francisco   Lisbon   London   Madrid   Mexico City
New Delhi   San Juan   Seoul   Singapore   Sydney   Toronto

The McGraw·Hill Companies

Current Diagnosis & Treatment of Sexually Transmitted Diseases

1 2 3 4 5 6 7 8 9 0   DOC/DOC   0 9 8 7

ISBN-13: 978-0-07-145606-7
ISBN-10 : 0-07-145606-6
ISSN: 1935-5017

Notice

Medicine is an ever-changing science. As new research and clinical experience broaden our knowledge, changes in treatment and drug therapy are required. The authors and the publisher of this work have checked with sources believed to be reliable in their efforts to provide information that is complete and generally in accord with the standards accepted at the time of publication. However, in view of the possibility of human error or changes in medical sciences, neither the authors nor the publisher nor any other party who has been involved in the preparation or publication of this work warrants that the information contained herein is in every respect accurate or complete, and they disclaim all responsibility for any errors or omissions or for the results obtained from use of the information contained in this work. Readers are encouraged to confirm the information contained herein with other sources. For example and in particular, readers are advised to check the product information sheet included in the package of each drug they plan to administer to be certain that the information contained in this work is accurate and that changes have not been made in the recommended dose or in the contraindications for administration. This recommendation is of particular importance in connection with new or infrequently used drugs.

This book was set in Adobe Garamond by International Typesetting and Composition.
The editors were James Shanahan and Harriet Lebowitz.
The production supervisor was Sherri Souffrance.
The illustration manager was Charissa Baker.
The designer was Eve Siegel; the cover designer was Mary Mckeon.
RR Donnelly was printer and binder.

This book is printed on acid-free paper.

Cover photo credits clockwise from top left: doctor, GettyImages; artistic depiction of AIDS treatment, JOUBERT/Photo Researchers Inc; hepatitis B virus, CMEABG-ACBL/Photo Researchers Inc.

INTERNATIONAL EDITION ISBN-13: 978-0-07-110461-6; ISBN-10: 0-07-110461-5

Contents

II. INFECTIONS

30. Commonly Encountered Genital Dermatoses
Laura Hinkle Bachmann, MD, MPH

31. The Sexual History
Jeffrey D. Klausner, MD, MPH

Appendix

Index

Authors

Renata Arrington-Sanders, MD, MPH
Adolescent Medicine Fellow
Division of General Pediatrics and Adolescent Medicine
Johns Hopkins University
Baltimore, Maryland
rarring3@jhmi.edu
Chapter 23, Sexually Transmitted Diseases in Adolescents

Michael Augenbraun, MD
Professor of Medicine
SUNY-Downstate Medical Center
Brooklyn, New York
michael.augenbraun@downstate.edu
Chapter 19, Syphilis

Natali Aziz, MD, MS
Clinical Fellow, Reproductive Infectious Diseases and
    Maternal-Fetal Medicine
Department of Obstetrics, Gynecology and Reproductive
    Sciences
University of California, San Francisco
naziz@stanford.edu
azizn@obgyn.ucsf.edu
Chapter 22, Sexually Transmitted Diseases in Pregnancy

Laura Hinkle Bachmann, MD, MPH
Assistant Professor of Medicine, Epidemiology, and
    International Health
Department of Medicine, Division of Infectious Diseases
University of Alabama at Birmingham
lbachmann@idmail.dom.uab.edu
Chapter 30, Commonly Encountered Genital Dermatoses

Peter V. Chin-Hong, MD
Assistant Professor
Division of Infectious Diseases
Department of Medicine
University of California, San Francisco
pvch@itsa.ucsf.edu
Chapter 15, External Genital Warts

Craig R. Cohen, MD, MPH
Associate Adjunct Professor
Department of Obstetrics, Gynecology and Reproductive
    Sciences
University of California, San Francisco
ccohen@globalhealth.ucsf.edu
Chapter 8, Pelvic Inflammatory Disease
Chapter 22, Sexually Transmitted Diseases in Pregnancy

Daniel E. Cohen, MD
Associate Medical Director
The Fenway Institute at Fenway Community Health
Instructor in Medicine
Harvard Medical School
Boston, Massachusetts
dcohen@fenwayhealth.org
Chapter 4, Genital Ulcer Disease

Myron S. Cohen, MD
J. Herbert Bate Distinguished Professor of Medicine,
    Microbiology and Immunology
Director, Division of Infectious Diseases
University of North Carolina at Chapel Hill
Chapel Hill, North Carolina
Myron_Cohen@med.unc.edu
Chapter 16, Gonorrhea

Jeri Dyson, MD
Assistant Professor of General Pediatrics and Adolescent
    Medicine
University of Florida
Jacksonville, Florida
jeri.dyson@jax.ufl.edu
Chapter 23, Sexually Transmitted Diseases in Adolescents

Jonathan Ellen, MD
Associate Professor of General Pediatrics and Adolescent
    Medicine
Johns Hopkins Hospital
Baltimore, Maryland
jellen@jhmi.edu
Chapter 23, Sexually Transmitted Diseases in Adolescents

William M. Geisler, MD, MPH
Assistant Professor of Medicine
Department of Medicine, Division of Infectious Diseases
University of Alabama at Birmingham
wgeisler@uab.edu
Chapter 6, Epididymitis & the Acute Scrotum Syndrome
Chapter 13, Genital Chlamydial Infections

Philip M. Grant, MD
Acting Instructor
University of Washington School of Medicine
Harborview Medical Center
Seattle, Washington
pmgrant@u.washington.edu
Chapter 7, Persistent & Recurrent Urethritis

Michael E. Hagensee, MD, PhD
Department of Medicine, Section of Infectious Disease
Louisiana State University Health Sciences Center
New Orleans, Louisiana
mhagen@lsuhsc.edu
Chapter 29, Management of Abnormal Pap Smears

Christopher S. Hall, MD, MS
Assistant Adjunct Professor, Division of Infectious
    Diseases
University of California San Francisco
Chief, Office of Clinical Affairs
California Department of Health Services STD Control
    Branch
California STD/HIV Prevention Training Center
Oakland, California
chall@dhs.ca.gov
Chapter 17, Lymphogranuloma Venereum

Thomas M. Hooton, MD
Professor of Medicine/Infectious Diseases
University of Miami Miller School of Medicine
Miami, Florida
thooton@med.miami.edu
Chapter 7, Persistent & Recurrent Urethritis

Edward W. Hook III, MD
Professor of Medicine, Microbiology, and Epidemiology
Department of Medicine, Division of Infectious Diseases
Director, STD Control Program
Jefferson County Department of Public Health
Birmingham, Alabama
ehook@uab.edu
Chapter 26, Principles of Serologic Testing for Syphilis

Richard H. Kahn, MS
Centers for Disease Control and Prevention
Division of Parasitic Diseases, Malaria Branch
Atlanta, Georgia
rkahn@cdc.gov
Chapter 28, Partner Notification & Management

Jeffrey D. Klausner, MD, MPH
Director, STD Prevention and Control Services
San Francisco Department of Public Health
Associate Clinical Professor of Medicine
Department of Medicine, Divisions of AIDS and
    Infectious Diseases
University of California, San Francisco
Jeff.Klausner@sfdph.org
*Chapter 1, Screening Guidelines for Sexually Transmitted
    Diseases, Including HIV*
Chapter 31, The Sexual History

John N. Krieger, MD
Professor of Urology
University of Washington School of Medicine
Chief of Urology
VA Puget Sound Health Care System
Attending surgeon
University of Washington Medical Center
Harborview Medical Center
Children's Orthopedic Hospital
Seattle, Washington
jkrieger@u.washington.edu
Chapter 6, Epididymitis & the Acute Scrotum Syndrome

Peter Leone, MD
Associate Professor of Medicine
University of North Carolina, Chapel Hill
Chapel Hill, North Carolina
Peter_Leone@med.unc.edu
Chapter 14, Genital Herpes
Chapter 16, Gonorrhea

Jeanne M. Marrazzo, MD, MPH
Associate Professor of Medicine
Division of Allergy and Infectious Diseases
University of Washington
Medical Director, Seattle STD/HIV Prevention Training
    Center
Seattle, Washington
jmm2@u.washington.edu
Chapter 10, Cervicitis
*Chapter 25, Sexually Transmitted Diseases in Women Who
    Have Sex with Women*

David H. Martin, MD
Harry E. Dascomb Professor of Medicine and
    Microbiology
Chief, Section of Infectious Diseases
Director, Gulf South STI TM Cooperative Research
    Center
Louisiana State University Health Sciences Center
New Orleans, Louisiana
dhmartin@lsuhsc.edu
Chapter 12, Chancroid

Kenneth Mayer, MD
Professor of Medicine
Brown University
Providence, Rhode Island
Kenneth_Mayer@Brown.edu
Chapter 4, Genital Ulcer Disease

Lisa A. Mills, MD
Infectious Diseases Fellow
Johns Hopkins Medical Institutions
Baltimore, Maryland
lmills7@jhmi.edu
*Chapter 21, Sexually Transmitted Diseases in
    HIV-infected Persons*

Joel M. Palefsky, MD
Professor of Medicine
Director of General Clinical Research Center
Associate Dean for Clinical and Translational Research
University of California, San Francisco
Joel.Palefsky@ucsf.edu
Chapter 15, External Genital Warts

Thomas A. Peterman, MD, MSc
Chief, Field Epidemiology Unit
Division of STD Prevention
Centers for Disease Control and Prevention
Atlanta, Georgia
tpeterman@cdc.gov
Chapter 28, Partner Notification & Management

Thomas C. Quinn, MD
Professor of Medicine
Johns Hopkins University
Baltimore, Maryland
tquinn@jhmi.edu
*Chapter 21, Sexually Transmitted Diseases in
    HIV-infected Persons*

Cornelis A. Rietmeijer, MD, PhD
Director, STD Control Program
Denver Public Health Department
Professor, Department of Preventive Medicine and
    Biometrics
University of Colorado at Denver and Health Sciences
    Center
Denver, Colorado
cornelis.rietmeijer@dhha.org
Chapter 27, Principles of Risk Reduction Counseling

Anne M. Rompalo, MD
Professor of Medicine
Johns Hopkins University School of Medicine
Baltimore, Maryland
arompalo@jhmi.edu
Chapter 9, Proctitis & Proctocolitis

Jane R. Schwebke, MD
Professor of Medicine
Division of Infectious Diseases
University of Alabama at Birmingham
schwebke@uab.edu
Chapter 2, Vaginal Discharge
Chapter 11, Bacterial Vaginosis
Chapter 18, Trichomoniasis

Arlene C. Sena, MD, MPH
Clinical Associate Professor of Medicine
University of North Carolina, Chapel Hill
Medical Director, Durham County Health Department
Durham, North Carolina
idrod@med.unc.edu
Chapter 16, Gonorrhea

Roger P. Simon, MD
Chair and Director
R S Dow Neurobiology Laboratories
Legacy Research
Adjunct Professor Neurology, Physiology &
    Pharmacology
Oregon Health & Sciences University
Portland, Oregon
rsimon@downeurobiology.org
Chapter 20, Neurosyphilis

Walter E. Stamm, MD
Professor of Medicine
Department of Medicine
University of Washington School of Medicine
Seattle, Washington
wes@u.washington.edu
Chapter 13, Genital Chlamydial Infections

Heidi Swygard, MD, MPH
Clinical Assistant Professor of Medicine
University of North Carolina, Chapel Hill
Heidi_Swygard@med.unc.edu
Chapter 16, Gonorrhea

Stephanie N. Taylor, MD
Medical Director, Delgado Personal Health Center
Associate Professor of Medicine and Microbiology
Section of Infectious Diseases
Louisiana State University Health Sciences Center
New Orleans, Louisiana
staylo2@lsuhsc.edu
Chapter 12, Chancroid

Harold C. Wiesenfeld, MDCM
Associate Professor of Obstetrics, Gynecology
    and Reproductive Sciences
University of Pittsburgh School of Medicine/
    Magee-Women's Research
Institute
Co-Director, Sexually Transmitted Diseases Program
Allegheny County Health Department
Pittsburgh, Pennsylvania
hwiesenfeld@mail.magee.edu
Chapter 5, Lower Abdominal Pain in Women

William Wong, MD
Medical Director
Division of STD/HIV/AIDS
Chicago Department of Public Health
Chicago, Illinois
wong_will@cdph.org
*Chapter 24, Sexually Transmitted Diseases in Men Who
Have Sex with Men*

Mark H. Yudin, MD, MSc, FRCSC
Department of Obstetrics and Gynecology
University of Toronto
Toronto, Ontario, Canada
yudinm@smh.toronto.on.ca
Chapter 5, Lower Abdominal Pain in Women

Jonathan M. Zenilman, MD
Chief, Infectious Diseases Division
Johns Hopkins Bayview Medical Center
Professor, Division of Infectious Diseases
Department of Medicine
Johns Hopkins University School of Medicine
Baltimore, Maryland
jzenilma@jhmi.edu
Chapter 3, Urethral Discharge

Preface

Sexually transmitted diseases (STDs) are common problems that have an impact on patients seen by many, if not all, clinicians, irrespective of their chosen practice. Family practitioners, internists, pediatricians, obstetrician-gynecologists, urologists, and dermatologists all regularly care for patients at risk for STDs. They are also common: the Centers for Disease Control and Prevention (CDC) estimates that nearly 20 million new STD cases occur each year, with about half among people less than 25 years of age. In addition, STD diagnosis and management is a dynamic area in medicine with significant recent advances in prevention, diagnosis, treatment, and clinical care. The advent of a vaccine for human papillomavirus, which is recommended for females aged 9–26, provides an important opportunity for clinicians to assess and discuss sexual activity with adolescents and their parents while offering a highly effective preventive intervention. Similarly, for the most common bacterial STDs, nucleic acid-based assays enable rapid and accurate identification of infections by clinicians, using noninvasively collected specimens (urine) and eliminating barriers to screening. Finally, multiple clinical trials have demonstrated the safety and efficacy of single-dose therapy for a number of common STDs and the widespread recognition that reinfection is common has led to important changes in partner management and recommendations for retesting. Each of these new elements for managing the infections caused by the nearly 30 organisms that are principally transmitted sexually provides clinicians with new tools for efficient, effective STD management.

We hope that the busy clinician, whether the experienced subspecialist, recently trained graduate, or *hard-working mid-level practitioner*, will find the up-to-date, practical, and evidence-based chapters in *Current Diagnosis Management of Sexually Transmitted Diseases* a useful and easy reference guiding the day-to-day clinical care of the patients they surely see who are at risk for STDs. Students of medicine and physicians in training will note the informative discussions of epidemiology and pathogenesis in certain chapters and tables summarizing the differential diagnosis of syndromes, lists of etiologic organisms, and clinical practice points.

Leading experts in medicine, surgery, obstetrics and gynecology, and pediatrics have joined together to create this first edition to further the appropriate and timely diagnosis and treatment of sexually transmitted diseases. Highlights of this edition include current U.S. STD and HIV screening guidelines, syndromic-based evaluations and rapid point-of-care tests, new evidence of the role of certain infections like *Mycoplasma genitalium*, and the renewed recognition of old diseases like lymphogranuloma venereum. Attention should be paid to chapters that focus on prevention—risk-reduction counseling and partner notification—which can enable the clinician to serve in his or her larger role as a potential agent of individual change and public health advocate. Lastly, recognizing the unique role of behavior and development in the risk and management of STDs, we have included specific chapters dedicated to special populations.

With the carefully composed chapters in this book, we hope that clinicians will be better able to manage sexually transmitted infections and, even more importantly, ally with their patients to prevent further infections and the continued spread of those diseases. As this is the first edition, we aim to continue to improve this text to increase its usefulness and welcome recommendations, comments, and criticism from our readers.

ACKNOWLEDGMENTS

We would like to acknowledge the hard work of the expert contributors whose dedication to the improvement of sexual health and knowledge was critical to the high quality of this text. We would like to acknowledge further our local administrative support staff, Joanne Carpio (San Francisco) and Sharron Hagy (Birmingham). Finally, we would like to acknowledge that without the support of our families (San Francisco: Tammy, Henry, Teddy, and Anna; and Birmingham: Kathy, Sarah, and Jessie) and their patience and tolerance of late nights and "working vacations," this text would not have been possible.

Jeffrey D. Klausner
San Francisco, California

Edward W. Hook III
Birmingham, Alabama

Introduction

Sexually transmitted diseases (STDs) are far too common and have an impact on the population in too many ways for them not to be of concern for most health care providers. Nearly all sexually active persons should now be considered at risk for STDs. Similarly, sexual activity should be assessed in every patient with resultant counseling and risk-appropriate STD screening. Dealing with STDs is not easy for patients or for providers.

For health care providers, the assumption that their patients are not at risk for STDs is now clearly incorrect. Old, unsubstantiated beliefs regarding the epidemiology, clinical manifestations, and management of STDs invited wrong assumptions about the impact that these common diseases have on patients in a wide variety of clinical settings. Population-based data demonstrating that more than 20% of Americans have genital herpes infection or that in excess of 50% of women will have human papillomavirus infection no longer allow clinicians to think that STDs involve persons other than their patients. Patients with STDs are present in private practices, in public and private clinics, and in virtually every other health care setting. This generalization is applicable to all those who provide primary care, as well as most specialists. Misperceptions that the clinical presentations of most STDs are readily apparent, that current treatment will resolve the problem when encountered, and perhaps most importantly, that STDs are not of great concern in a clinician's day-to-day practice, each contribute to the continuing unacceptable high rates of infection and their potential life-threatening consequences.

In addition, STDs are frequently asymptomatic or, if symptoms are present, they may not be sufficiently distinctive to lead infected persons to seek expeditiously evaluation and treatment. As a result in the majority of instances STDs are spread by persons who are unaware of their infections (ie, they are either asymptomatic or symptoms are attributed to other causes). With respect to therapy, incorrect diagnoses may lead to disease recurrence or failure of symptoms to resolve and, in the case of many of the most common STD syndromes (eg, vaginal discharge due to bacterial vaginosis in women, nongonococcal urethritis in men, and genital warts in both sexes), even recommended therapy results in clinical cure in 70–90% of infected persons.

For patients on the receiving end of both STD transmission and care, the appreciation that one is at risk is often difficult to acknowledge. STDs are stigma laden. As a result, many persons fail to seek STD screening or diagnosis because they are "not the sort of person" who is at risk for STDs. This in turn provides the basis for circular reasoning leading them not to seek evaluation and care and serving to reinforce the all too common misperception that others are somehow "the kind of person" who get STDs. As described above, data generated in the past two decades now provide the facts to challenge those misperceptions.

Putting together the needs of both patients and the health care providers who care for them, it is clear that STD management skills and clinical competency in STD care are essential in most health care settings. The task of providing STD assessment and management for all appropriate patients has been simplified by recent technological advances, but still presents clinicians with challenges. The large number of pathogens that may be sexually transmitted, the large variety of STD syndromes, and the complexity accompanying a broad range of sexual behaviors make it difficult for clinicians who wish to provide comprehensive sexual health care for their patients. At the same time, recent technologic progress has provided new opportunities. In June 2006, the approval by the United States Food and Drug Administration of a vaccine to prevent the STD (caused by human papillomavirus) that accounts for nearly all cervical cancer makes discussion of STDs and their prevention simultaneously more imperative and easier than ever before. Similarly, the advent of reliable sero-logic tests for herpes simplex virus and nucleic acid amplification tests, which allow screening for the most common bacterial STDs (*Chlamydia trachomatis* and *Neisseria gonorrhoeae* infections), using minimally inva-sive specimens such as voided urine or self-obtained vaginal swab specimens provides mechanisms for easier, more accurate STD screening. We hope that this book will provide useful, up-to-date information to clinicians about all facets of day-to-day STD management, from risk assessment and specimen collection to the treat-ment and followup of patients with STDs detected in the course of routine medical practice.

Screening Guidelines for Sexually Transmitted Diseases, Including HIV Infection

1

Jeffrey D. Klausner, MD, MPH

ESSENTIAL FEATURES

- *Most sexually transmitted diseases (STDs) are asymptomatic. Persons with asymptomatic STDs are at risk for complications and transmission of infection to others.*

- *In some cases, screening is the only means to detect and treat infection to prevent adverse outcomes.*

- *The judicious use of screening tests relies on appreciation of disease epidemiology and accurate assessment of a patient's sexual risk behavior.*

Most sexually transmitted diseases are asymptomatic. Patients often acquire infection from sex partners who exhibit no symptoms. Persons with asymptomatic infection may develop complications or sequelae without knowledge of being infected. The epidemiology of STDs—how those diseases are distributed within a population—is not random; risk factors that include age, gender, and sexual activity dictate who is likely to be infected. Screening and timely treatment have been shown to reduce the consequences of infection. National organizations, including the US Preventive Services Task Force and the Centers for Disease Control and Prevention (CDC), as well as professional medical societies, regularly review the current scientific literature and make evidence-based recommendations for STD and HIV screening. Individuals are advised to undergo STD testing not only to identify and treat asymptomatic infection (screening) but to monitor trends in the population (surveillance) and

confirm a diagnosis. Table 1–1 summarizes current STD and HIV screening recommendations.

Guidelines for Women's Health Care. American College of Obstetricians and Gynecologists, 1996.

Hauth JC, Merenstein GB (editors): *Guidelines for Perinatal Health Care,* 4th ed. American Academy of Pediatrics and the American College of Obstetricians and Gynecologists, 1997.

NONPREGNANT WOMEN

Routine screening for *Chlamydia trachomatis* has been shown to reduce the incidence of pelvic inflammatory disease (PID) and, on a population level, such screening may be associated with reductions in PID and ectopic pregnancy. All sexually active women aged 25 years and younger should be screened annually for *C trachomatis*, as should older women whose behaviors may place them at risk (ie, those with multiple or new sex partners). Recently some experts have suggested that the age range for *C trachomatis* screening should be expanded to encompass all sexually active women up to age 30 years. In addition to routine screening, new CDC guidelines recommend that women who test positive for chlamydia should be retested at 3 months to rule out reinfection.

Currently the most sensitive diagnostic assays are nucleic acid amplification tests (NAATs). Each available NAAT uses slightly different technology: polymerase chain reaction, strand displacement amplification, and transcription-mediated amplification. Overall these NAATs are significantly more sensitive than culture and more sensitive than nonamplified DNA probe assays. Specificity of these assays is very high (>99%). An additional advantage of these tests for screening is their simplified method of specimen collection. Obviating the need for pelvic examination, all currently available NAATs can be used on first-void urine specimens, and transcription-mediated amplification (APTIMA assays,

Table 1–1. Recommendations for sexually transmitted disease (STD) screening.[a]

Disease	Recommending Group	Population	Frequency	Considerations
Cervical cancer	Centers for Disease Control and Prevention (CDC), US Preventive Services Task Force (PSTF)	All women who have been sexually active and have a cervix	Within 3 y of onset of sexual activity or age 21 (whichever comes first) and screening at least every 3 y	Routine screening for cervical cancer is not recommended in women older than 65 y if they have had adequate recent screening with normal Pap smears and are not otherwise at high risk for cervical cancer
Chlamydia	CDC, PSTF	All sexually active women aged 25 y and younger, and other asymptomatic women at increased risk for infection (Age important risk marker. Other patient characteristics associated with a higher prevalence of infection include being unmarried, African-American race, having a prior history of STD, having new or multiple partners, having cervical ectopy, and using barrier contraceptives inconsistently); sexually active men who have sex with men (MSM) should be screened at relevant anatomic sites (rectum) every 3–12 months	Yearly	More frequent screening may be required in those with increased risk, recent partners with chlamydia, and recent prior history of chlamydia. CDC recommends that all women treated for chlamydia undergo repeat testing 3 mo after treatment.
Genital herpes	CDC, PSTF	Persons with HIV infection and at increased risk for acquiring HIV infection,[b] and those with a sex partner known to have genital herpes	Yearly	Although serologic screening is not recommended in asymptomatic pregnant women at any time during pregnancy to prevent neonatal HSV infection, the American College of Obstetricians and Gynecologists and state of California recommend obtaining a history of genital herpes disease or potential exposure in all pregnant women

Gonorrhea	CDC, PSTF	All sexually active women, including those who are pregnant, with increased risk for infection (ie, young age or other individual or population risk factors)[b]; sexually active MSM should be screened at relevant anatomic sites (throat and rectum) every 3–12 mo	
Hepatitis			
A or C	CDC, PSTF	None	
B	CDC, PSTF	Pregnant women at their first prenatal visit	
HIV	CDC, PSTF	All adolescents and adults seeking evaluation and treatment for STDs or those at increased risk for HIV infection[c]; All 13–64 year olds at least once; repeat based on risk behaviour	Yearly, but no optimal frequency clearly defined	CDC recommends routine testing in medical settings (ie, without required written informed consent or specific pre- or post-test counseling); results may be disclosed over the telephone. State laws regarding HIV testing requirements may vary.
Human papillomavirus	CDC, PSTF	None	
Syphilis	CDC, PSTF	Persons at increased risk for syphilis infection (MSM and those who engage in high-risk sexual behavior, commercial sex workers, persons who exchange sex for drugs, and those in adult correctional facilities); all pregnant women at their first prenatal visit, with testing repeated in the third trimester and at delivery in those in high risk groups	Yearly

(Continued)

Table 1-1. Recommendations for sexually transmitted disease (STD) screening.[a] *(Continued)*

Disease	Recommending Group	Population	Frequency	Considerations
Trichomonas vaginalis	CDC	None		Some experts recommend screening of pregnant women with a history of adverse outcomes in pregnancy (eg, premature rupture of membranes; preterm labor; low-birth-weight infant)

[a]Recommendations are for US adults as of 2006.

[b]Women and men younger than 25 years of age, including sexually active adolescents, are at highest risk for genital gonorrhea infection. Risk factors for gonorrhea include a history of previous gonorrhea infection, other sexually transmitted infections, new or multiple sexual partners, inconsistent condom use, sex work, and drug use. Risk factors for pregnant women are the same as for nonpregnant women. Prevalence of gonorrhea infection varies widely among communities and settings. African Americans and MSM have a higher prevalence of infection than the general population in many communities and settings.

[c]Persons at risk for HIV infection include men who have had sex with men after 1975; men and women having unprotected sex with multiple partners; past or present injection drug users; men and women who exchange sex for money or drugs or have sex partners who do; individuals whose past or present sex partners were infected with HIV; bisexual, or injection drug users; persons being treated for STDs; and those with a history of blood transfusion between 1978 and 1985. Persons who request an HIV test despite reporting no individual risk factors may also be considered at increased risk, because this group is likely to include individuals not willing to disclose high-risk behaviors. Others at risk include patients seen in high-risk or high-prevalence clinical settings, including STD clinics, correctional facilities, homeless shelters, tuberculosis clinics, clinics serving MSM, and adolescent health clinics with a high prevalence of STDs. High-prevalence settings are defined by the CDC as those known to have a 1% or greater prevalence of infection among the patient population being served.

GenProbe, Inc) is cleared by the Food and Drug Administration (FDA) for use on self-collected vaginal swabs.

In 2005 the US Preventive Services Task Force issued guidelines for gonorrhea screening in young women with select risk factors (eg, women with multiple partners, prior history of an STD, and black race). In areas where gonorrhea is relatively common, screening is likely to be beneficial and can be readily accomplished, because the same specimen collected for nucleic acid amplification testing for *C trachomatis* can also be used to test for *Neisseria gonorrhoeae*.

Beginning at age 21 or no later than 3 years after the onset of sexual activity, nonpregnant women should be screened annually for cervical disease using Papanicolaou (Pap) smears. The use of type-specific human papillomavirus testing remains under consideration as a screening tool. In women older than 30 years of age who have a history of normal results on three recent Pap smears, the frequency of screening can be reduced to every 2 or 3 years.

Syphilis screening using serologic tests for syphilis (rapid plasma reagin [RPR] or Venereal Disease Research Laboratories [VDRL] test) is not routinely recommended in nonpregnant women, nor is serologic screening for herpes simplex virus (HSV) infection. However, in women with select risk factors (eg, those who have multiple partners, exchange money or drugs for sex, have partners with other partners, have partners with an STD, or are at increased risk for HIV infection), some expert groups recommend syphilis testing and testing for HSV type 2 (HSV-2) antibody.

Routine screening in asymptomatic women is not recommended for trichomoniasis, bacterial vaginosis, or vaginal yeast infection.

PREGNANT WOMEN

Pregnant women are screened more aggressively for STDs than nonpregnant women because of the increased risk for adverse outcomes, including preterm delivery (resulting in low-birth-weight infants) and premature rupture of membranes (resulting in increased risk for chorioamnionitis). At the first prenatal visit all women should be screened for chlamydia and gonorrhea with an NAAT, and blood should be tested for syphilis (RPR or VDRL). Although HSV-2 antibody screening is not routinely recommended, a thorough history assessing risk for genital herpes—including prior episodes of genital ulcer disease, vesicular lesions, or recurrent urogenital symptoms of burning, pain, or erythema—is strongly recommended. If a current or prior sex partner has or had genital herpes, HSV-2 antibody screening is recommended. In most states, pregnant women must be offered HIV testing with the option to decline ("opt-out" testing). In asymptomatic pregnant women, evaluation

of vaginal fluid for the presence of trichomoniasis or bacterial vaginosis is recommended in women who are at increased risk for an adverse pregnancy outcome, primarily defined as women with a history of preterm delivery. Two studies have demonstrated no benefit and perhaps harm in asymptomatic low-risk pregnant women who were screened and treated for bacterial vaginosis or trichomoniasis.

HETEROSEXUAL MEN

There are no guidelines recommending routine STD screening of sexually active asymptomatic men. Although numerous studies have demonstrated high rates (5–15%) of asymptomatic chlamydial infections in select men (age younger than 25 years, incarcerated, urban residents), no national organization currently recommends routine chlamydia screening. In specific settings (eg, detention facilities and STD clinics), however, screening of asymptomatic men younger than 25 years of age is useful and has been associated with decreased rates of infection in the local community. Screening in that regard serves as a public health disease control strategy rather than a medical strategy to prevent the consequences of infection in an individual. Given the current low rates of asymptomatic gonococcal and syphilitic infections in much of the United States in men without specific risk factors (eg, men who have sex with men), screening for those infections is not routinely recommended. The prevalence of HSV-2 infection in some segments of the general adult population exceeds 20%; however, no recommendation currently exists for routine HSV-2 screening in persons without symptoms or known exposure to a partner with genital herpes. Screening for human papillomavirus infection is also not recommended.

New evidence suggests that screening for HIV infection should be routine in all sexually active adults, and the CDC recommends HIV screening for populations in which the prevalence is greater than 1%. The frequency of routine screening, however, remains unclear.

MEN WHO HAVE SEX WITH MEN

Men who have sex with men (MSM) with multiple partners are at increased risk for STDs and HIV infection. Several organizations recommend routine screening for rectal chlamydia, rectal and pharyngeal gonorrhea, syphilis, HIV infection, and HSV-2 infection in MSM as a public health measure to decrease the continued community-level transmission of those infections. Ample evidence also exists to support routine STD screening and treatment as an individual measure to reduce the risk of HIV acquisition and transmission. The optimal frequency of screening is unclear, and recommendations range from every 3–6 months in men with "many" partners to annually in those with "few" partners. Unfortunately, data are limited on which to form strong evidence-based guidelines about the frequency of screening.

STD SCREENING IN HIV-INFECTED PERSONS

In HIV care settings, it has been recommended that syphilis tests be conducted every 3 months, with routine immunologic and virologic monitoring and gonorrhea and chlamydia screening every 6 months. It is important to recognize that gonorrhea and chlamydia screening should be performed at each potentially exposed anatomic site where infection can occur. Thus, gonorrhea and chlamydia screening of the throat and rectum is recommended. NAATs have been proven to have superior sensitivity and comparable specificity to traditional culture of the throat and rectum. Nucleic acid amplification testing with strand displacement amplification or transcription-mediated amplification of specimens from those sites is also easier for the clinician and less laborious and time consuming for the laboratory. Although routine screening for cervical cancer caused by human papillomavirus infection is strongly recommended in HIV-infected women, the data are less robust in men and there are no national recommendations for anal cancer screening. The rates of anal cancer in men are similar to the rates of cervical cancer in women before the advent of routine cervical cancer screening (40–50 cases per 100,000 population); for this reason, some HIV care experts recommend routine anal cancer screening in HIV-infected men with annual or biannual anal Pap smears.

PRACTICE POINTS

- Obviating the need for pelvic examination, all currently available NAATs can be used on first-void urine specimens, and transcription-mediated amplification is cleared by the FDA for use on self-obtained vaginal swabs.

Relevant Web Sites

[Updated web-based guidelines are available at:]
http://www.ahrq.gov/clinic/uspstf/uspstopics.htm
http://www.cdc.gov/std/default.htm

SECTION I
Syndromes

Vaginal Discharge

2

Jane R. Schwebke, MD

ESSENTIALS OF DIAGNOSIS

- *Patient complaints and sexual history.*
- *Appearance of the discharge (character and color).*
- *Vaginal pH higher than 4.5.*
- *Presence of motile trichomonads, yeast or pseudohyphae, or clue cells on light microscopy.*
- *Positive "whiff" test.*

General Considerations

Vaginal discharge is a common complaint that is often considered trivial and thus incorrectly managed by the clinician. Empiric diagnosis and treatment based on either history or appearance of the discharge alone is inadequate and frequently results in inappropriate treatment and repeated visits by the patient. When considering the etiology of vaginitis it is important to take into account the patient's age and sexual history. Lactobacilli, the predominant bacteria in the vagina of a healthy premenopausal woman, are typically absent in women who are menopausal and not receiving estrogen replacement therapy. The estrogen-deficient vaginal epithelium in postmenopausal women is also thinner; thus, atrophic vaginitis is a consideration in this age group. For sexually active women, sexually transmitted diseases (STDs) such as trichomoniasis, genital herpes, gonorrhea, and chlamydia should be considered.

Pathogenesis

The three major causes of vaginal discharge during the reproductive years are candidiasis, bacterial vaginosis, and trichomoniasis. The latter is the only one of the three that is known to be sexually transmitted; however, bacterial vaginosis is clearly associated with sexual activity. In addition, vaginal candidiasis is frequently seen in the setting of increased sexual activity, likely due to colonizing organisms that gain entry to the epithelium via microabrasions from sexual intercourse. In older women, as previously mentioned, atrophic vaginitis should be considered.

Other STDs, such as gonorrhea, chlamydia, and genital herpes, may lead to vaginal complaints. However, the physical signs of gonorrhea and chlamydia are cervical inflammation, not vaginal discharge. Genital herpes may cause discharge along with ulceration.

Some other causes of vaginal discharge include retained foreign body, cytolytic vaginosis, and desquamative inflammatory vaginitis. It should be noted that some women perceive their vaginal discharge to be abnormal when it is simply physiologic.

Prevention

Use of condoms is protective against STDs and also appears to protect against acquisition of bacterial vaginosis. If an STD is diagnosed, the patient's sex partners should be treated to avoid reinfection. Episodes of recurrent bacterial vaginosis may be prevented by use of twice weekly intravaginal metronidazole gel. Similarly, recurrent vaginal candidiasis can be controlled with use of once weekly fluconazole (150 mg). Estrogen replacement therapy will prevent atrophic vaginitis.

Clinical Findings

A. SYMPTOMS AND SIGNS

Patients should be asked about the consistency and color of the discharge and whether it is accompanied by pruritus (internal and external), irritation, or a fishy odor. Another useful question is whether a fishy odor is present after unprotected intercourse (a characteristic finding in bacterial vaginosis). During the examination, the clinician should note the presence or absence of vaginal ulcerations, erythema, characteristics (color and consistency) of the discharge, and the appearance of the cervix (mucopus at the os may suggest gonorrhea or chlamydia).

B. LABORATORY FINDINGS

The most widely used tests for the diagnosis of vaginitis are vaginal pH evaluation, the so-called "whiff" test, and light microscopy (see Table 2–1). Light microscopy is the most helpful of the three tests.

1. Vaginal pH—The vaginal pH is best measured using pH paper strips (ColorpHast indicator strips, EM Science, Gibbstown, NJ). The color resulting from contact of the vaginal fluid with the indicator paper can be compared directly with the color chart on the container. When collecting specimens for pH evaluation, care should be taken to avoid cervical secretions. These are normally more alkaline than secretions from the healthy vagina and may falsely influence the pH reading. Other factors that can influence the pH result are semen and blood in the sample. Semen is alkaline, and blood obscures the color change on the indicator paper.

The vaginal pH is normally ≤4.5 in the presence of predominantly lactobacillus flora; this includes the healthy vagina as well as one in which yeast infection is present. An elevated pH is indicative of bacterial vaginosis or trichomoniasis, although in some patients with trichomoniasis, the pH may be normal.

2. "Whiff" test—The most expeditious way to collect the vaginal specimen for both the "whiff" test and microscopy is to place a generous amount of vaginal discharge collected from the lateral vaginal wall into a small glass tube containing 0.3 mL of normal saline. This method allows for preparation of cover-slipped slides at the microscope, and for multiple preparations if required. The "whiff" test is performed by mixing a drop of the vaginal saline mixture with 10% potassium hydroxide (KOH) and then sniffing for a fishy smell. The fishy odor indicates the presence of volatilized amines associated with the anaerobic flora typical of bacterial vaginosis; however, the test is highly subjective.

3. Light microscopy—The cover-slipped specimen is examined at 400 × magnification under reduced light. When examining the fluid, the clinician should note the presence of white blood cells, parabasal cells, motile trichomonads, budding yeast and pseudohyphae, clue cells, and bacteria (specifying the type, if present). White blood cells are frequently present in vaginal secretions of patients with candidiasis and trichomoniasis. They may also be present, along with parabasal cells, in women with atrophic vaginitis or desquamative inflammatory vaginitis. White blood cells may also be seen in patients with bacterial vaginosis as a result of a vaginal or cervical coinfection. Although direct microscopic examination of the vaginal fluid for motile trichomonads is the fastest, least expensive diagnostic method for trichomoniasis, the sensitivity of this test compared with culture is only 60%.

Perhaps the most difficult diagnosis to confirm microscopically is that of candidiasis. The presence of budding yeast without the report of symptoms compatible with a yeast infection may simply represent colonization. On the other hand, clumps of pseudohyphae in vaginal secretions of a patient with candidiasis can be difficult to visualize and may require examination of multiple preparations. The addition of KOH, which dissolves other cellular elements, may be helpful.

4. Amsel criteria—The most commonly used diagnostic method for bacterial vaginosis is the Amsel criteria, which comprises four findings: (1) a homogenous vaginal discharge, (2) vaginal pH higher than 4.5, (3) positive "whiff" test, and (4) clue cells on direct microscopic examination of the vaginal fluid (wet mount). If three of these four findings are present, the diagnostic criteria for bacterial vaginosis are met. Clue cells, defined as squamous epithelial cells covered with bacteria to the extent that the edges of the cell are obscured, are also subject to the interpretation of the microscopist. The careful observer, however, will go beyond the Amsel criteria to note the amount and morphotypes of the vaginal bacteria in the wet mount. In bacterial vaginosis, there will be many coccobacillary morphotypes and a paucity of large rods, which represent the lactobacilli. Motile curved rods, which represent *Mobiluncus,* are pathognomonic for bacterial vaginosis.

C. SPECIAL TESTS

Additional tests are commercially available for point-of-care testing of vaginitis. Several rapid card tests are available. One test detects proline aminopeptidase, an enzyme found in the vaginal secretions of women with bacterial vaginosis (QuickVue Advance *G vaginalis* Test, Quidel Corporation, San Diego, CA). A second test detects elevated pH and amines (QuickVue Advance pH and Amines Test Card, Quidel Corporation, San Diego, CA) and may be a useful screening tool for determining patients who should receive a more thorough evaluation. A third, rapid colorometric test for the diagnosis of bacterial vaginosis detects sialidase in the vaginal fluid (Osom BVBlue Test, Genzyme Corporation, Cambridge, MA). A semiautomated test for vaginitis, which includes trichomoniasis, candidiasis, and bacterial vaginosis, is also

Table 2-1. Laboratory and other studies for vaginitis.

Test	Sensitivity (%)	Specificity (%)	Comments
Vaginal pH	89 (for diagnosis)	73 (for diagnosis of bacterial vaginosis)	Normal pH is <4.5. Blood, semen, cervical secretions may interfere with test. pH is usually normal in candidiasis and >4.5 in bacterial vaginosis and trichomoniasis; however, trichomoniasis may be present with a normal pH.
"Whiff" test of vaginal secretions	43 (for diagnosis of bacterial vaginosis)	91 (for diagnosis of bacterial vaginosis)	Add 10% KOH to vaginal secretions; test is positive if a fishy smell is present (volatilization of amines produced by anaerobes); positive in bacterial vaginosis and sometimes in trichomoniasis.
Microscopic examination of vaginal fluid (wet mount)	65–85 (for yeast infection) 60 (for trichomoniasis) 80 (for bacterial vaginosis)	—	Mix secretions in small amount of saline and observe using "high dry" 40 × lens. Note presence of budding yeast and pseudohyphae, motile trichomonads, and clue cells (squamous epithelial cells covered with bacteria whose edges are obscured). Observe number and type of bacteria: moderate numbers of large rods represent lactobacilli (normal flora); large numbers of coccobacilli or motile curved rods are highly suggestive of bacterial vaginosis. Use of KOH prep may be helpful in identifying yeast infection because KOH dissolves the other cellular elements; demonstration of yeast infection is subject to sampling error; examination of repeated slide preparations can be helpful. **Note:** Mixed infections can occur.
Amsel criteria for bacterial vaginosis	70 (compared with Gram stain)	94 (compared with Gram stain)	3 of the following 4 signs must be present: vaginal pH > 4.5, positive "whiff" test, presence of clue cells, homogenous vaginal discharge.
Gram stain of vaginal secretions for bacterial vaginosis	89 (compared with Amsel criteria [22])	83 (compared with Gram stain)	Nugent method is the most widely used; determines quantities of 3 different bacterial morphotypes: large gram-positive rods (lactobacilli), small gram-variable coccobacilli (*Gardnerella, Prevotella*), and curved rods (*Mobiluncus*). Score ranges from 1 to 10; 0–3 = normal, 4–6 = intermediate, and 7–10 = bacterial vaginosis.

(Continued)

Table 2–1. Laboratory and other studies for vaginitis. (*Continued*)

Test	Sensitivity (%)	Specificity (%)	Comments
Culture for yeast or *Gardnerella vaginalis*	—	—	Not routinely indicated; may detect colonization as opposed to infection.
InPouch TV culture for *Trichomonas vaginalis*	90–95	100	Commercially available culture media inoculated at beside is currently the "gold standard"; compared with culture, wet mount has a sensitivity of 60%. A self-obtained specimen may be used with culture in special settings. Vaginal specimen may be transported to laboratory on an Amies gel transport swab before inoculation into culture pouch.
Osom Trichomonas Rapid Test	80 (compared with InPouch TV)	98.6	ELISA strip test for vaginal samples CLIA complexity: waived
Affirm VPIII	94 (for bacterial vaginosis) 80 (for trichomoniasis)	81 (for bacterial vaginosis) 98 (for trichomoniasis)	Semiautomated office-based test to distinguish between etiologic agents of vaginitis
QuickVue Advance pH and Amines Test Card	87	92	Rapid card test for pH and amines; if positive, consistent with bacterial vaginosis but further testing is needed to rule out mixed infections CLIA complexity: waived
QuickVue Advance *G vaginalis* Test	90	97	Rapid card test for bacterial vaginosis; detects proline iminopeptidase CLIA complexity: moderate
Osom BVBlue	90.3	96.6	Rapid colorometric test for sialidase production by anaerobes associated with bacterial vaginosis; limited data on performance CLIA complexity: moderate

CLIA, Clinical Laboratories Improvement Act; ELISA, enzyme-linked immunosorbent assay.

available (Affirm VPIII, Becton Dickinson, Sparks, MD). A point-of-care enzyme-linked immunosorbent assay (ELISA)–based test for trichomonas has recently been licensed (Osom Trichomonas Rapid Test, Genzyme Corporation, Cambridge, MA). This strip test is used with vaginal secretions, has a sensitivity of approximately 80% compared with culture, and is easy to perform.

Routine bacterial culture of vaginal secretions is not helpful and can be misleading. Culturing for *Trichomonas vaginalis* may be helpful in patients without a confirmed diagnosis, because culture is more sensitive for the diagnosis of trichomoniasis than the wet mount.

Sobel JD. Vaginitis. *N Engl J Med* 1997;337:1896–1903. [PMID: 9407158] (Useful review of vaginitis.)

Differential Diagnosis

Other causes of vaginal discharge include atrophic vaginitis, retained foreign body, cytolytic vaginitis, desquamative inflammatory vaginitis, genital herpes, physiologic discharge, and perhaps gonorrhea or chlamydia. Vaginal complaints should never be diagnosed without analyzing objective laboratory data except, perhaps, in the case of recurrent infections that have been previously documented.

Complications

Bacterial vaginosis is associated with obstetric and gynecologic complications. In cross-sectional studies, bacterial vaginosis is a risk factor for preterm birth and low birth weight. However, prospective treatment studies have yielded inconsistent results as to the benefit of screening and treating for bacterial vaginosis in pregnancy. Gynecologic complications include postoperative infections following gynecologic surgery; acquisition of sexually transmitted diseases, including pelvic inflammatory disease; acquisition and transmission of HIV; and recurrent urinary tract infections. Screening and treating for bacterial vaginosis prior to elective gynecologic procedures is recommended.

Trichomoniasis has also been associated with preterm birth and acquisition and transmission of HIV.

Treatment

Table 2–2 summarizes drug treatment for vaginal infections. Treatment should be targeted specifically at the cause of the vaginal discharge; empiric therapy should always be avoided. In the case of trichomoniasis, sex partners should also be treated.

Centers for Disease Control and Prevention; Workowski KA, Berman SM. Sexually transmitted diseases treatment guidelines, 2006. *MMWR Recomm Rep* 2006;55(RR-11):1–94. [PMID: 16888612] (Most recent published treatment guidelines from the CDC.)

Joesoef MR, Schmid GP, Hillier SL. Bacterial vaginosis: Review of treatment options and potential clinical indications for therapy. *Clin Infect Dis* 1999;28:S57–S65. [PMID: 10028110] (Review of treatment for bacterial vaginosis.)

Lossick JG. Treatment of sexually transmitted vaginosis/vaginitis. *Rev Infect Dis* 1990;12:S665–S681. [PMID: 2201078] (Review of treatment for infectious vaginitis.)

When to Refer to a Specialist

Women with recurrent or persistent infections may be referred to an infectious disease specialist or gynecologist for additional management. If the cause of the vaginal discharge cannot be identified, consultation with those specialists may also be helpful.

Prognosis

The overall prognosis is excellent; however, bacterial vaginosis cure rates are 70–80%, and recurrence rates may be as high as 50% within 6 months.

PRACTICE POINTS

- *When collecting specimens for pH evaluation, care should be taken to avoid cervical secretions. These are normally more alkaline than secretions from the healthy vagina and may falsely influence the pH reading.*

Relevant Web Sites

[American Social Health Association STD information page:] http://www.ashastd.org

[Centers for Disease Control and Prevention fact sheet on bacterial vaginosis:]

http://www.cdc.gov/std/bv/STDFact-Bacterial-Vaginosis.htm [Information about trichomoniasis, sponsored by Presutti Laboratories:]

http://www.trichomoniasis.net

Table 2-2. Drug treatment for vaginal infections.

Agent	Dosage	Benefits	Side Effects	Comments
Imidazoles (cream and suppository)	1–7 d intravaginal dosing for candidiasis	Effective and safe; some are available OTC	Local irritation	For vaginal candidiasis; yeast balanitis may occur in male partners.
Fluconazole	150 mg PO as a single dose for vaginal candidiasis 150 mg/wk PO to prevent recurrent infection	1 oral dose	GI upset	Equal in efficacy to topical medication and may be used prophylactically for recurrent candidiasis. Contraindicated in pregnancy—topical therapy is preferred. Generic formulation is now available.
Metronidazole				
Oral	500 mg PO twice daily for 7 d for bacterial vaginosis; 2 g as a single dose for trichomoniasis	Inexpensive	GI upset, metallic taste, peripheral neuropathy, dizziness; disulfiram-like reaction is possible	Efficacy is ~70–85% for bacterial vaginosis, and recurrences are common. Resistant strains of *Trichomonas* are usually cured with increased doses. Treat sex partners if trichomonas.
Gel	1 applicator intravaginally daily or twice daily for 5 d for bacterial vaginosis	Topical therapy with little systemic absorption	Avoids usual side effects of metronidazole; can cause vaginal candidiasis	Efficacy is same as oral formulation for bacterial vaginosis; not effective for trichomoniasis. Some data exist for twice-weekly prophylactic use of metronidazole gel for recurrent bacterial vaginosis; longer duration of therapy (10–14 d) may be helpful for persistent bacterial vaginosis.
Clindamycin				
Oral	300 mg PO twice daily for 7 d for l bacteria vaginosis	Alternative to metronidazole for bacterial vaginosis	Colitis	Expensive; can be used in pregnancy.
2% cream	1 applicator intravaginally at bedtime for 7 d for bacterial vaginosis	Alternative to metronidazole, equal efficacy for bacterial vaginosis	Vaginal yeast infections	Generic formulation is now available.

Ovules	1 vaginal suppository daily for 3 d for bacterial vaginosis	Alternative to metronidazole for bacterial vaginosis	Vaginal yeast infections	
Single-dose bioadhesive formula	1 applicator intravaginally	Single dose but sustained levels	Vaginal yeast infections	
Tinidazole	2 g as a single dose for uncomplicated trichomoniasis; longer duration for resistant strains	Effective against some strains of *Trichomonas* that are resistant to metronidazole	GI upset but may be less severe than with metronidazole	Recently approved by the FDA.

GI, gastrointestinal; OTC, over the counter.

Urethral Discharge

3

Jonathan M. Zenilman, MD

ESSENTIALS OF DIAGNOSIS

- *Spontaneous urethral discharge.*
- *Burning with urination.*
- *Purulent or mucoid exudate with urethral stripping.*
- *More than 5 white blood cells (WBCs) per high-power field of urethral exudate.*

General Considerations

Urethral discharge is characterized by abnormal purulent or mucoid secretions from the penis or, rarely, the female urethra. Urethral discharge reflects inflammation of the urethra usually caused by infection. Urethritis is defined as the presence of leukorrhea and urethral inflammation. Clinically, urethritis in men is characterized by urethral discharge and is often accompanied by dysuria. Leukorrhea has been defined as the presence of more than 5 WBCs per high-power field in a urethral swab specimen, using either Gram stain or other cellular stain (eg, Wright or methylene blue).

Epidemiology & Pathogenesis

Urethral discharge can occur in sexually active persons of all ages but is most common in young adults, the age group in which the prevalence of *Chlamydia trachomatis* and *Neisseria gonorrhoeae* infection is highest. High rates of urethritis also occur in men who have sex with men. Urethral discharge occurs after urethral infection in persons exposed to infectious agents during oral, vaginal, or anal intercourse.

The most common etiology of urethral discharge is *N gonorrhoeae*, followed by *C trachomatis*. These two organisms account for about 40% of cases of urethritis. Although historically urethritis has been differentiated

into gonococcal urethritis versus nongonococcal urethritis (NGU), with the discovery of additional causes of urethritis that dichotomy has little clinical relevance. The other major putative organisms that have been associated with sexually transmitted NGU include *Mycoplasma genitalium, Trichomonas vaginalis,* herpes simplex virus, and adenovirus (see Table 3–1). The role that *Mycoplasma hominis* and *Ureaplasma urealyticum* play in urethritis remains unproven.

A. N GONORRHOEAE

Urethral discharge is most commonly associated with gonorrhea. Infection with these gram-negative diplococci can occur after oral, vaginal, or anal intercourse, with symptoms developing between 1 and 3 days after exposure.

B. C TRACHOMATIS

In early studies that largely relied on culture methods, *Chlamydia* was found to account for a relatively small proportion of cases of NGU. In three large studies performed at STD clinics in the 1980s and 1990s, *Chlamydia* was identified in 19–31% of patients. On average one third but in some studies up to 60% of patients with gonococcal urethritis may have coinfection with *C trachomatis.*

C. M GENITALIUM

This organism was first identified as a cause of NGU in 1981. It is very difficult to grow in culture, and diagnostic surveys have been performed in research settings with nucleic acid amplification tests. Some investigators have suggested that *M genitalium* is responsible for 15–25% of cases of NGU; others cite a much lower percentage. A large review of the literature conducted in 2002 found that patients with NGU were 2.5 times more likely to have *M genitalium* isolated from their genitourinary tract than patients without urethritis (20% compared with 8%). However, it is difficult to determine the exact relationships between this organism and other urethral pathogens. Although diagnosis of *M genitalium* infection is currently limited to research settings, commercial assays for *M genitalium* are in development.

Table 3–1. Pathogens that can cause sexually transmitted urethritis.[a]

Common causes
Neisseria gonorrhoeae
Chlamydia trachomatis
Mycoplasma genitalium
Trichomonas vaginalis
Herpes simplex virus
Rare causes
Ureaplasma urealyticum
Escherichia coli
Anaerobic bacteria
Adenovirus

[a]Listed from most to least common.

D. T VAGINALIS

Urethritis accompanying *Trichomonas* infection is usually associated with minimal discharge. Not surprisingly, men with trichomonas-related urethritis are much more likely to have been exposed to women with trichomonas-related vaginitis. One of the more intriguing questions in understanding the epidemiology of *Trichomonas* infection in men is identification of the anatomic source. *Trichomonas* infection is very difficult to identify in the urethra in male contacts of women who have trichomoniasis. Several investigators have proposed that *Trichomonas* is sequestered in the prostate gland and may be a cause of prostatitis.

E. HERPES SIMPLEX VIRUS

Up to sixty percent of men with primary herpes infection have associated herpes NGU. A clinical clue to herpes as an etiology is that the urethral inflammatory cells are lymphocytes, and patients present with pain on urination and minimal discharge. Often, patients are treated empirically for NGU; however, because of the natural history of genital herpes (resolution within 5–7 days), the resolution of symptoms is often attributed to treatment for other organisms. Intraurethral herpes infection should be suspected when the primary manifestation is severe dysuria. In these patients, a urethral culture or, if available, a nucleic acid amplification test (polymerase chain reaction) for herpes may be positive. Occasionally, herpetic lesions are seen at the meatus.

F. M HOMINIS AND U UREALYTICUM

These species have had a putative association with urethritis for more than 30 years. Although both organisms are associated with sexual activity, few well-controlled studies have demonstrated that they are isolated more frequently from individuals with urethritis than from normal controls. Therefore, whether these species represent true pathogens or urethral colonizers has yet to be determined.

G. OTHER ETIOLOGIES

Because of the large number of cases of NGU that are not associated with an identifiable pathogen, there has been substantial interest in a nonherpetic viral cause. Adenovirus has been associated with NGU, especially in persons who have had insertive oral sexual exposure. However, one criticism in such cases is the possibility that, similar to the situation with *Mycoplasma* and *Ureaplasma,* the isolation of an organism does not confirm that the organism is pathogenic.

In men who have sex with men who have had insertive rectal intercourse, anaerobic bacteria and enteric organisms (eg, *Escherichia coli*) occasionally cause urethritis.

Finally, some cases of NGU do not appear to be associated with the traditional sexually transmitted organisms; possible underlying etiologies include contact dermatitis and immunologic disorders.

Anagrius C, Lore B, Jensen JS. Mycoplasma genitalium. Prevalence, clinical significance and transmission. *Sex Transm Infect* 2005;81:458ñ-462. [PMID: 16326846] (Current review of the epidemiology and clinical manifestations of *M genitalium.*)

Bradshaw CS, Tabrizi SN, Read TR, et al. Etiologies of nongonococcal urethritis: Bacteria, viruses, and the association with orogenital exposure. *J Infect Dis* 2006;193:336–345. [PMID: 8480958] (Comprehensive clinical assessment demonstrating that herpes simplex virus type 1 and adenovirus are major causes of NGU, especially in patients with orogenital exposure.)

Krieger JN, Jenny C, Verdon M, et al. Clinical manifestations of trichomoniasis in men. *Ann Intern Med* 1993;118:844–849. [PMID: 16388480] (Classic article describing the role of trichomonas in NGU.)

Clinical Findings

A. SYMPTOMS AND SIGNS

All patients who are evaluated for sexually transmitted diseases should be evaluated for urethritis. Urethral evaluation should occur a minimum of 2 hours after the last voided urine, because recent voiding can reduce the sensitivity of microbiologic testing.

The typical presenting symptoms of urethritis are dysuria or discharge. With gonococcal urethritis, the discharge is more likely to be purulent, although this should not be used alone to either rule in or rule out gonococcal infection. The discharge of NGU is typically mucoid or watery. If no spontaneous discharge is evident, the clinician should perform urethral stripping ("milking" the urethra three to four times from the base of the penis distally to the meatus), which will yield urethral exudate in a majority of patients with asymptomatic NGU.

B. LABORATORY FINDINGS

Ideally, a smear of urethral exudates and Gram stain should be performed. If no spontaneous or induced discharge is present, a urethral smear is prepared by inserting a narrow swab (eg, calcium alginate swab) 2 cm into the urethra, rotating the swab, and withdrawing it. Exudate from the swab is then rolled onto a glass slide for staining and examination. In settings where Gram stain is not available, an alternative means to identify urethral inflammation is leukocyte esterase testing performed on 15 mL of the first-voided urine, using a criterion of +1 leukocytes on the leukocyte esterase test strip.

Unfortunately, microscopy and rapid testing are not available in most clinical settings in which acute urethritis is seen, thus precluding an on-site diagnosis.

In clinical practice, most of the organisms associated with NGU, such as *Chlamydia* and *Mycoplasma*, are susceptible to macrolide (eg, erythromycin), azalide (azithromycin), or tetracycline (eg, doxycycline) antibiotics. Results of organism-specific diagnostic tests typically are not available for several days. With the lack of on-site diagnostic testing, *syndromic* clinical management is common practice. This approach is outlined in Figure 3–1. As with all STD evaluations, obtaining a thorough history is essential.

C. DIAGNOSTIC TESTS

With the advent of highly sensitive nucleic acid amplification tests, diagnostic testing can be performed using urine as the testing substrate, obviating the need to collect a urethral swab specimen. Ideally testing should include assays for *N gonorrhoeae* and *C trachomatis*. All patients evaluated for sexually transmitted diseases should also undergo serologic testing for syphilis, as well as HIV testing. Despite the increased logistical problems, costs, and follow-up issues involved in diagnostic testing, such testing is essential to assure proper treatment and to facilitate partner management. Because gonococcal and chlamydial infections are exclusively sexually acquired, partner notification for these infections should be based on a confirmed laboratory result.

Differential Diagnosis

The major differential diagnosis is between gonorrhea, chlamydia, urethritis due to *Mycoplasma, T vaginalis,* and herpes simplex. If microscopy is available, gonococcal urethritis can be excluded on the basis of a Gram stain of the urethral exudate. Noninfectious causes of urethritis should also be considered; these causes may be suggested by the history and include urethral trauma

from recent catheterization or sex play, and autoimmune conditions such as Reiter syndrome.

As a general rule, urethritis in men younger than 40 years of age who have not undergone invasive urologic procedures (eg, catheterization, cystoscopy) can be presumed to be sexually acquired. Older men, especially those with systemic diseases such as diabetes and prostatic hypertrophy, are susceptible to urinary tract infections, which can mimic urethritis. In all cases, however, a careful sexual history and evaluation should be obtained in patients who are sexually active.

Complications

Epididymitis can result from urethral infection with *Chlamydia* or *N gonorrhoeae* and must be differentiated from testicular torsion. Acute prostatitis is often considered to be a potential complication of urethral infection in patients with persistent or recurrent urethritis. Prostatitis can often be excluded by a normal prostate examination. Rarely, chronic urethritis can result in urethral stricture. Complications specific to individual organisms may occur in patients with untreated gonorrhea who progress to disseminated gonococcal infection or those with chlamydial infection who have immune-mediated reactive arthritis (formerly known as Reiter syndrome); however, these complications are rare.

Treatment

A. PHARMACOTHERAPY

Patients who present with a purulent discharge or who reside in or have visited an area that is endemic for gonorrhea should be offered treatment for both gonorrhea and chlamydia. Areas that are hyperendemic for gonorrhea include many urban environments, the southeastern United States, and developing countries. Current treatment recommendations for gonorrhea include ceftriaxone, 125 mg intramuscularly, or cefixime, 400 mg orally once. Cefixime, however, is not commercially available in the United States and many authorities recommend another third-generation cephalosporin, cefpodoxime, 400 mg once orally instead. Because of the increased incidence of fluoroquinolone-resistant gonorrhea (almost 40%) on the East and West coasts of the United States in men who have sex with men, these drugs should not be used in the treatment of that population. As of 2006, fluoroquinolones continue to be recommended for treatment of gonorrhea in heterosexuals, except in Hawaii and California. If fluoroquinolones are used in populations where quinolone resistance is common, a "test of cure" is recommended.

If the patient is a homosexual man or has a history of insertive rectal intercourse, the clinician should consider the possibility of enteric or anaerobic infection. Treatment

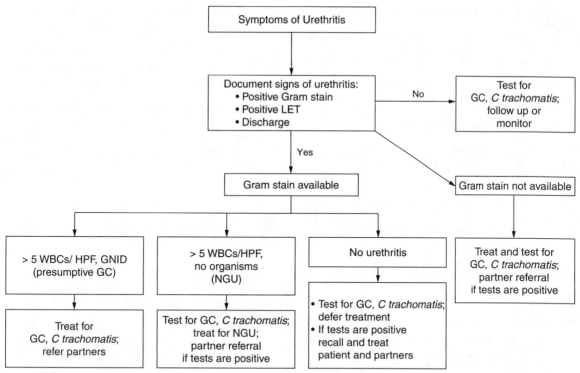

Figure 3–1. Algorithm for the diagnosis and management of urethritis. GC = gonococcal infection; GNID = gram-negative intracellular diplococci; HPF = high-power field; LET = leukocyte esterase test; NGU = nongonococcal urethritis. (Reproduced with permission from Burstein G, Zenilman JM. Non-gonococcal urethritis—A new paradigm. *Clin Infect Dis* 1999;28:S72.)

for those infections is similar to treatment for gonorrhea. All patients should be treated presumptively for the other causative agents of urethritis (see earlier discussion and Table 3–1) with azithromycin, 1 g as a single dose. An alternative regimen is to administer doxycycline, 100 mg twice daily for 7 days. Azithromycin is preferred for patients with NGU because clinical trial data suggest that treatment success rates for *M genitalium* are higher when azithromycin rather than a tetracycline is used. Azithromycin, however, does not treat incubating syphilis, so some public health authorities recommend the use of tetracycline (doxycycline) in the treatment of NGU in populations at high risk for syphilis.

Partners of patients with gonococcal or chlamydial infection must be treated. Patient-delivered partner therapy has been shown to be safe and highly effective in heterosexual men and women, and this option, if available, should be used.

In addition, patients with gonococcal or chlamydial urethritis should return at 3 months for repeat testing to rule out reinfection. Some studies have shown rates of reinfection in adequately treated patients to be as high as 20% at 3 months.

B. Clinical Challenges

One of the biggest challenges to the clinician is presented by the patient who reports urethral "tingling" without discharge. Approximately one third of patients with clinically demonstrable urethritis do not have discharge. If the results of diagnostic evaluation are negative, these patients should be informed that no infection is present and that the urethral discomfort will resolve spontaneously. It is not uncommon for patients to experience urethral symptoms after sexual experiences they later regret, suggesting a psychological cause to their physical complaints. Testing and informing the patient of the negative test results is often associated with resolution of symptoms. Empiric treatment for urethral symptoms without objective evidence of urethritis is not recommended

Burstein G, Zenilman JM. Non-gonococcal urethritis—-A new paradigm. *Clin Infect Dis* 1999;28(suppl 1):S66–S73. [PMID: 10028111] (Comprehensive review of the diagnosis and treatment of NGU, which served as the background paper for the 1999 STD treatment guidelines. Includes algorithms for diagnosis and management.)

Horner PJ. European guideline for the management of urethritis. *Int J STD AIDS* 2001;12(suppl 3):63–67. [PMID: 11589800]

(Comprehensive European guidelines for the management of urethritis.)

Kissinger P, Mohammed H, Richardson-Alston G, et al. Patient-delivered partner treatment for male urethritis: A randomized controlled trial. *Clin Infect Dis* 2005;41:623–629. [PMID: 16080084] (Seminal article that describes the use of patient-delivered therapy for treating partners of patients with gonococcal or chlamydial infection, using reinfection as the outcome.)

When to Refer to a Specialist

If objective signs of urethritis persist after proper treatment and reinfection or nonadherence is unlikely, then referral to an infectious disease specialist or urologist may be necessary. Those specialists often have access to additional diagnostic tests for less common or antimicrobial-resistant pathogens. Rarely, cystoscopy may be indicated to rule out structural urethral or bladder disease. In cases of urethritis complicated by epididymitis or disseminated disease, referral may be indicated to exclude testicular torsion or initiate intravenous therapy, respectively.

Prognosis

Most cases (95%) of urethritis are adequately treated with the recommended antibiotics, leading to rapid resolution of symptoms. Urethral discharge generally resolves within 24–48 hours; however, dysuria and urethral discomfort may persist for up to 7 days. Although antimicrobial treatment usually renders patients noninfectious within 1–2 days, it is recommended that they abstain from sexual intercourse for 7 days following the initiation of treatment to prevent further transmission.

Despite appropriate diagnosis and treatment, many clinicians will encounter patients who have chronic urethral symptoms of unknown etiology. These patients often have associated affective or obsessive-compulsive disorders, in which the presence of chronic urethral complaints represents expression of the underlying psychological disorder.

PRACTICE POINTS

- *Urethral evaluation should occur a minimum of 2 hours after the last voided urine, because recent voiding can reduce the sensitivity of microbiologic testing.*
- *All patients evaluated for sexually transmitted diseases should also undergo serologic testing for syphilis, as well as HIV testing.*

Genital Ulcer Disease

4

Daniel E. Cohen, MD, & Kenneth Mayer, MD

ESSENTIALS OF DIAGNOSIS

- *Diagnosis is based on the finding of one or more mucocutaneous ulcers involving the genitalia, perineum, or anus.*
- *Careful inspection of all genital mucosa is important, as lesions may be inside the foreskin, labia, vagina, or rectum, and may be painless.*
- *Genital herpes is the most common cause, followed by syphilis.*
- *A specific pathogen often cannot be identified based on clinical findings alone; laboratory testing should include culture or polymerase chain reaction (PCR) amplification for herpes simplex virus (HSV), and serologic testing for syphilis.*
- *Despite appropriate testing, no pathogen is identified in up to 50% of patients.*

General Considerations

Genital ulcer disease (GUD) is a syndrome characterized by ulcerating lesions on the penis, scrotum, vulva, vagina, perineum, or perianal skin. In general usage the term refers to genital ulcerations from a sexually transmitted disease (STD), which is the most common etiology; however, nonsexually acquired illnesses, including infectious (bacterial skin infections, fungi) or noninfectious etiologies (fixed drug eruption, Behçet syndrome, sexual trauma), can present with similar ulcers. The clinician should bear in mind that nonvenereal dermatoses (eg, psoriasis) resulting from a variety of causes also can present with anogenital lesions.

The annual global incidence of GUD probably exceeds 20 million cases. The most commonly identified pathogens are HSV types 1 and 2 (HSV-1, HSV-2), syphilis, and chancroid. As recently as 20 years ago, the predominant causes of GUD in much the developing world were bacterial pathogens, especially *Haemophilus ducreyi*, the etiologic agent of chancroid. However, since the early 1990s the prevalence of chancroid in sub-Saharan Africa has decreased dramatically, while HSV-2 infection has increased. Although this change may be related to more widespread use of antibiotics and syndromic treatment of STDs, the HIV epidemic and behavioral changes in response may have played an equally important role. As a result, genital herpes now constitutes the most common infectious cause of GUD worldwide.

Regardless of the cause, GUD has assumed increased importance in view of its well-recognized role in facilitating HIV transmission. Surveys of HIV prevalence among patients seeking treatment for STDs have found a higher prevalence of coexisting HIV infection in those with genital ulcers than in those without, both in the United States and in the developing world. The presence of GUD in an individual not infected with HIV makes that person more susceptible to HIV infection by breaching the integumentary barrier and by recruiting macrophages and T-helper cells to the genital tract, where they may more readily be infected. Conversely, GUD in an HIV-infected individual increases his or her likelihood of transmitting HIV to a sex partner. HIV-infected patients with GUD who present for care at STD clinics actually have a higher plasma HIV viral load than similar patients without GUD. In a 2001 study of 174 HIV-serodiscordant couples in Uganda, the presence of GUD was associated with an almost fourfold increase in the probability of HIV transmission. A similar magnitude of increased risk of HIV acquisition (hazard ratio of 3.8) was associated with new onset of HSV-2 infection in the prior 6 months in a cohort of over 2700 patients in Pune, India.

Gray RH, Wawer MJ, Brookmeyer R, et al. Probability of HIV-1 transmission per coital act in monogamous, heterosexual, HIV-1-discordant couples in Rakai, Uganda. *Lancet* 2001; 357:1149–1153. [PMID: 11323041] (The landmark study documenting the role of GUD and HIV viral load in transmission risk.)

Paz-Bailey G, Rahman M, Chen C, et al. Changes in the etiology of sexually transmitted diseases in Botswana between 1993 and 2002: Implications for the clinical management of genital ulcer disease. *Clin Infect Dis* 2005;41:1304–1312. [PMID: 16206106] (A good account of the changes in GUD etiology over a 10-year period in a representative sub-Saharan African county.)

Prevention

A. RISK COUNSELING

The mainstay of prevention of GUD, as for prevention of STDs in general, is risk reduction counseling. Topics of counseling include limiting the number of sex partners, use of condoms (either male or female), and regular testing for asymptomatic disease. However, there are some ways in which GUD differs from other STDs. For example, condom use is somewhat less efficacious in preventing GUD. Because causative pathogens may be transmitted by skin-to-skin contact, contact with skin that is not covered by a condom may transmit infection. Furthermore, patients may only put on a condom preparatory to penetrative sex, whereas transmission may occur via nonpenetrative contact. Finally, despite counseling messages, few patients routinely use condoms for oral sex. Some patients engage more frequently in oral sex than in anal or vaginal penetrative sex, perceiving oral sex as a lower risk activity. However, the three most common pathogens implicated in GUD (HSV-2, HSV-1, and *Treponema pallidum*) can be transmitted efficiently by oral sex, a fact that may be underappreciated by patients.

B. CHEMOPROPHYLAXIS

Among other potential prevention strategies, chemoprophylaxis is available for genital herpes in the form of daily suppressive medication such as acyclovir. Daily suppressive therapy not only reduces the frequency and severity of herpes outbreaks, but also reduces asymptomatic viral shedding and transmission. This strategy may be appropriate for many patients and is discussed in more detail in Chapter 14. In many parts of the developing world where bacterial pathogens are prevalent, mass anti-infective treatment of populations has been attempted as a prevention strategy.

C. CIRCUMCISION

Interest has recently been raised in circumcision as a possible strategy for prevention of HIV infection, and large, well-controlled studies in Africa have demonstrated significant reductions in infection rates among circumcised versus uncircumcised adults. Because some ulcerative diseases (eg, chancroid) are more common in uncircumcised men and tend to occur in the preputial sulcus and inside surface of the prepuce, circumcision may also provide some protection against these diseases; however, this hypothesis has not been studied, and the magnitude of any protective effect is unknown.

Clinical Findings

A. HISTORY

In the diagnosis of GUD, the first consideration is whether or not the condition is sexually acquired; that is, whether a potential sexual exposure has occurred. Thus, an accurate sexual history is essential to diagnosis and management. Many clinicians may not readily elicit a sexual history in busy clinical practices, and many patients are unwilling to broach the subject of their sexual practices if they are not fully comfortable with their health care provider. Nevertheless, because accurate information about potential sexual exposures is essential to a diagnosis, it is incumbent on any health care provider who sees sexually active patients to become proficient in this area of history taking. Details about obtaining an accurate sexual history are found in Chapter 31.

Once a potential sexual route of infection has been established, the history can sometimes help differentiate between different pathogens. The interval between a high-risk sexual exposure and the onset of symptoms may suggest the diagnosis. A primary genital herpes infection most often produces symptoms within a week of exposure. Symptoms of primary syphilis generally appear after 2–3 weeks, and more uncommon pathogens may have a longer incubation period. The patient's description of the initial stages of the lesion (eg, as small blisters [vesicles]) may be helpful; however, these earlier stages may not have been noticed by the patient, particularly if the lesions are in an area that is difficult for the patient to inspect, such as the perineum, labia majora or minora, or perianal region. In addition, patients may not reliably distinguish an initial lesion as papular, vesicular, or pustular; thus, the patient's description is frequently not contributory. A history of travel to an endemic area may increase the likelihood of a more exotic pathogen, such as chancroid or donovanosis.

If sexually acquired GUD has been ruled out, a more detailed history may be helpful in pointing toward certain less common diagnoses. An appropriate exposure history in an endemic area, for example, may suggest tularemia; likewise, a history of oral ulcers can suggest Behçet syndrome, an uncommon disease of unknown etiology whose hallmarks are recurrent oral and genital ulcers. However, most of the nonvenereal causes of genital ulceration are less common than sexually transmitted GUD. As a general rule, whenever there is doubt as to the etiology, it is safest to assume that genital ulcers are sexually acquired. Even a highly experienced provider with expertise at obtaining an accurate sexual history will frequently be given unreliable information about sexual risk.

B. SYMPTOMS AND SIGNS

1. Description of ulcer(s)—Classic textbook descriptions would have the clinician believe that herpes, syphilis, and chancroid can be easily distinguished on the basis of physical presentation and symptoms. In fact, diagnosis of specific etiologies of GUD on the basis of clinical presentation alone is often impossible. Nevertheless, it is helpful to be familiar with the "textbook" distinguishing characteristics, which are summarized in Table 4–1. Important findings to note include whether the ulcer is single or multiple, painless or painful, tender or nontender, and indurated or soft. The base of the ulcer may be necrotic (as in chancroid) or clean (as in a syphilitic chancre); it may appear shallow or have raised or rolled margins. The location of the ulcers also should be noted, because conditions such as chancroid are most often confined to the prepuce and glans in men and the labia majora and minora in women. Ulcers seen on the scrotum in men or the cervix in women should raise suspicion for herpes or syphilis.

2. Lymphadenopathy—The presence of inguinal lymphadenopathy can provide a clue to the etiology of GUD. Enlarged inguinal lymph nodes are a common finding

in many ulcerating conditions. In primary genital herpes the enlarged lymph nodes are frequently tender, whereas the classic adenopathy of syphilis is firm and nontender. Less common diseases such as chancroid and lymphogranuloma venereum usually present with tender, fluctuant inguinal lymph nodes (buboes). In lymphogranuloma venereum the primary ulcer may be transient, and lymphadenopathy, most often unilateral, is the predominant finding. The lymph nodes in patients with lymphogranuloma venereum become large and matted, and may erode through the skin to produce draining sinus tracts. Donovanosis, described in more detail below (see Differential Diagnosis), is one of the few causes of genital ulcer disease that does not characteristically include inguinal lymphadenopathy, although it can produce firm subcutaneous swellings called pseudobuboes.

3. Systemic findings—Physical examination should include a thorough inspection of the oral cavity and a

Table 4–1. Characteristics of genital ulcers.

Disease	Incubation Period	Pain and Tenderness	Lymphadenopathy	Description
Genital herpes	2–7 d for primary infection, not applicable for recurrence	Present, along with tingling and itching	Bilateral and tender in primary infection	Clusters of small shallow ulcers that may coalesce; vesicles are often not seen in women
Syphilis	10–90 d; usually 2–3 wk	Painless, nontender	Bilateral, firm, nontender	Firm, cartilaginous induration; heaped-up margins; clean base with serous exudate
Chancroid	3–10 d	Painful in men; may be painless in women	Painful, tender, usually unilateral	"Soft chancre" (no induration); may be multiple, especially in women; ragged border; necrotic base that bleeds easily
Lymphogranuloma venereum	3–30 d	Varies, usually painless	Very tender, usually unilateral; most often the predominant finding in male penile disease; usually absent in vaginal or anal disease	Exquisitely tender adenopathy is predominant; ulcer is small (≤1 cm) and transient
Donovanosis (granuloma inguinale)	8–80 d	Painless	Absent; firm, subcutaneous granulomas (pseudobuboes) may be present	Hypertrophic, beefy red, or verrucous; may resemble squamous cell carcinoma or condylomata lata

general skin examination. The presence of fever, malaise, headaches, or other constitutional findings in conjunction with a genital ulcer strongly suggests either primary genital herpes or a nonvenereal systemic disease such as Behçet syndrome or tularemia. In general, primary syphilis, chancroid, donovanosis, and the ulcerative stage of lymphogranuloma venereum are not associated with systemic symptoms. Rarely, a chancre will persist until the onset of secondary syphilis.

C. LABORATORY TESTING

Because clinical findings are not reliable for diagnosis of GUD, the appropriate choice of diagnostic tests and collection of samples is critical. Even in optimal circumstances, however, laboratory testing may fail to produce a diagnosis. In fact, in research studies of GUD, laboratory investigation fails to identify a pathogen in up to one third of cases.

1. Darkfield microscopy—The most reliable way of diagnosing a syphilitic chancre at the time of presentation is to identify live treponemes in a microscopic examination of the ulcer exudate, using darkfield microscopy. The organisms are abundant and have a characteristic appearance and motility. Visualizing spirochetes from a genital ulcer is pathognomonic for primary syphilis; darkfield examination of oral or intrarectal ulcers must be interpreted with more caution, because they may be contaminated by commensal spirochetes that are part of the resident flora.

Although visual inspection using darkfield examination is a mainstay of classic venereology, this test is no longer practical for most clinicians, because accurate visual identification of treponemes requires some experience, and most clinicians have not performed enough of these examinations to be proficient. Additionally, most clinical practices do not have access to darkfield microscopy.

2. Serology—Serologic testing for syphilis is the major method by which syphilis is diagnosed and comprises a generally inexpensive nontreponemal screening test (eg, rapid plasma reagin, RPR), with reactive tests confirmed by a more specific treponemal assay, such as the fluorescent treponemal antibody absorbed (FTA-ABS) or *T pallidum* particle agglutination (TP-PA) assay. Although highly sensitive for syphilis in secondary and early latent disease, syphilis serologies may be nonreactive in a large proportion of acute, primary infections. Furthermore, previous syphilis infection can confound the diagnosis, because positive findings on both the RPR and treponemal tests can persist for long periods of time despite successful treatment. Finally, syphilis may coexist with other causes of GUD; therefore, serologic testing for syphilis should be performed in all patients presenting with GUD, even if an alternative diagnosis is strongly suspected, unless such testing has been done recently.

The measurement of changes in syphilis serologic responses is helpful in differentiating recurrent from chronic infections. Individuals in whom serial syphilis serologies do not decrease by at least fourfold within 6 months after appropriate clinical treatment may be diagnosed with recurrent infection, if the clinical history is corroborative. In some individuals serologic responses remain reactive more than 6 months after successful antitreponemal therapy, a condition referred to as "serofast." These individuals are generally at low risk for recurrent infection and may have other predisposing conditions (eg, HIV infection or autoimmune diseases).

Serologic testing for type-specific HSV antibodies can be helpful in supporting a diagnosis of genital herpes. However, because 30–40% of genital herpes infections are caused by HSV-1, the absence of HSV-2 antibodies does not rule out such infections. Furthermore, although the presence of HSV antibodies can support the diagnosis, it cannot rule out other proximate causes or distinguish between active genital herpes and prior history of genital herpes. HSV antibody testing thus plays very little role in the etiologic diagnosis of GUD.

3. Viral culture—HSV-1 and HSV-2 are easily grown in cell culture, and with current technology a presumptive positive culture can be read in as little as 2 days. However, viral culture is of limited sensitivity in later disease and is not likely to be positive after crusting or scabbing of lesions has occurred. Nevertheless, given its ease of performance and high positive predictive value, viral culture should be considered a test of first choice for diagnosis of genital herpes, especially in patients in whom the etiology is not obvious.

4. Nucleic acid amplification tests—A PCR assay has been developed for the detection of HSV DNA from a genital ulcer swab. This assay can be performed in real time, with results often available within hours, and can distinguish HSV-1 from HSV-2. PCR is at least as sensitive as viral culture and is clearly superior to culture later in the course of genital herpes disease after lesions have ulcerated. Drawbacks of the test include cost and availability; although most commercial laboratories perform HSV PCR.

5. Biopsy—If an etiology has not been determined by other laboratory testing and an ulcer has failed to respond to empiric antimicrobial therapy directed against the most likely pathogens, a biopsy may be appropriate. Besides identifying a causative agent, a biopsy of a nonhealing ulcer should be pursued to rule out cancer. When donovanosis is suspected, a crush preparation can be examined to look for the characteristic Donovan bodies in cells from the ulcer base. For this purpose, a scraping, curettage, or excisional biopsy specimen is crushed between two glass slides, then air-dried and stained.

6. Bacterial culture—*H ducreyi* is fastidious and not easily grown in culture; however, a bacterial culture using select media is still recommended if chancroid is suspected, because isolation of *H ducreyi* in culture establishes the diagnosis with certainty. Although antibiotic resistance is not common in chancroid, bacterial culture also permits confirmation of antimicrobial susceptibility. Nevertheless, a negative culture should not be relied upon to exclude chancroid. Other bacterial causes of GUD (syphilis, lymphogranuloma venereum, donovanosis) are not routinely diagnosed by culture.

7. Gram stain—A swab of the exudative base of a suspected chancroid ulcer can also be examined with Gram stain for the presence of typical gram-negative coccobacilli. This test is also less useful for the practicing clinician than might be hoped; Gram-negative bacilli of a variety of morphologies may be seen from superficially colonized or secondarily infected wounds, and the textbook "school of fish" arrangement that is considered suggestive of chancroid on Gram stain requires interpretation by a microscopist familiar with the disease.

8. Tzanck preparation—A Tzanck preparation is a scraping from the base of a skin lesion, smeared on a slide and stained with Giemsa or Wright stain. The presence of multinucleated giant cells establishes the causative agent as a herpesvirus. In real-world settings most clinical practices are not set up for same-day preparation and interpretation of Tzanck smears. In addition, the sensitivity of a Tzanck smear diminishes considerably after vesicular lesions have ulcerated. For these reasons, and with the availability of technologies such as shell vial culture and PCR, which permit rapid diagnosis of genital herpes, the Tzanck preparation has no role in the diagnosis of GUD.

Differential Diagnosis

The differential diagnosis of GUD includes the previously described sexually transmitted pathogens, as well as several other causes of ulcerative disease.

A. GENITAL HERPES

A history of similar episodes of genital ulcers in the past suggests a diagnosis of genital herpes, as does a sex partner with known genital herpes. Most often the ulcers of genital herpes are tender and shallow; they also may be multiple and clustered. If the typical clusters of small vesicles are seen on external genital skin or mucosa the diagnosis is obvious; however, patients often present for care after ulceration has occurred. Men with penile or scrotal herpes are more likely to present with vesicles still intact, whereas in women, vaginal or vulvar disease is often ulcerative and frequently associated with discharge. Primary genital herpes is often significantly painful and accompanied by constitutional symptoms such as fever, malaise, and headaches, but these symptoms are usually absent from recurrent episodes. The diagnosis of GUD

resulting from HSV may be made by a positive viral culture or PCR test.

B. SYPHILIS

As mentioned, a disproportionate number of cases of primary and secondary syphilis occur among men who have sex with men (MSM), particularly among those who are infected with HIV. Indeed, virtually all of the increase in primary and secondary syphilis incidence in the United States over the past decade is probably attributable to infection among MSM; the rate of primary and secondary syphilis has actually decreased among women. Thus, a history of male-male sexual activity or HIV infection in a patient with GUD increases the likelihood of syphilis.

The classic chancre of primary syphilis is a single painless, nontender, indurated ulcer, with a clean base, a heaped-up or "rolled" margin, and accompanying inguinal adenopathy. Although all of these descriptors are true in general, many cases are atypical in appearance. For instance, multiple chancres may occur, especially in HIV-infected patients. Furthermore, up to 30% of chancres are described as painful. It is also important to remember that many causes of GUD are relatively painless when the vagina or cervix is involved, and supposedly painless ulcers can become secondarily infected with staphylococci or other bacteria and become tender when first brought to clinical attention. The clinician who has access to a darkfield microscope can examine ulcer exudate after abrading the ulcer (the preferred diagnostic test for primary syphilis). Otherwise he or she must rely on clinical impression and serologic testing, which is negative in approximately 30% of patients with chancres. Finally, a patient with GUD from another cause may have a positive serologic response for syphilis because of preexisting undiagnosed latent syphilis.

C. CHANCROID

Chancroid is rare in the United States (54 cases were reported in 2003, mostly in the Southeast), and it usually occurs in the setting of a sporadic outbreak. It shows a striking male-to-female predominance, on the order of 10:1, although this may be due to greater identification of disease in men. In the developing world, chancroid is associated with intercourse with commercial sex workers. In contrast to genital herpes and syphilis, untreated chancroid ulcers can persist for many months.

In the United States, patients with chancroid typically seek care for an ulcer that has been present for 1–3 weeks. Chancroid ulcers are usually painful, generally larger than chancres or herpes lesions, and likely to be multiple. The "soft chancre" of chancroid is classically described as well circumscribed and nonindurated, with ragged edges and a necrotic base with purulent exudate, which bleeds when scraped. If the constellation of a painful genital ulcer with associated tender lymphadenopathy is seen, the diagnosis of chancroid can be made with some confidence. In fact, this "classic" presentation occurs in fewer than half of patients. Diagnosis is best established by obtaining a swab for culture on selective medium (notify the testing laboratory that chancroid is suspected), or presumptively in patients with a typical presentation in the setting of a local outbreak.

D. Lymphogranuloma Venereum

Lymphogranuloma venereum is caused by three serotypes (L1, L2, and L3) of *Chlamydia trachomatis,* and its presentation varies depending on the site of infection. Rectal lymphogranuloma venereum was recently reported in MSM in the Netherlands and has now been identified in some gay communities in the United States. However, rectal lymphogranuloma venereum almost never presents with external ulcers. Infection on the male external genitalia is characterized by a small, transient ulcer in the earliest phase of illness; subsequently very large, tender inguinal lymphadenopathy and constitutional symptoms predominate. In cases of rectal or female genital involvement, the infection drains to pelvic lymph nodes, and inguinal lymphadenopathy is usually not apparent.

Only about 10% of patients with lymphogranuloma venereum present with a complaint of a genital ulcer, which has usually resolved by the time the patient seeks care. Diagnosis can be made by a positive culture or molecular testing of appropriate clinical specimens for *C trachomatis* in the setting of an appropriate syndrome. Some laboratories can analyze an isolate to confirm that it is a lymphogranuloma serotype or genotype, but a presumptive diagnosis can be made merely by isolating *C trachomatis* from a lesion in a patient with a typical presentation.

E. Donovanosis

Donovanosis, a rare condition also known as granuloma inguinale, is caused by infection with the gram-negative bacterium *Calymmatobacterium granulomatis*. It is endemic to certain geographic "hot spots," most notably Papua New Guinea and parts of South Africa, as well as Australia, Brazil, and parts of the Caribbean. Donovanosis is rarely reported in the United States. The typical ulcerative form of donovanosis is beefy red and bleeds easily when touched. The lesions of donovanosis may also be hypertrophic, often raised above the surrounding skin, and can become dry and verrucous in appearance. In its exuberant hypertrophic form, donovanosis can be mistaken for carcinoma, tuberculosis, or condylomata lata. It is generally not painful. "Kissing lesions" (ie, on areas of the skin in contact with each other, such as bilateral labia) or autoinoculation of other body sites may occur. The lesions of donovanosis do not resolve unless treated appropriately.

O'Farrell N. Donovanosis. *Sex Transm Infect* 2002;78:452–457. [PMID: 12473810] (An excellent review of an uncommon disease.)

F. Cancer

Although the vast majority of genital ulcers are not neoplastic, cancers and premalignant lesions may present as GUD and can carry considerable morbidity and mortality if not diagnosed early. Thus, all practitioners should be able to recognize a suspicious lesion. A large percentage of squamous cell carcinomas of the vulva, vagina, and penis are associated with human papillomavirus infection, as are virtually all cervical and anal squamous cell cancers. Thus, the patient with a history of sexually transmitted infections may be at increased risk of genital malignancy. A prior history of an abnormal Pap smear or anogenital warts may be helpful but is not always present in such cases. Physical findings suggestive of cancer include hyperpigmentation, tenderness, and induration. If the provider does not have the capability of performing a detailed examination under high magnification (ie, colposcopy) and biopsy in the office, patients with these findings should be referred to an experienced surgeon expeditiously.

G. Other Causes of Genital Ulcers

1. Fixed drug eruption—A fixed drug eruption is a localized skin lesion that occurs in response to a medication, generally an oral medication that is used intermittently. Fixed drug eruptions may involve any part of the skin, and the genitalia are sometimes affected They are most often solitary, well-circumscribed plaques, but they occasionally become ulcers, which may be painful and may mimic genital herpes. The most common genital sites of involvement are the glans and shaft of the penis. Tetracyclines and nonsteroidal anti-inflammatory drugs have been implicated in this regard, as have less commonly used medications such as hydroxyurea and foscarnet.

2. Behçet syndrome—Behçet syndrome is an idiopathic inflammatory multisystem disease characterized by oral and genital ulcerations and ocular disease. The genital lesions of Behçet syndrome are painful except when the vagina or cervix is involved, and they tend to heal with scarring. Although these lesions may be confused with genital herpes, the diagnosis can be made by taking note of the multisystem nature of the disease.

3. Other genital and systemic infections—Severe candidiasis can lead to skin breakdown and should be considered in the differential diagnosis. In addition to specific genital infections, several systemic illnesses can present with genital ulcers, including infections such as tuberculosis, histoplasmosis, and tularemia. Tularemia acquired from a tick bite may present with an ulcer in the genital region, perineum, or lower trunk (reflecting the site of inoculation) and inguinal adenopathy. The ulcer of tularemia is frequently tender and has a raised border. When it occurs on the genitalia it can be confused with syphilis, lymphogranuloma venereum, or chancroid. Genitourinary tuberculosis is well known historically but rarely presents with lesions mimicking STDs; in women, an ulcerating mass may be seen on the cervix, and in men, a painful mass in the scrotum may be associated with a draining sinus.

4. Primary HIV infection—Patients with primary HIV infection frequently present with a constellation of symptoms that may include oral and genital ulcers in up to 15% of cases. Although the presence of mucocutaneous ulcers in the setting of a recent exposure to an HIV-infected source is considered highly predictive of acute HIV disease by some experts, ulcers are not the predominant manifestation of this disease. More common signs and symptoms are most often present in acute HIV infection, including fevers, sweats, malaise, lymphadenopathy, and an evanescent maculopapular eruption.

5. Sexual trauma—External genital ulcers occur occasionally in men due to sexual trauma (eg, vigorous masturbation, biting during fellatio, etc) or nonsexual injury. The etiology may be obvious to the patient and can often be elicited by taking a sensitive and thorough history. Likewise, women may have internal genital ulcerations after a traumatic sexual assault.

Complications

Although genital ulcers are not generally life-threatening, some of the pathogens of GUD are associated with significant complications if untreated. The sequelae of untreated syphilis are considered elsewhere (see Chapter 19). Perhaps the gravest complication of GUD, overall, is its role in facilitating HIV infection. Given the high prevalence of HIV coinfection in patients with GUD, all such patients should be strongly counseled to undergo testing for HIV.

A. Scarring, Strictures, and Genital Deformity

Untreated chancroid can result in phimosis, balanoposthitis, and formation of fistulous tracts or nonhealing ulcers from draining buboes. Lymphogranuloma venereum that is not treated early in the course of the infection can progress to scarring, rectal strictures, genital deformity and fistula formation. Donovanosis is a progressive destructive granulomatous infection that can result in considerable tissue destruction and deformity if untreated.

B. Systemic Complications

Both lymphogranuloma venereum and donovanosis can spread systemically if not treated promptly. Systemic spread of lymphogranuloma venereum is most common

in women and may result in arthritis, ocular disease, aseptic meningitis, hepatitis or perihepatitis, or pulmonary disease. Donovanosis can involve multiple organs, including viscera and bone.

Treatment

When no pathogen has been identified, the provider may have to resort to empiric treatment. It is probably wisest to treat for both HSV and syphilis in such circumstances. Additional coverage for the more exotic pathogens should be added only if suggested by the patient's history. Table 4–2 summarizes preferred and alternative treatments for the most common causes of GUD. Laboratory "test of cure" is not required except for syphilis, where the RPR should be repeated to confirm a decline in titer (if positive initially). However, it is advisable to follow up cases of chancroid, lymphogranuloma venereum, and donovanosis clinically to confirm an appropriate response to therapy.

When to Refer to a Specialist

Evaluation by a dermatologist or infectious disease specialist is warranted when diagnostic tests for HSV, *T pallidum,* and *H ducreyi* have been negative, particularly if the patient has failed to respond to empiric anti-infective therapy directed toward these common pathogens. Early referral is particularly important if cancer is suspected; a patient with an ulcerating lesion that is raised or indurated, especially if also painful, should be referred promptly for biopsy if the lesion does not respond to anti-infective treatment.

Prognosis

With appropriate treatment, GUD is always either treatable or curable. Some causes of GUD (syphilis, lymphogranuloma venereum, chancroid, and donovanosis) may have long-term complications if untreated.

 PRACTICE POINTS

- As a general rule, whenever there is doubt as to the etiology, it is safest to assume that genital ulcers are sexually acquired.
- When no pathogen has been identified, the provider may have to resort to empiric treatment. It is probably wisest to treat for both HSV and syphilis in such circumstances.

Table 4–2. Recommended and alternative treatments for causes of genital ulcer disease.

Diagnosis	Treatment	Comments
Genital herpes		
Primary episode	Acyclovir, 400 mg PO 3 times daily for 7–10 d[a] *or* Famciclovir, 250 mg PO 3 times daily for 7–10 d[a] *or* Valacyclovir, 1000 mg PO twice daily for 7–10 d[a]	
Recurrence	Acyclovir, 400 mg PO 3 times daily for 5 d[a] *or* Acyclovir, 800 mg PO twice daily for 5 d[a] *or* Famciclovir, 125 mg PO twice daily for 5 d[a] *or* Valacyclovir, 500 mg PO twice daily for 3–5 d[a] *or* Valacyclovir, 1 g PO daily for 5 d[a]	In HIV, episodes may be prolonged or severe; acyclovir, 5–10 mg/kg IV q 8 h may be necessary
Syphilis (primary)	Benzathine penicillin G, 2.4 million U IM[a] *For penicillin allergy:* Doxycycline, 100 mg PO twice daily for 14 d *or* Ceftriaxone, 1 g IM or IV daily for 8–10 d (limited studies)	Penicillin should be used *whenever possible;* use of ceftriaxone has not been studied in HIV; azithromycin, 2 g PO as a single dose, has been used, but azithromycin resistance has been reported, limiting its usefulness
Chancroid	Azithromycin, 1 g PO as a single dose[a] *or* Ceftriaxone, 250 mg IM as a single dose[a] *or* Ciprofloxacin, 500 mg PO twice daily for 3 d[a] *or* Erythromycin base, 500 mg PO 3 times daily for 7 d[a]	Reexamine 3–7 d after treatment; buboes may require drainage
Lymphogranuloma venereum	Doxycycline, 100 mg PO twice daily for 21 d[a] *or* Erythromycin base, 500 mg PO 4 times daily for 21 d	
Donovanosis (granuloma inguinale)	Doxycycline, 100 mg PO twice daily[a] *or* Trimethoprim-sulfamethoxazole, 800 mg/160 mg PO twice daily[a] *or* Ciprofloxacin, 750 mg PO twice daily *or* Erythromycin base, 500 mg PO 4 times daily *or* Azithromycin, 1 g PO weekly	Treat until complete resolution occurs; minimum of 3 wk required

[a]First-line treatment.

Lower Abdominal Pain in Women | 5

Mark H. Yudin, MD, MSc, FRCSC, & Harold C. Wiesenfeld, MDCM

ESSENTIALS OF DIAGNOSIS

- *Lower abdominal pain in women is a common presenting complaint; pain characteristics (duration, location, quality, and severity) may be helpful in determining the diagnosis.*
- *Pain may be caused by gynecologic disorders, but also by disorders of the gastrointestinal, urinary, and musculoskeletal systems.*
- *Pain on abdominal or pelvic examination may signal peritoneal irritation.*
- *History, physical examination, and laboratory tests should be used to arrive at a diagnosis.*
- *Ultrasound may aid in the diagnosis; diagnostic laparoscopy can provide a definitive diagnosis and may be considered when the diagnosis is uncertain.*

General Considerations

Lower abdominal pain is a common presenting complaint and one of the most difficult problems to evaluate in women. Arriving at the correct diagnosis when a woman of reproductive age presents with acute pelvic pain remains a challenge in clinical medicine—a fact that has been confirmed by numerous studies. A comprehensive evaluation leading to a timely diagnosis will reduce the morbidity associated with delayed diagnosis.

Pelvic pain is a common presenting symptom of many gynecologic disorders. However, it also may occur with disorders of the gastrointestinal, urinary, and musculoskeletal systems. To determine the etiology of the pain, the clinician must use the history, physical examination, and diagnostic tests as tools.

Clinical Findings

A. SYMPTOMS AND SIGNS

1. Pain characteristics—Characteristics of the pain may aid in determining the diagnosis. Important characteristics include timing of onset, location, quality, and severity.

a. Onset—Pain of sudden onset suggests an acute event such as hemorrhage, rupture, or torsion of an ovarian cyst, whereas pain that is more gradual may be present in subacute or progressive conditions. The differential diagnosis of lower abdominal pain grouped by time of onset is presented in Table 5–1.

b. Location—The location of the pain may also be helpful, although different disease processes can lead to pain in the same region. The uterus, cervix, and adnexae share visceral innervation with the lower ileum, sigmoid, and rectum (T10–L1), and pain from any of these structures may be felt in the same place. This is one of the dilemmas when trying to distinguish acute appendicitis from pelvic inflammatory disease (PID), although typically the pain of appendicitis is localized in the right lower quadrant whereas that of PID is more diffuse. Diffuse and generalized pain should alert the clinician to the possibility of peritonitis, which may be seen following intra-abdominal hemorrhage or sepsis.

c. Quality and severity—Although pain quality and severity are nonspecific symptoms, they may provide some clue to the etiology of the pain. Abrupt and severe pain is typically associated with perforation (ectopic pregnancy), strangulation (ovarian torsion), or hemorrhage (ovarian cysts). Crampy pain is often seen with dysmenorrhea or spontaneous abortion. Pain that is colicky in nature is typical of ovarian torsion or nephrolithiasis. Burning or aching pain often occurs with inflammatory processes such as appendicitis or PID.

2. Associated symptoms—Associated symptoms are often helpful when trying to narrow the diagnosis. Pain with fever suggests an infectious or inflammatory etiology, such as appendicitis, PID, or a tubo-ovarian abscess.

Table 5–1. Differential diagnosis of lower abdominal pain by time of onset.

Acute onset (seconds to minutes)
  Aortic dissection
  Nephrolithiasis
  Ovarian cysts
    Rupture
    Hemorrhage
    Torsion
  Rupture
    Tubo-ovarian abscess
    Abdominal aortic aneurysm
    Ectopic pregnancy
Gradual onset (hours to days)
  Abortion
  Appendicitis
  Diverticulitis
  Ectopic pregnancy
  Gastroenteritis
  Herpes zoster
  Mittelschmerz (midcycle ovulatory pain)
  Pelvic inflammatory disease (PID)
  Primary dysmenorrhea
Slow onset (days to weeks)
  Abdominal aortic aneurysm
  Abortion
  Cystitis
  Diverticulitis
  Ectopic pregnancy
  Neoplasms
  PID
  Pyelonephritis
Chronic onset (weeks to months)
  Chronic pelvic pain
  Diverticular disease
  Domestic violence or sexual abuse
  Endometriosis
  Inflammatory bowel disease
  Neoplasms
  Irritable bowel syndrome

Nausea, vomiting, and anorexia are nonspecific symptoms of peritoneal irritation that may be present in patients with inflammatory conditions and hemoperitoneum. Vaginal discharge can occur with infectious conditions of the female genital tract, such as cervicitis or PID. Vaginal bleeding may be associated with pregnancy-related disorders, abnormalities of the menstrual cycle, PID, or pathology of the uterus or cervix.

3. Aggravating and alleviating factors—Depending on the etiology, changes in pain may occur in relation to menses, coitus, activity, diet, bowel movements, or voiding.

4. Vital signs—In women who present with lower abdominal pain, vital signs must be obtained as part of the evaluation. The presence of fever is a key feature that can help to identify an inflammatory process but may not help to specify which one. One study, for example, found no significant difference between oral temperatures in patients with PID and appendicitis. Women with acute PID or tubo-ovarian abscess may be afebrile; therefore, the absence of fever should not exclude these conditions. In conditions that raise suspicion of hemorrhage, such as ruptured ectopic pregnancy or hemorrhagic ovarian cysts, orthostatic pulse and blood pressure should be measured to evaluate for hypovolemia.

5. Abdominal examination—The important components of the abdominal examination include inspection, auscultation, percussion, and palpation. Bowel sounds may be decreased in the presence of peritoneal irritation. Percussion and palpation can help to identify masses and peritoneal irritation. Peritoneal irritation is confirmed by the presence of rebound tenderness, involuntary guarding, and increased pain with motion or cough.

6. Pelvic examination—The pelvic examination is most easily organized to proceed from external to internal structures.

    a. External structures—The external genitalia should be carefully inspected for lesions. The presence of inguinal adenopathy is suggestive of a local infectious process such as genital ulcer disease. On speculum examination, the vagina and cervix should be visualized. Lesions, blood, or discharge should be noted. The presence of cervical discharge, erythema, or friability should alert the clinician to the possibility of cervicitis or PID. Grossly purulent cervical discharge (mucopus) reflects a high concentration of polymorphonuclear leukocytes in the mucus, but the presence of mucopus has not been shown to accurately predict PID.

    b. Internal structures—On internal pelvic examination, the first step should be an assessment for cervical motion tenderness. Its presence is nonspecific and may indicate PID, ectopic pregnancy, endometriosis, or appendicitis. Next, a bimanual examination should be performed, with assessment of the uterus and adnexae. An enlarged uterus may indicate fibroids or pregnancy. A uterus that is fixed and immobile may occur as a result of adhesions from endometriosis or PID. Adnexal enlargement may be seen with ovarian cysts, torsion, tubo-ovarian abscess, or ectopic pregnancy. Pain on bimanual examination may occur with endometritis, degenerating uterine fibroids, endometriosis, PID, ovarian cysts or torsion, ectopic pregnancy, or appendicitis. Finally, digital rectal and rectovaginal examinations should be performed. These parts of the examination can be especially useful when abdominal examination is unremarkable. Nodularity in the cul-de-sac or on the uterosacral ligaments as a result of endometriosis may be appreciated this way. Also, a tender mass may be palpated in certain gastrointestinal disorders, such as appendicitis or diverticulitis.

When interpreting the pelvic examination, it is important to remember that movement of the pelvic organs will be painful if peritoneal irritation is present, regardless of the cause. Therefore, cervical motion tenderness and adnexal tenderness may be found with a variety of disorders, not only pelvic infection. In one study that compared findings in patients with PID and appendicitis, cervical motion tenderness was found significantly more often in patients with PID, but was still found in 28% of patients with appendicitis. Adnexal tenderness was found with equal frequency in both groups but was usually limited to the right side in patients with appendicitis and was usually, but not always, bilateral in patients with PID.

B. LABORATORY FINDINGS

Laboratory and diagnostic imaging tests may help in the differential diagnosis of acute pelvic pain but should be interpreted cautiously. Baseline tests should include at least a complete blood count (CBC) and pregnancy test. The white blood cell (WBC) count may be elevated in inflammatory conditions, and the hematocrit may be low in the setting of hemorrhage. In one study, the total WBC count was significantly higher in patients with appendicitis than in those with PID (15.3 cells/ mm^3 vs 12.7 cells/mm^3, $P < .01$). It is important to note, however, that the CBC has a low sensitivity and specificity. The hematocrit is low in roughly one third of patients with ectopic pregnancy but normal in the remainder. In studies, a normal WBC count has been found in over half of patients with PID and in one third of patients with acute appendicitis, whereas an elevated WBC count is commonly seen in patients with ectopic pregnancies and bleeding corpus luteum cysts. The erythrocyte sedimentation rate is another nonspecific sign of inflammation. It is classically elevated in PID, but can be normal in up to 25% of patients.

A urinalysis should be performed on every patient with acute pelvic pain to rule out the presence of a urinary tract infection or kidney stone. Care must be taken with specimen collection to avoid contamination by vaginal or cervical discharge. Cervical specimens should be obtained to test for *Neisseria gonorrhoeae* and *Chlamydia trachomatis*. Vaginal fluid should be collected for saline (wet mount) and potassium hydroxide (KOH) preparation, for the diagnosis of bacterial vaginosis, *Trichomonas vaginalis,* and yeast infection. The finding of leukocytes on wet mount is very useful for making the diagnosis of PID, and the presence of 3 or more leukocytes per high-power field has a high sensitivity. Furthermore, the absence of leukocytes has a high negative predictive value for excluding PID as a diagnosis.

C. IMAGING STUDIES

Imaging studies, especially ultrasound, may be very useful in making the diagnosis. Ultrasound is invaluable in the evaluation of ovarian cysts and their complications. Ultrasound, especially when performed transvaginally, is often the most useful imaging modality for the gynecologic organs. Nonetheless, computed tomography and magnetic resonance imaging scanning may also be helpful in the evaluation of women presenting with lower abdominal pain, especially when a nongynecologic cause is higher up on the differential diagnosis.

D. SPECIAL TESTS

Diagnostic laparoscopy is perhaps the most definitive way to arrive at a diagnosis in a patient with acute pelvic pain. It is the best and most reliable method to achieve a complete evaluation of the pelvic structures, and allows direct visual access to the peritoneal cavity. It must be remembered, however, that although laparoscopy is minimally invasive, it carries with it some risks. Vascular injuries, as well as injuries to the gastrointestinal and urinary tracts, have been reported. The overall risk of injury to a vital structure has been estimated at between 2 and 3 per 1000. The high cost associated with diagnostic laparoscopy limits its utility in many cases of abdominal pain. Finally, although laparoscopy can be helpful, it requires the involvement of a gynecologist. Consultation may be useful in cases where the diagnosis remains unclear after investigation, or where the chosen treatment regimen is not resulting in the patient's improvement.

Differential Diagnosis

To assist in the diagnosis of acute pelvic pain, it is convenient to divide the causes into pregnancy-related, gynecologic, and nongynecologic. The gynecologic causes can be further subdivided into infectious and noninfectious. This classification is presented in Table 5–2.

When considering the diagnosis in a female patient with lower abdominal or pelvic pain, it is important to remember that this is a nonspecific symptom, with a wide variety of causes. Although lower abdominal pain is the most consistent symptom in patients with confirmed PID, it is seen with many other conditions as well. Similarly, pain on abdominal, pelvic, or bimanual examination can be a result of many conditions. Movement of the pelvic organs during examination will be painful if peritoneal irritation is present, regardless of the cause. Cervical motion tenderness can be found in up to 97% of patients with PID but is also commonly found in those with other disorders, such as ectopic pregnancy and appendicitis.

Of particular importance is the patient who presents with pelvic pain following an episode of **domestic violence** or **sexual assault**. It is estimated that up to 44% of all women have been the victims of an actual or attempted assault at some time in their lives. Women who have suffered abuse may account for 22–35% of

Table 5–2. Differential diagnosis of acute pelvic pain.

Pregnancy-related causes
Ectopic pregnancy
Spontaneous abortion (threatened, complete, incomplete, septic)
Gynecologic causes
Infectious
  Endometritis
  Pelvic inflammatory disease or salpingitis
  Tubo-ovarian abscess
Noninfectious
  Domestic violence or sexual abuse
  Dysmenorrhea
  Endometriosis
  Mittelschmerz
  Ovarian cancer or tumor
  Ovarian cysts (rupture, hemorrhage, torsion)
  Ovarian hyperstimulation syndrome following assisted reproductive technologies
  Uterine fibroids
Nongynecologic causes
Gastrointestinal
  Abdominopelvic adhesions
  Appendicitis
  Bowel obstruction
  Constipation
  Diverticulitis
  Gastroenteritis
  Inflammatory bowel disease
  Irritable bowel syndrome
  Mesenteric lymphadenitis
Urinary
  Interstitial cystitis
  Lower urinary tract infection or cystitis
  Nephrolithiasis
  Pyelonephritis
Musculoskeletal
  Hernia
  Joint infection or inflammation
  Strained tendons or muscles
Other
  Aortic aneurysm
  Aortic dissection
  Porphyria

women seeking care for any reason in an emergency department. Finally, it has been estimated that two million cases of domestic violence occur each year in the United States. The patient may present with vague symptoms and pain that is not well localized, and may not volunteer that she has been the victim of assault. Abuse may not be raised by the patient, and probing may be necessary. If a woman presenting with pain seems extremely nervous, anxious, or uneasy during the evaluation, it is appropriate to ask if she has been the victim of any unwanted sexual activity or physical violence. These patients need to be evaluated by clinicians familiar with the appropriate counseling and specimen collection techniques. Most hospitals have an assault or crisis team with a protocol for evaluating and managing these patients. Physical examination is tailored to a systematic search for injuries and to the collection of samples. Appropriate workup includes screening for sexually transmitted diseases (STDs), and pregnancy and HIV testing. Consideration must also be given to emergency contraception and prophylaxis for HIV and other infections.

Certain patient characteristics may assist in narrowing the differential diagnosis. The **age** of the patient can be useful, as infectious causes of pain such as PID and appendicitis are more common in younger women (adolescents and women younger than 30 years of age), whereas disorders such as diverticulitis are more commonly seen in women older than 40. The differential diagnosis of pain grouped by patient age is presented in Table 5–3. The **menstrual history,** including last normal menstrual period, can also be helpful. If the patient has missed any menstrual periods or if the last period was atypical, the diagnosis of pregnancy must be considered. If the patient is at midcycle, her pain may be related to ovulation (mittelschmerz). If the patient is menstruating, she may be suffering from dysmenorrhea.

Table 5–3. Differential diagnoses of pelvic pain by age.[a]

Menarche to age 21
  Appendicitis
  Dysmenorrhea
  Inflammatory bowel disease
  Ovarian cysts (rupture, hemorrhage, torsion)
  Pelvic inflammatory disease (PID)
  Pregnancy (spontaneous abortion, ectopic pregnancy)
Ages 21–35
  Endometriosis
  Irritable bowel syndrome
  Ovarian cysts
  PID
  Pregnancy (spontaneous abortion, ectopic pregnancy)
Age 35 to menopause
  Diverticulitis
  Endometriosis
  Hernias
  Irritable bowel syndrome
  Nephrolithiasis
  Ovarian cancer or tumor
  PID
  Pregnancy (abortion, ectopic pregnancy)
  Uterine fibroids

[a]There is considerable overlap between age groups.

The results of some studies have suggested that PID is more likely to occur in the first half of the menstrual cycle, whereas appendicitis is randomly distributed.

A **contraceptive history** is also of diagnostic value. Women not using reliable contraception are at risk for pregnancy. Women not using barrier methods of contraception are at increased risk for STDs and PID, whereas those using barrier methods or combined oral contraceptives have a reduction in the risk of PID of approximately 50%. The presence of an intrauterine contraceptive device (IUD) increases the risk for developing acute PID, particularly around the time of insertion. Historically, IUD users were at an overall increased risk for PID, but with currently available IUDs this risk is limited to the time of insertion. IUD use does not increase the absolute risk for developing an ectopic pregnancy. However, an IUD is more effective at preventing intrauterine versus extrauterine gestation, so a pregnancy that occurs with an IUD in place has a 10-fold increased risk of being ectopic.

Finally, a **sexual history** is important. Information about sexual habits and risky behavior, current partners, and number of lifetime partners helps the clinician to estimate the patient's risk of STDs and PID.

A complete **medical and surgical history** may assist with the differential diagnosis. A history of urinary or gastrointestinal tract disorders may be a clue to the current problem. The surgical history may help to rule out certain disorders (eg, appendicitis) or heighten awareness of the possibility of other problems (eg, ectopic pregnancy in a patient with previous pelvic or tubal surgery).

To establish a working diagnosis in the woman of reproductive age with acute pelvic pain, the clinician must use all tools available. Clinical history, physical examination, laboratory tests, and imaging procedures are useful in providing diagnostic clues, but they may lack adequate sensitivity or specificity to make a final diagnosis. For example, abnormal uterine bleeding is part of the classic triad of symptoms for ectopic pregnancy but is absent in up to 50% of patients with this diagnosis. Similarly, up to 50% of patients with ectopic pregnancy have no palpable mass, and 43% have cervical motion tenderness. Despite a comprehensive history and physical examination, a significant proportion of patients with acute pelvic pain will continue to have an unclear diagnosis.

Bongard F, Landers DV, Lewis F. Differential diagnosis of appendicitis and pelvic inflammatory disease. *Am J Surg* 1985; 150:90–96. [PMID: 3160252] (A classic article describing the differences in clinical presentation between appendicitis and PID.)

Hewitt GD, Brown RT. Acute and chronic pelvic pain in female adolescents. *Med Clin North Am* 2000;84:1009–1025. [PMID: 10928199] (A discussion of the differential diagnosis of acute pelvic pain in adolescents.)

Robertson C. Differential diagnosis of lower abdominal pain in women of childbearing age. *Lippincotts Prim Care Pract* 1998;2:210–229. [PMID: 9644437] (A review of the causes of lower abdominal pain in women.)

Complications

Many causes of lower abdominal pain in women are not associated with long-term complications, provided they are managed quickly and effectively. However, some of these conditions may lead to sequelae. Spontaneous abortion is common and usually not associated with long-term problems. Ectopic pregnancy may result in tubal damage or loss of the fallopian tube if rupture occurs. Endometritis can progress to myometritis, parametritis, or peritonitis.

PID may lead to both short-term and long-term consequences as a result of upper genital tract infection. Short-term sequelae include perihepatitis or Fitz-Hugh-Curtis syndrome (occurring in 15–30% of women with acute PID), tubo-ovarian abscess (occurring in 15–34% of women with acute PID), and death (occurring very rarely). Long-term sequelae include infertility (with the risk increasing with the number and severity of episodes of PID), ectopic pregnancy (with the risk 7- to 10-fold higher compared with women who have no history of PID), and chronic pelvic pain (occurring in 17–24% of women after acute PID). Chronic pelvic pain after PID is usually a result of pelvic adhesions caused by the inflammatory response to the infection. Similar to other sequelae after PID, the rate of chronic pelvic pain is proportional to the number and severity of episodes of PID. Pain can sometimes be severe enough to require analgesia, and may lead to the need for surgery.

Endometriosis may lead to pelvic adhesive disease, chronic pelvic pain, and infertility.

Treatment

The management of lower abdominal or pelvic pain in the female patient depends on the cause. The first step in management is, in fact, narrowing the wide differential diagnosis to come to a working diagnosis, using the previously described tools (history, physical examination, and laboratory tests). The differential should first be narrowed by system. That is, the clinician should first determine whether the pain has a gynecologic or nongynecologic cause. Determining whether the patient is pregnant is paramount in aiding with the diagnosis. Referral to a specialist is appropriate when the diagnosis is unclear.

A. ACUTE PELVIC PAIN

The most common pregnancy-related causes of acute pelvic pain are **abortion** and **ectopic pregnancy**. Some spontaneous abortions require no treatment, but some women may require medical or surgical intervention to complete the process. Ectopic pregnancy is a condition that requires medical or surgical management depending on several factors, including the size of the ectopic gestation, stability of the patient, and patient reliability. Medical management is accomplished with methotrexate, and surgical options include salpingostomy or salpingectomy via either laparoscopy or laparotomy. Referral to a gynecologic specialist is essential.

B. Infectious Gynecologic Causes of Pain

Infectious gynecologic causes of acute pelvic pain include endometritis, PID, and tubo-ovarian abscess. **Endometritis** is a polymicrobial infection, and treatment must therefore be with an antibiotic regimen covering a broad spectrum of bacteria. **PID** can also be caused by a wide spectrum of bacteria, both sexually and nonsexually transmitted, and management by a gynecologist is essential. The treatment regimens currently recommended by the Centers for Disease Control and Prevention are discussed in Chapter 8. **Tubo-ovarian abscess** is usually associated with PID and requires broad-spectrum antibiotics with anaerobic coverage (eg, metronidazole) and, depending on the size of the abscess, surgical drainage.

C. Noninfectious Gynecologic Causes of Pain

There are many noninfectious gynecologic causes of acute pelvic pain, each requiring different treatment strategies. The typical treatment of **dysmenorrhea** is with prostaglandin synthase inhibitors such as nonsteroidal anti-inflammatory drugs (NSAIDs) or combined oral contraceptives. Management of **uterine fibroids** is either medical (ie, NSAIDs or hormonal suppression) or surgical (ie, myomectomy or hysterectomy). Treatment of **endometriosis** is either medical or surgical. Medical therapy includes oral contraceptives, progestins, danazol, or gonadotropin-releasing hormone agonists. The objective of surgical therapy is to restore normal anatomy and to remove or ablate as much abnormal tissue as possible; this can be accomplished with laparoscopy or laparotomy.

For physiologic **cysts of the ovary** such as follicular and corpus luteum cysts, management should be expectant as they usually resolve spontaneously within 4 to 8 weeks. Complications such as rupture, hemorrhage, or torsion may require surgical intervention. Rupture of a follicular cyst leads to release of fluid, which may irritate the peritoneum and cause pain. This pain is typically sudden in onset and may be severe but is self-limited and resolves without treatment. Corpus luteum cysts have an extensive vascular supply and rupture can lead to severe hemorrhage and pain that can be indistinguishable from that of a ruptured ectopic pregnancy. If the diagnosis of a ruptured corpus luteum cyst is confirmed and the patient is stable, expectant management may be appropriate. If significant hemorrhage is suspected or the patient is unstable, surgery is required.

Adnexal torsion is an acute surgical emergency because the blood supply to the adnexa is interrupted, and this can lead to necrosis and infarction. Surgical management is usually accomplished via laparoscopy. The current surgical approach involves untwisting the adnexa and assessing its viability, and removing the ovary if it is not viable. If an ovarian cyst is present, a cystectomy should be done to obtain a histologic diagnosis.

D. Nongynecologic Causes of Pain

Nongynecologic causes of acute pelvic pain include disorders of the gastrointestinal, urinary, and musculoskeletal systems. Treatment should be directed to the cause. Acute appendicitis is managed surgically with appendectomy, either laparoscopically or through an incision over McBurney's point. The treatment of gastroenteritis is usually supportive care with fluids and bowel rest. Diverticulitis, inflammatory bowel disease, and bowel obstruction may all be managed medically or surgically depending on the severity. Treatment of lower urinary tract infections can usually be accomplished with oral antibiotics. Pyelonephritis may require hospital admission and parenteral antibiotics, as these patients are typically unwell and may have high fevers with chills. Management of nephrolithiasis is usually expectant and involves analgesia and hydration; surgical treatment is occasionally required. For musculoskeletal causes of lower abdominal, pelvic, or back pain, management is usually medical, with muscle relaxants or NSAIDs.

Centers for Disease Control and Prevention; Workowski KA, Berman SM. Sexually transmitted diseases treatment guidelines, 2006. *MMWR Recomm Rep* 2006;55(RR-11):1–94. [PMID: 16888612] (Outlines the current treatment regimens for STDs.)

When to Refer to a Specialist

Because the diagnosis of lower abdominal pain in women has such a wide variety of causes, it is helpful to narrow the differential diagnosis before referral to a specialist is made. Once the diagnosis has been categorized by organ system (gynecologic, gastrointestinal, urinary, or musculoskeletal), referral may be considered.

Another circumstance that warrants referral occurs when the practitioner has made a diagnosis and begun treatment, but the treatment regimen does not seem to be resulting in cure. In complicated cases such as these, consultation with a specialist may be helpful.

PRACTICE POINTS

• *The finding of leukocytes on wet mount is very useful for making the diagnosis of PID, and the presence of 3 or more leukocytes per high-power field has a high sensitivity. Furthermore, the absence of leukocytes has a high negative predictive value for excluding PID as a diagnosis.*

Epididymitis & the Acute Scrotum Syndrome

6

William M. Geisler, MD, MPH, & John N. Krieger, MD

ESSENTIALS OF DIAGNOSIS

- *Scrotal pain and swelling is typically unilateral in epididymitis.*
- *Epididymitis is typically characterized by the presence of urethritis or bacteriuria.*
- *An abnormally high position of the testicle may indicate testicular torsion.*
- *Have a low threshold to obtain a doppler ultrasound or radionuclide scanning to rule out testicular torsion in adolescents or young adults, because prompt surgical intervention is essential to save the involved testicle.*

General Considerations

Epididymitis, an inflammatory process involving the epididymis, is one of the primary etiologies of the acute scrotum syndrome. Epididymitis is common and can cause substantial short-term morbidity (eg, suffering and loss of time from work) and long-term complications (eg, infertility, chronic epididymitis, etc). The incidence of epididymitis may range from 1 to 4 per 1000 men per year. The inflammatory process causes a gradual onset of scrotal pain and swelling that is characteristically unilateral.

With the improved understanding of the etiology of epididymitis, the diagnosis and management of this condition is becoming more rational, leading to decreased morbidity and, possibly, to prevention of recurrences. Epididymitis usually results from infection. There are two main infectious causes: (1) urethral infection with *Neisseria gonorrhoeae* or *Chlamydia trachomatis,* and (2) genitourinary tract infection with coliform bacteria or *Pseudomonas aeruginosa* (see Table 6–1). Age is an important predictor of

the etiology, with heterosexual men younger than 35 years of age more likely to have a sexually transmitted pathogen, and older individuals more likely to have a pathogen associated with bacteriuria. In rare cases, epididymitis may occur as a complication of systemic infection with various bacterial, fungal, viral, or parasitic pathogens, or may be due to noninfectious causes (see Table 6–1). In prepubertal boys, epididymitis may be related to concomitant presence of structural, functional, or neurologic abnormalities of the genitourinary tract. Men who have sex with men and who practice insertive anal intercourse are at greater risk for epididymitis caused by coliform bacteria. Cases for which no etiologic agent can be determined after thorough investigation are referred to as idiopathic.

Pathogenesis

The epididymis is a sausage-shaped structure positioned on the posterior aspect of the testicle. It consists of a single, delicate convoluted tubule 12–15 feet long. During passage through the epididymis, sperm become motile and achieve the potential to fertilize an ovum. Hence, inflammation and fibrosis from epididymitis can impair the passage and maturation of sperm, leading to infertility. In epididymitis associated with urethritis or bacteriuria, there is a retrograde spread of infection intraluminally to the epididymis. In contrast, systemic infections spread to the epididymis by a hematogenous route. Reflux of sterile urine does not cause epididymitis.

Clinical Findings

Clinical manifestations, laboratory results, and imaging findings may differ, depending on the etiology of the acute scrotum syndrome. In epididymitis, clinical findings are influenced by whether the etiology is infectious versus noninfectious, and in the case of the former, by whether the presentation is local versus systemic.

Table 6–1. Etiology of epididymitis.

Associated with urethritis
  Gonorrhea
  Chlamydia
  Trichomoniasis
Associated with bacteriuria
  Coliform bacteria (eg, *Escherichia coli*)
  Pseudomonas aeruginosa
Associated with funguria
  Candida spp
Associated with systemic infection
  Bacterial
    Tuberculosis
    Mycobacterium other than *M tuberculosis* (MOTT)
    Brucellosis
    Haemophilus influenzae
  Fungal
    Histoplasmosis
    Coccidioidomycosis
    Blastomycosis
    Cryptococcosis
  Viral
    Mumps
    Cytomegalovirus
  Parasitic
    Schistosomiasis
    Sparganosis
    Bancroftian filariasis
Associated with drugs
  Amiodarone
Associated with systemic vasculitis
  Behçet syndrome
  Henoch-Schönlein purpura
  Polyarteritis nodosa
  Wegener granulomatosis
Associated with postinfectious etiology
  Upper respiratory tract infections
Associated with trauma

A. SYMPTOMS AND SIGNS

Patients with epididymitis characteristically complain of testicular or scrotal pain and may also complain of inguinal pain. In severe cases, acute swelling of the spermatic cord may result in flank pain from obstruction of the ureter as it crosses over the spermatic cord. More than two thirds of patients with epididymitis describe a gradual onset of pain.

Symptoms typical of the underlying cause, such as urethral discharge associated with sexually transmitted epididymitis or symptoms of urinary urgency and frequency associated with urinary tract infection, are discussed in detail below. Rarely, epididymitis may present with nonspecific symptoms such as fever or malaise, especially in patients with epididymitis associated with chronic catheterization or neurogenic bladder associated with a spinal cord injury.

On examination, the scrotum on the involved side may be red and edematous. The testicle tends to lie in the normal position in the scrotum. Shortly after the onset of inflammation, the tail of the epididymis, which connects with the vas deferens near the lower pole of the testes, is swollen. Later, swelling spreads to the head of the epididymis, near the upper pole of the testes. The groove between the epididymis and the testicle should be examined, as this will help to demonstrate whether the maximum swelling is in the testicle or in the epididymis. The spermatic cord may be swollen and tender (a condition termed *funiculitis*). A hydrocele may be present; characteristically this results from secretion of fluid by the inflamed tunica vaginalis. Signs and symptoms more specific for a particular etiology of epididymitis are discussed below.

1. Findings associated with urethritis—Men with epididymitis secondary to sexually transmitted pathogens often have a history of dysuria or urethral itching or discharge. Usually, they have a history of recent sexual exposure. If the patient has not voided recently, spontaneous urethral discharge may be apparent on examination. It is important to recognize that asymptomatic urethral infection without discharge may occur. Such asymptomatic urethral infections have been estimated for up to 50% of gonococcal infections and over 75% of chlamydial infections. If no spontaneous discharge is noted, then the urethra should be stripped from the base of the penis to the urethral meatus ("milked") and examined again. In some patients, digital rectal examination may reveal abnormalities suggestive of bacterial prostatitis. The degree of scrotal erythema and epididymal edema may be less in patients with chlamydial epididymitis compared with those in whom epididymitis is a result of other etiologies. However, massive erythema and edema may also occur with untreated *C trachomatis epididymitis*.

2. Findings associated with bacteriuria—In patients with coliform or pseudomonal epididymitis, a history of bacteriuria or symptoms suggesting urinary tract infection may or may not be present. Symptoms include urinary frequency, urgency, or dysuria. Patients may have a history of symptoms suggestive of urinary tract obstruction (eg, hesitancy or slow urinary stream), indicating conditions that predispose them to urinary tract infection (eg, urethral stricture and benign prostatic hypertrophy). Others may have a history of conditions predisposing them to bacteriuria, including prostatic calculi, recent genitourinary or prostate instrumentation, neurogenic bladder, an indwelling catheter, or chronic bacterial prostatitis.

3. Findings associated with systemic infectious or inflammatory diseases—Bilateral epididymal involvement is more common in epididymitis caused by systemic diseases; in contrast, epididymitis associated with urethritis or bacteriuria is nearly always unilateral. Symptoms or signs relating to systemic infection or inflammation may be present. For example, in tuberculous epididymitis, patients can present with clinical disease involving the kidneys, adrenal glands, lymphatics (retroperitoneal, abdominal, or mediastinal), or all of these structures. Patients with tuberculous epididymitis often have a prior history of pulmonary tuberculosis or a history of exposure to tuberculosis. Another example is epididymitis occurring with Behçet syndrome, in which patients may have oral or genital ulcers, other cutaneous lesions, eye involvement (eg, iritis, uveitis, etc), arthritis, and central nervous system involvement. Genitourinary examination findings in systemic infectious or inflammatory disorders otherwise tend to resemble the findings in epididymitis associated with urethritis or bacteriuria. One exception is that in tuberculous epididymitis, a "string of beads" may be noted on palpation of the vas deferens due to presence of granulomas. An additional,

less specific, finding is prostatic calculi that may be detected on digital rectal examination.

4. Findings associated with amiodarone—Sterile epididymitis has been recognized as a complication of amiodarone therapy, especially at high dosages. Although amiodarone-associated epididymitis is usually bilateral, it may be unilateral.

B. LABORATORY FINDINGS

Because the vast majority of cases of epididymitis result from urethritis or bacteriuria, laboratory evaluation should target these entities, unless the history or clinical findings suggest a different entity. Recommended evaluations are discussed below and summarized in Figure 6–1.

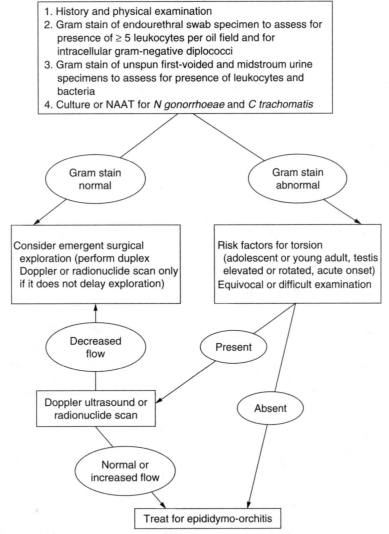

Figure 6–1. Algorithm for initial evaluation of the acute scrotum syndrome.

1. Urethral Gram stain—Either urethral Gram stain or urine microscopy, and preferably both of these evaluations, are indicated routinely in the initial evaluation of suspected epididymitis (see Figure 6–1).

In cases of suspected urethritis, Gram-stained smear of an endourethral swab specimen will often indicate the presence of urethritis (≥5 polymorphonuclear leukocytes per oil field). The Gram stain can also establish, with a high degree of certainty, whether the etiology is gonococcal (ie, demonstrating gram-negative diplococci) or nongonococcal.

2. Urine microscopy—Ideally, first-voided and midstream urine specimens should be examined for bacteria and white blood cells. Comparison of the urinary sediments in the first-voided and midstream specimens may reveal the source of pyuria (ie, urethra or bladder); higher concentrations of leukocytes are typically found in the first-voided urine of patients with urethritis.

A midstream urine Gram stain should be performed, which can be used to presumptively establish the diagnosis of bacteriuria. Presence of more than 1 gram-negative rod per high-power field of unspun midstream urine correlates with presence of more than 10^5 organisms per milliliter.

If microscopy is not available, then dipstick urinalysis can be performed on a first-voided urine specimen. A positive leukocyte esterase test is consistent with an etiology of urethritis or bacteriuria but does not distinguish between these two possibilities.

3. Testing for *N gonorrhoeae* and *C trachomatis*—All urethral specimens should be tested for *N gonorrhoeae* and *C trachomatis*. Culture has been the traditional diagnostic standard for chlamydia and gonorrhea; however, tests of first-voided urine for *N gonorrhoeae* and *C trachomatis* using highly sensitive and specific nucleic acid amplification tests may prove just as or even more useful, although some experts believe more experience with these tests is needed in men with epididymitis.

4. Urine culture—Quantitative midstream urine culture should be obtained in all cases of acute epididymitis in which bacteriuria is suspected. Culture identifies the responsible pathogen and also provides antimicrobial susceptibility data.

5. Other considerations—Finding so-called sterile pyuria in individuals with negative gonococcal and chlamydial tests who have not recently received antimicrobial therapy should prompt the clinician to consider alternative infectious or inflammatory etiologies, such as mycobacterial, other bacterial, or fungal epididymitis. Pyuria is absent in drug-associated epididymitis and in most cases of epididymitis associated with autoimmune disorders.

C. IMAGING STUDIES

Imaging is not indicated in routine cases of epididymitis. However, in the selected situations considered below, imaging procedures may prove very helpful.

1. Diagnosis of testicular torsion or complications of epididymitis—The most common indication for imaging studies is to distinguish epididymitis from alternative diagnoses such as testicular torsion (see Differential Diagnosis, below). Imaging to rule out testicular torsion is especially important in adolescents and young men who have no history or risk factors suggesting possible sexually transmitted urethritis or urinary tract infection. Imaging is also valuable in patients who do not respond to therapy. Such patients may have possible complications of epididymitis, such as testicular abscess, testicular infarction, or pyocele of the scrotum. In these settings, Doppler ultrasound is our preferred imaging study.

2. Diagnosis of anatomic abnormalities associated with epididymitis—Anatomic abnormalities are most common in two populations of patients with epididymitis: children and older men. Men with epididymitis associated with bacteriuria merit urologic evaluation. This may include imaging of the lower or upper urinary tract, or both. Additional studies such as cultures to diagnose bacterial prostatitis, urine flow studies, or determination of residual urine volumes by ultrasound may be indicated by the clinical findings.

Imaging of the upper and lower urinary tract, usually starting with gray-scale ultrasound, is indicated in children who present with epididymitis. This population has a very high prevalence of anatomic congenital abnormalities, including many that merit consideration of surgical correction. This is the least common population of patients with epididymitis.

Berger RE, Alexander ER, Harnisch JP, et al. Etiology, manifestations and therapy of acute epididymitis: Prospective study of 50 cases. *J Urol* 1979;121:750–754. [PMID: 379366] (This article emphasizes the presentation of epididymitis in different age groups. For men older than 35 years, *E. coli* was the most important pathogen, whereas *C trachomatis* and *N gonorrhoeae* were the predominant pathogens in men younger than 35.)

Differential Diagnosis

The main considerations in the differential diagnosis of epididymitis include torsion of the testes and testicular tumor. The clinical history, physical examination, and results of imaging are important in distinguishing among these entities. An algorithm for the initial diagnostic evaluation of the patient with the acute scrotum syndrome is presented in Figure 6–1. In general, in adolescents and adults, the initial evaluation will include microscopy and diagnostic testing for pathogens causing epididymitis. The history and physical examination determine whether other studies (eg, Doppler ultrasound) are indicated to exclude conditions such as testicular torsion or complications of epididymitis. In infants and prepubertal children, torsion of the testicle is a much more common cause of the acute scrotum syndrome than acute epididymitis or testicular cancer, and an acute scrotum in this group must be presumed to be torsion of the testicle unless proven otherwise.

A. TESTICULAR TORSION

Acute epididymitis must always be differentiated from torsion of the testicle, which requires urgent surgical exploration to perform detorsion and orchidopexy to preserve testicular viability. A history of previous scrotal pain is more common in testicular torsion than in epididymitis, presumably reflecting previous intermittent torsion. A history of a sudden onset of scrotal pain is also more common in testicular torsion. A history of trauma to the testicle or lifting or straining at the onset of pain may occur with either epididymitis or torsion and is probably not significant in differentiating the etiology of the acute scrotum syndrome.

Unless physical examination is performed early in the course of the acute scrotum syndrome, findings may be very similar in torsion and epididymitis. In torsion, the testicle is often high in the scrotum (due to shortening that occurs with twisting of the spermatic cord), whereas in epididymitis this is unusual. Also in torsion, examination of the involved testicle may reveal that the epididymis is anterior to the testis, rather than in the usual posterior orientation. In epididymitis, the spermatic cord in the inguinal canal may be quite tender, whereas in torsion tenderness is generally limited to the scrotal contents.

Examination of the urine and urethral smear may prove helpful in differentiating epididymitis from torsion. Patients with epididymitis usually have either urethral inflammation or bacteriuria or leukocytes in their urine, whereas in torsion these findings are usually absent.

Cases of suspected epididymitis in adolescents or young adults should be confirmed by Doppler ultrasound or radionuclide scanning, because the incidence of torsion is also higher than the incidence of epididymitis for most populations in this age group. Doppler ultrasound may demonstrate increased blood flow to the acutely inflamed epididymis and decreased blood flow to a testicle that has undergone torsion, cutting off its blood supply. False-negative ultrasound findings can occur in some cases of testicular torsion (eg, hyperemia surrounding a necrotic testicle may produce a false-positive signal for epididymitis), and a strong clinical suspicion for torsion in the absence of consistent ultrasound findings should prompt the clinician to consider surgical exploration. Radionuclide testicular scanning is another useful imaging modality that is also based on finding increased blood flow in epididymitis. Magnetic resonance imaging has also been reported in a few small studies to be accurate in differentiating among the causes of the acute scrotum syndrome. Thus, magnetic resonance merits further study.

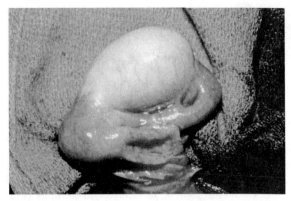

Figure 6–2. Epididymitis in a 28-year-old man who underwent surgical exploration for a presumed testicular torsion. An inflamed tunica vaginalis and spermatic cord were present, along with an indurated, engorged epididymis (lower left). The testis and spermatic cord did not demonstrate findings consistent with testicular torsion. An aspiration culture of the epididymis grew *Chlamydia trachomatis*. This case illustrates the difficulties sometimes encountered in distinguishing acute epididymitis from testicular torsion.

In summary, multiple imaging modalities are available to assist in distinguishing torsion from epididymitis. In all cases, unless the examiner and imaging can unequivocally rule out torsion of the testicle, scrotal exploration should be considered. (See Figure 6–2, which illustrates such a scenario.) Some experts believe surgical exploration without prior imaging is appropriate for presumed torsion, because after 4 hours of complete torsion, there is a significant risk of irreversible testicular damage.

Wilbert DM, Schaerfe CW, Stern WD, et al, Evaluation of the acute scrotum by color-coded Doppler ultrasonography. *J Urol* 1993;149:1475–1477. [PMID: 8501791] (This article confirms earlier reports suggesting that color Doppler ultrasonography is the preferred method for noninvasive imaging of arterial and venous blood vessels in patients with acute scrotal pain.)

B. TESTICULAR TUMOR

Testicular tumor is another important consideration in the differential diagnosis of the acute scrotum syndrome. The peak incidences for epididymitis and testicular tumors occur in similar age groups. The presentation of a painless or persistent testicular mass suggests the possibility of testicular tumor. However, approximately one quarter of patients with testicular tumors present with testicular or scrotal pain. Therefore, the presence of testicular or scrotal pain does not rule out a tumor, especially because hemorrhage or rapid tumor growth may, on occasion, cause such pain.

In the early stages of epididymitis, swelling is limited to the epididymis, and differentiation from testicular tumor usually is not difficult. However, as epididymitis progresses and involvement of the testicle increases, the limits of inflammation are not easily defined. Further, testicular tumors may invade the epididymis and, on physical examination, mimic exactly the findings of acute epididymitis. Reactive hydrocele formation may further limit the usefulness of physical examination. In testicular tumors, the urine and urethral smear should show no evidence of inflammation.

Failure of improvement in the size of swelling or pain in any young man being treated for epididymitis should lead to the suspicion of an incorrect diagnosis or complication of epididymitis. Imaging, and possibly scrotal exploration through an inguinal incision, should be considered to rule out carcinoma of the testicle. Transscrotal open or needle biopsy should never be performed when carcinoma of the testicle is suspected to avoid spreading the tumor to the inguinal lymph nodes, which are rarely involved by testicular tumors (the usual lymphatic drainage of the testis is to the nodes at the level of the renal hilum, not to the inguinal nodes).

C. COMMON INTRASCROTAL CONDITIONS

Other common intrascrotal conditions included in the differential diagnosis of the acute scrotum include spermatocele, hydrocele, varicocele, and hernia. **Spermatocele** and **hydrocele** are easily differentiated by transillumination or by ultrasound. The dilated scrotal veins characteristic of a **varicocele** disappear on assuming the supine position and are accentuated by the Valsalva maneuver (straining). These appear as a "bag of worms" on physical examination. A **hernia** protruding into the scrotum may sometimes present difficulties in diagnosis. Usually, such a scrotal hernia is palpable as a mass protruding through the inguinal canal. Hernias may be reducible as the patient lies down or with pressure. Hernias are not transilluminable, and bowel sounds may occasionally be heard in the hernia contents.

Complications

An accurate diagnosis with early intervention may prevent long-term complications of epididymitis.

A. SURGICAL COMPLICATIONS

Since the availability of effective antimicrobial therapy, the incidence of surgical complications from epididymitis has decreased. The most serious local complications of epididymitis are abscess formation and infarction of the testicle, and both should be considered when a patient fails to improve clinically after 72 hours of appropriate antibiotic therapy, scrotal support, and bed rest. In many cases, abscess or testicular infarction may be identified by ultrasound or a radionuclide scan. Treatment requires surgical drainage and, often, orchiectomy.

B. INFERTILITY

Another complication of acute epididymitis, although poorly documented, is decreased fertility. Infertility rates are high in patients with bilateral epididymitis and bilateral occlusion of the vas deferens or epididymis. In some cases of sexually transmitted epididymitis (eg, especially with *C trachomatis* infection), symptoms may be absent or minimal (ie, subclinical) and may lead to asymptomatic scarring and, possibly, decreased fertility. This intriguing observation may be analogous to the well-documented finding that many infertile women with bilateral tubal obstruction have serologic evidence of past *C trachomatis* infection, although only about half have a past history of salpingitis.

Because transit through the epididymis is necessary for development of normal sperm function, it is possible that acute inflammation and damage to the epididymis could lead to decreased fertility even in the absence of epididymal tubule occlusion. However, epididymal obstruction reverses spontaneously in some patients. Whether unilateral epididymitis, subclinical epididymitis, or epididymitis without occlusion, can result in infertility remains unproven.

C. CHRONIC EPIDIDYMITIS

Chronic epididymitis is a poorly defined clinical syndrome. Patients labeled as having chronic epididymitis account for a significant number of outpatient urology visits. Until recently, there was no clear definition of this syndrome or its clinical course. A 2002 study by Nickel and colleagues began to address the unclear aspects of chronic epididymitis, starting with the clinical definition. Based on the available literature, chronic epididymitis was defined as symptoms of discomfort or pain at least 3 months in duration in the scrotum, testicle, or epididymis localized to one or both epididymides on clinical examination. These investigators also performed a comprehensive clinical survey of 50 men meeting this definition and compared findings with a control group. From their survey, a classification system for chronic epididymitis (inflammatory, obstructive, and epididymalgia) and a symptom assessment index (based on pain and quality of life) were developed that may provide a basis for further epidemiologic and clinical studies.

It remains unclear whether chronic epididymitis is related to persistence of bacteria or bacterial antigens in the epididymis or whether this syndrome reflects an ongoing immunologic reaction, scarring, neurologic injury, or other factors. Chronic epididymitis is generally considered idiopathic and traditionally felt to be unresponsive to antimicrobial therapy, which in some instances has lead to epididymectomy or other surgical procedures for pain relief. Our clinical experience includes numerous patients who have not responded to such surgical procedures. Thus, our current approach to chronic epididymitis is to evaluate possible contributing anatomic and infectious causes. We then evaluate the response to anti-inflammatory therapy; spermatic cord blocks using local anaesthetics or steroids, or both; and other measures. To our knowledge, little evidence-based data are available to suggest that a substantial proportion of patients benefit from more invasive therapies.

Nickel JC, Siemens DR, Nickel KR, et al. The patient with chronic epididymitis: Characterization of an enigmatic syndrome. *J Urol* 2002;167:1701–1704. [PMID: 11912391] (This comprehensive clinical survey of men diagnosed with chronic epididymitis defined and characterized this particular population, setting the stage for further studies in the etiology, epidemiology, and management of chronic epididymitis.)

Padmore DE, Norman RW, Millard OH. Analyses of indications for and outcomes of epididymectomy. *J Urol* 1996;156:95–96. [PMID: 8648848] (This report from a series of 57 patients who underwent epididymectomy found greater satisfaction among patients having excision of epididymal cysts (92%) than among patients with epididymitis or epididymalgia (43%, *P* < .001). Furthermore, more patients in the latter group complained of subsequent problems that they considered related to the procedure. The authors conclude that epididymectomy should avoided for patients with epididymitis or epididymalgia unless they have been carefully counseled regarding the likelihood of poor results.)

Treatment

Effective management of epididymitis depends on accurate etiologic diagnosis. The responsible infectious causes must be identified and treated, and attention must be directed toward correction of any contributing anatomic, physiologic, and behavioral factors. The management of infectious epididymitis thus includes antimicrobial therapy directed against the most likely pathogens, combined with analgesics, scrotal support, and clinical follow-up (see Table 6–2).

A. Antimicrobial Therapy

Because most cases of acute epididymitis are caused by infections, antimicrobial agents represent the cornerstone of therapy. Appropriate empiric therapy can be selected based on whether initial Gram stain evaluation of an endourethral specimen and urine microscopy suggest urethritis or bacteriuria as the inciting event.

1. Epididymitis caused by urinary tract infection— In patients with bacteriuria, broad-spectrum antimicrobial therapy appropriate for a urinary tract infection should be initiated promptly. For ambulatory treatment of epididymitis associated with bacteriuria, the 2006 treatment guidelines from the Centers for Disease Control and Prevention recommend either oral ofloxacin, 400 mg twice daily, or levofloxacin, 500 mg once daily for a 10-day course. If *P aeruginosa* is a concern, then levofloxacin would be more appropriate.

Table 6–2. Initial management of epididymitis.

Epididymitis associated with urethritis
1. Scrotal support
2. Bed rest
3. Analgesics
4. Antibiotics to empirically treat chlamydia and gonorrhea
   Recommended regimen:
      Ceftriaxone, 250 mg IM as single dose
        plus
      Doxycycline, 100 mg PO twice daily for 10 d
   Alternative regimen in patients with allergies to recommended regimen:
      Ofloxacin, 300 mg PO twice daily for 10 d
        or
      Levofloxacin, 500 mg PO daily for 10 d
5. Contact sex partners for evaluation and treatment
6. Follow results of chlamydial and gonococcal testing
7. Reevaluate patient at 72 h

Epididymitis associated with bacteriuria
1. Scrotal support
2. Bed rest
3. Analgesics
4. Antibiotics to empirically treat coliform bacteria and *Pseudomonas* (if at risk)
   Recommended regimen:
      Ofloxacin, 300 mg PO twice daily for 10 d
        or
      Levofloxacin, 500 mg PO daily for 10 d
5. Follow results of urine culture, antimicrobial susceptibility testing and chlamydial and gonococcal testing
6. Reevaluate patient at 72 h
7. Consider correction of underlying urogenital structural abnormalities

Ciprofloxacin is not recommended as first-line therapy because it is less effective against *C trachomatis* than ofloxacin or levofloxacin. Traditionally, trimethoprim-sulfamethoxazole was recommended as an empiric option for uncomplicated epididymitis attributed to coliform infection. However, trimethoprim-sulfamethoxazole is no longer an empiric antimicrobial option because of increasing resistance in *E coli* and other coliform bacteria. For febrile individuals or those with more severe or complicated epididymitis, intravenous broad-spectrum therapy directed against coliforms and *P aeruginosa*, including the addition of an aminoglycoside, should be considered. Therapy can be modified based on susceptibility testing results for organisms cultured from the urine. Antibiotic treatment may need to be prolonged in more complicated cases.

2. Epididymitis caused by sexually transmitted diseases— In patients with epididymitis associated with urethritis or a suspected sexually transmitted pathogen, antimicrobial therapy directed against both *N gonorrhoeae* and *C trachomatis* should be initiated promptly. Treatment for both organisms is necessary because chlamydiae can be isolated from the urethra in approximately 20% of patients with gonorrhea and theoretically could cause epididymitis even when *N gonorrhoeae* is isolated. The recommended treatment regimen is a single dose of ceftriaxone, 250 mg intramuscularly (which is active against β-lactamase–producing *N gonorrhoeae* strains), followed by 10 days of oral doxycycline, 100 mg twice daily, to adequately cover chlamydial infection.

3. Other considerations—If microscopy is unavailable, then history and physical examination findings may guide treatment selection, depending on whether the most likely etiology is related to urethritis or bacteriuria. In cases that are unclear, the general recommendations are that men older than 35 years of age should be treated for bacteriuria-associated pathogens while younger men should be treated for urethritis-associated pathogens. However, those age-specific guidelines should be reconsidered in adults older than 35 years of age with recent or new sex partners and in men who have sex with men. Recommended treatment for men with urethritis who report an allergy to penicillins, cephalosporins, or tetracyclines includes either the ofloxacin or the levofloxacin regimen, discussed earlier, for 10 days.

Although most individuals with epididymitis can be treated in the outpatient setting, hospitalization should be considered in the following instances: febrile persons, concerns about antibiotic nonadherence, a suspected complication of epididymitis, or clinical findings suggesting alternative diagnoses that require more immediate attention.

B. NONANTIMICROBIAL MEDICAL THERAPY

Symptomatic treatment of the patient with epididymitis is always indicated. Analgesics should be given as necessary for pain. Scrotal elevation, which provides for maximum lymphatic and venous drainage, is also recommended. Elevation may also provide pain relief. The patient should be placed on bed rest with the scrotum elevated on a towel between the legs. The use of constricting scrotal support while the patient is supine often only holds the scrotal contents between the patient's legs in a dependent position and is not recommended routinely. If the patient is standing, gravity limits proper drainage of the tissues and may increase swelling. Bed rest is also recommended until the scrotal contents are no longer tender. If the pain returns after ambulation, the patient should return to bed rest and scrotal elevation.

C. SURGICAL THERAPY

Surgery is seldom necessary for acute epididymitis in patients who receive early appropriate therapy. Many patients do not begin to show improvement for 48–72 hours but then do well without surgical intervention. Some experts advocate that epididymectomy should be considered for older patients after unsuccessful conservative treatment, although we have rarely found this to be necessary.

Surgical therapy (generally orchiectomy) may prove necessary for complications of severe epididymo-orchitis, such as testicular infarction, abscess formation, or development of a pyocele of the scrotum (ie, an infected hydrocele).

D. FOLLOW-UP

Patients should be reevaluated 72 hours after initiation of antimicrobial therapy. Failure to improve clinically within 72 hours of the initiation of medical treatment requires further investigation (see Table 6–3), including reevaluation of the initial diagnosis and the current therapy. Swelling and tenderness that persist following completion of antimicrobial therapy should be evaluated more comprehensively through other means, including imaging or surgical exploration. The differential diagnosis includes testicular tumor, abscess or infarction, or a different infectious etiology (eg, tuberculosis or fungal epididymitis).

E. ADDITIONAL MANAGEMENT ASPECTS

In patients with sexually transmitted epididymitis, treatment is not complete without evaluation and treatment of sex partners. This limits the risk of reinfection of the patient and treats or prevents disease in the partner. Epididymitis secondary to bacteriuria always requires urological investigation, if such an evaluation has not

Table 6–3. Treatment considerations for epididymitis that does not improve or clinically worsens following initial therapy.

Address treatment compliance

Ensure that sex partners of patients with urethritis were treated

Review culture and susceptibility data and adjust antimicrobial regimen, if necessary

Consider alternative diagnoses and proceed with necessary history taking, laboratory testing, and imaging studies:
- Epididymitis due to other infectious agents (eg, tuberculosis, histoplasmosis, etc)
- Epididymitis due to noninfectious process (eg, systemic vasculitis, drug associated, etc)
- Etiology of acute scrotum syndrome other than epididymitis (eg, testicular torsion or testicular cancer)

Consider referral to specialist for further evaluation and management already been performed. Some patients with epididymitis secondary to bacteriuria, such as those with lower urinary tract outflow obstruction, may benefit from correction of the underlying genitourinary abnormality.

Recurrence of acute epididymitis usually reflects a lack of adequate treatment, failure to identify factors predisposing to recurrence (eg, untreated sex partners, persisting genitourinary abnormality, etc), or inadequate suppression of a source of chronic infection (eg, chronic bacterial prostatitis). Evaluation should address these factors.

Centers for Disease Control and Prevention; Workowski KA, Berman SM. Sexually transmitted diseases treatment guidelines, 2006. *MMWR Recomm Rep* 2006;55(RR-11):1–94. [PMID: 16888612] (Current recommendations from the CDC.)

Davis BE, Noble MJ, Weigel JW, et al. Analysis and management of chronic testicular pain. *J Urol* 1990;143:936–939. [PMID: 329609] (This series included 45 patients with chronic unilateral or bilateral orchialgia, defined as intermittent or constant testicular pain 3 months or longer in duration that significantly interfered with daily activities. Of 15 patients who underwent inguinal orchiectomy 11 (73%) reported complete relief of pain. This compared with complete pain relief for 5 (55%) of 9 patients who underwent scrotal orchiectomy, suggesting that inguinal orchiectomy is the procedure of choice for management of chronic testicular pain when conservative measures are unsuccessful.)

Hoppner W, Strohmeyer T, Hartmann M, et al. Surgical treatment of acute epididymitis and its underlying diseases. *Eur Urol* 1992;22:218–221. [PMID: 1468479] (This report describes findings in 270 (26%) of 1031 patients with acute epididymitis who underwent surgery for treatment of the disease. Surgery was almost exclusively diagnostic in young patients [exclusion of testicular torsion] and almost always therapeutic in older patients [abscess, prolonged disease].)

Vordermark JS. Acute epididymitis: Experience with 123 cases. *Milit Med* 1985;150:27–30. [PMID: 3920554]

When to Refer to a Specialist

Patients in whom the etiologic agent responsible for epididymitis is unclear or who have not fully responded to therapy may benefit from referral to a specialist. This includes patients with indwelling urethral catheters, failure to respond to initial antimicrobial therapy, epididymitis identified on surgical exploration for torsion of the testicle, and recurrent epididymitis in which the etiologic agent is uncertain. In such difficult cases, diagnosis may be facilitated by epididymal aspiration cultures. Such cultures may be useful in patients with indwelling urethral catheters who may have multiple organisms isolated from the urine and in patients who have been started on antibiotics or recently completed antibiotics because the urine may be sterile, and the use of epididymal aspiration cultures may identify the causal pathogen and also provide needed antimicrobial sensitivity information.

Another indication for referral to a specialist is for management of pain from epididymitis that does not respond to conservative measures. Some specialists believe that anesthetic infiltration of the spermatic cord with procaine or lidocaine hydrochloride and the use of oxyphenbutazone in addition to antibiotics and oral analgesics may increase the comfort of a patient with epididymitis. However, it is not clear whether these other forms of treatment provide better symptomatic relief than the use of analgesics with antibiotics. The effect of such adjuvant therapy on the long-term sequelae of epididymitis also remains uncertain.

Finally, referral to a specialist is warranted if clinical suspicion or imaging studies suggest a complication of epididymitis or an alternative diagnosis that needs further evaluation.

Prognosis

Timely initiation of appropriate antimicrobial therapy, scrotal support, and bed rest leads to a successful clinical outcome in the vast majority of patients with acute epididymitis. Follow-up in 72 hours is necessary to ensure such expected clinical improvement.

The keys to preventing recurrent and chronic epididymitis are (1) ensuring patient adherence with treatment, (2) appropriate evaluation and treatment of sex partners in patients with urethritis, (3) providing education and risk reduction counseling to prevent future sexually transmitted diseases, and (4) correcting genitourinary abnormalities if possible in patients with bacteriuria. Individuals with chronic pain following acute epididymitis or who seem to have chronic epididymitis respond poorly to conservative measures and in some cases will benefit from referral to a specialist. Early surgical intervention (ie, within 4 hours from the onset of testicular pain) in testicular torsion provides the best opportunity for salvaging testicular function. A "wait-and-see" attitude is never justified in any case in which testicular torsion is suspected.

PRACTICE POINTS

• Imaging to rule out testicular torsion is especially important in adolescents and young men who have no history or risk factors suggesting possible sexually transmitted urethritis or urinary tract infection.

Persistent & Recurrent Urethritis

Philip M. Grant, MD, & Thomas M. Hooton, MD

ESSENTIALS OF DIAGNOSIS

- *Requires objective signs of urethral inflammation.*

Nongonococcal Urethritis
- *Absence of gram-negative intracellular diplococci on Gram stain.*
- *Mucopurulent or purulent discharge, Gram stain of urethral secretions indicating ≥5 white blood cells (WBCs) per high-power field (HPF), positive leukocyte esterase test, or ≥10 WBCs per HPF on spun urine sediment.*

Persistent Urethritis
- *No standard definition; has been defined as urethritis that fails to resolve or substantially improve within 1 week of initiating therapy.*

Recurrent Urethritis
- *No standard definition; has been defined as the return of urethritis within 6 weeks following an initial response to therapy.*

General Considerations

An estimated two million cases of nongonococcal urethritis (NGU) occur in the United States each year. Approximately 30–50% of these cases are caused by *Chlamydia trachomatis,* although in some studies the proportion caused by chlamydia is lower. Many etiologies have been proposed for the remaining cases of NGU, but the most consistent associations have been found with *Mycoplasma genitalium, Ureaplasma urealyticum,* herpes simplex virus (HSV), and *Trichomonas vaginalis.* Even with extensive evaluations, in 25–30% of cases of NGU, no microbiologic cause can be identified. The association between *Ureaplasma* and NGU has

not been clearly established and remains controversial; however, it has been suggested that serovars 2, 5, 8, and 9 of *U urealyticum* are associated with NGU whereas other serovars are not.

Following treatment for chlamydial urethritis, 10–20% of patients have persistent or recurrent urethritis. However, in nonchlamydial NGU, failure rates in excess of 50% often are reported. When a patient returns with symptoms consistent with urethritis following treatment for NGU, urethritis must be objectively documented. Furthermore, it is important to confirm adherence with previous therapy and to assess the possibility the patient has been reinfected by a new or untreated sex partner.

There are no widely accepted definitions for persistent or recurrent NGU (PRNGU), and none are provided in the 2006 treatment guidelines for sexually transmitted diseases provided by the Centers for Disease Control and Prevention. For the purposes of this chapter, we define **persistent urethritis** as urethritis that has not substantially improved within 1 week of initiating therapy for NGU. This definition was chosen because the majority of cases of NGU respond to therapy within this time. **Recurrent urethritis** is defined as urethritis occurring within 6 weeks of a previous episode of NGU. Some men have persistent or recurrent episodes of nonchlamydial NGU over a long period of time. However, the longer the duration between episodes of urethritis in a sexually active man, the greater is the likelihood that reinfection is the cause.

A. INFECTIOUS CAUSES

The causes of PRNGU are poorly understood. After reinfection and poor adherence to treatment have been ruled out, the clinician should consider other infectious causes. Possible infectious causes of PRNGU include genital mycoplasmas (eg, *U urealyticum* or *M genitalium*), *T vaginalis,* HSV, an antimicrobial-resistant strain of *Chlamydia,* and a prostatic nidus of infection. However, in only a minority of cases is a microbiologic cause found, even after extensive investigation.

M genitalium, detected by polymerase chain reaction (PCR), is reported to cause 7–50% of cases of NGU. Although the microbiology of PRNGU is less well defined, in one report 21% of patients were infected with *M genitalium.* Data are sparse, but it appears that macrolide antibiotics, in particular azithromycin, are more effective than tetracyclines in eradicating *M genitalium* in men with urethritis and women with cervicitis. Such clinical data correspond with in vitro data demonstrating that *M genitalium* is less susceptible to tetracyclines than macrolides. Some fluoroquinolones have bacteriocidal activity against mycoplasmas; however, in one study a 14-day course of levofloxacin at a dose of 100 mg three times daily failed to eradicate *M genitalium* in 67% of cases as detected by PCR. Although the best results in treating *M genitalium* have been reported with macrolides, relapses still occur. In one study, after erythromycin treatment of *M genitalium* PRNGU, symptomatic relapses occurred both in the presence and absence of *M genitalium* infection at baseline. These observations raise questions as to the role of *M genitalium* in the pathogenesis of PRNGU but may also be explained by a lack of sensitivity of detection techniques for *M genitalium,* intermittent shedding of organisms, or an immunologic basis for urethritis following *M genitalium* infection.

T vaginalis is an established cause of acute NGU, but there are few data on its role in PRNGU. Not surprisingly, if trichomonas were causing NGU it would not be expected to respond to conventional NGU therapy and thus could result in PRNGU. The reported prevalence of trichomonas in cases of NGU varies from 1% to 68%, with a median prevalence of 11%. The large variation in the prevalence of trichomonas in cases of NGU is likely due to the differences in the study populations and the detection methods used. In men, detection of trichomonas is difficult and the direct microscopic examination of a wet mount preparation has poor sensitivity. Although culture and PCR are superior to the wet mount, neither method is widely available. In one study of PRNGU, trichomonas was isolated in 6% of cases using culture techniques. However, given the scarcity of reports detailing the microbiology of PRNGU, the actual percentage of cases caused by trichomonas may differ greatly from this estimate.

HSV types 1 and 2 can cause NGU, even in the absence of genital lesions. Researchers have documented HSV types 1 and 2 in 2–12% of cases of NGU, more commonly in primary HSV than with recurrences of HSV.

Less likely causes of PRNGU include antimicrobial-resistant chlamydial infections. One report in 2000 described three patients with NGU caused by chlamydia resistant to doxycycline, azithromycin, and ofloxacin and subsequent treatment failure. Further cases have not been reported, but no systematic surveillance for antimicrobial resistance in chlamydia exists. Another possible cause of PRNGU is infection of the prostate, which can serve as a persistent nidus of infection. Prostatic infection is usually associated with symptoms and signs of prostatitis—urinary hesitancy, urgency, incomplete voiding, and prostatic tenderness—and requires a longer duration of treatment (6 or more weeks).

B. NONINFECTIOUS CAUSES

Noninfectious causes of PRNGU include an immunologic reaction to chlamydial heat-shock protein, Reiter syndrome, Kawasaki disorder, urethral strictures, foreign bodies, and periurethral fistulas. Generally, however, there is no reason to consider such possible causes in the absence of other manifestations associated with such syndromes.

Corey L, Adams HG, Brown ZA, Holmes KK. Genital herpes simplex virus infections: Clinical manifestations, course, and complications. *Ann Int Med* 1983;98:958–972. [PMID: 6344712] (Classic article describing a case series of 648 patients with genital HSV followed prospectively in King County, Washington.)

Madeb R, Nativ O, Benilevi D, et al. Need for diagnostic screening of herpes simplex virus in patients with non-gonococcal urethritis. *Clin Infect Dis* 2000;30:982–983. [PMID: 10880323] (Suggests HSV can be an important cause of NGU.)

Maeda S, Tamaki M, Kojima K, et al. Association of Mycoplasma genitalium persistence in the urethra with recurrence of nongonococcal urethritis. *Sex Transm Dis* 2001;28:472–476. [PMID: 11473221] (Reveals an association between recurrent NGU and *M genitalium.* Levofloxacin, at 100 mg three times daily for 14 days, frequently does not eradicate this pathogen.)

Somani J, Bhullar VB, Workowski KA, et al. Multiple drug-resistant Chlamydia trachomatis associated with clinical treatment failure. *J Infect Dis* 2000;181:1421–1427. [PMID: 10762573] (Case study of three patients with chlamydia resistant to doxycycline, azithromycin, and ofloxacin. Two of the patients in the study failed to respond to therapy.)

Taylor-Robinson D, Gilroy CB, Thomas BJ, Hay PE. Mycoplasma genitalium in chronic non-gonococcal urethritis. *Int J STD AIDS* 2004;15:21–25. [PMID: 14769166] (Case series of 11 patients with *M genitalium* revealed that patients receiving long courses of antimicrobial agents frequently had relapses of urethritis despite only intermittent isolation of *M genitalium* by PCR techniques.)

Totten PA, Schwartz MA, Sjostrom KE, et al. Association of Mycoplasma genitalium with non-gonococcal urethritis. *J Infect Dis* 2001;183:269–276. [PMID: 11120932] (Case control study evaluating the associations of various pathogens with NGU in King County, Washington.)

Yoshida T, Ishiko H, Yasuda M, et al. Polymerase chain reaction-based subtyping of Ureaplasma parvum and Ureaplasma urealyticum in first-pass urine samples from men with or without urethritis. *Sex Transm Dis* 2005;32:454–457.[PMID: 15976604] (A case-control study that suggests serovars 2, 5, 8 and 9 of *U urealyticum* are associated with NGU while other serovars of *U urealyticum* and *U parvum* are not associated with NGU. This study clarifies the inconsistent relationship in previous studies—many of which did not perform subtype analysis of *Ureaplasma*—between ureaplasmas and NGU.)

Clinical Findings

A. SYMPTOMS AND SIGNS

Patients with PRNGU generally complain of dysuria and may report clear, mucoid, mucopurulent, or purulent discharge. They may also have nonspecific genital complaints, similar to those described in men with chronic prostatitis. Objective evidence of urethritis is most likely to be present before the first void in the morning. "Milking" the urethra (ie, manually stripping the penis from its base to the meatus) may be necessary to demonstrate discharge; however, discharge is not present in all patients with PRNGU.

B. LABORATORY FINDINGS

Nongonococcal urethritis is diagnosed by absence of gram-negative diplococci on Gram stain and presence of any of the following signs: mucopúrulent or purulent discharge, Gram stain of urethral secretions indicating 5 or more WBCs per HPF, positive leukocyte esterase test, or 10 or more WBCs per HPF on spun urine sediment.

C. SPECIAL TESTS

It is recommended that identification of chlamydia and gonorrhea be pursued by nucleic acid amplification tests in men with PRNGU, regardless of whether a pathogen was identified at the time of initial presentation with NGU. Tests for *Ureaplasma* and *M genitalium* are not routinely available, and the results generally would not change management. Urethral culture or PCR for *T vaginalis,* if available, may be helpful. However, given the lack of availability of these tests in most clinics, we recommend treating men with PRNGU empirically with metronidazole as described later in this chapter. Testing for HSV is generally not recommended. However, culture or PCR of a urethral specimen for HSV is a reasonable step if the patient has clear discharge, a recent history of contact with an HSV-positive source, or a clinical syndrome otherwise consistent with HSV.

Repeated microbiologic evaluations in PRNGU have low yield and are not recommended unless the patient gives a history of continued sexual exposures to new or untreated partners.

Differential Diagnosis

The differential diagnosis of PRNGU is limited. When a patient has persistent or recurrent symptoms of dysuria, the importance of objectively documenting urethritis cannot be overemphasized. Not infrequently in such men, no objective evidence of urethritis can be found, and multiple examinations may be necessary to convince the patient. For those with evidence of urethritis, additional considerations include prostatitis, urinary tract infections, and anatomic urethral abnormalities.

A. PROSTATITIS

Although urethritis is not typical of prostatitis syndromes, evidence of prostatitis can be found in some men with PRNGU. The current National Institutes of Health classification divides prostatitis into the following categories: acute prostatitis; chronic bacterial prostatitis; chronic prostatitis/pelvic pain syndrome; inflammatory, chronic prostatitis/pelvic pain syndrome; noninflammatory and asymptomatic inflammatory prostatitis. No more than 5% of men with prostatitis have an identifiable bacterial cause, and the bacteria known to cause urethritis have not been shown to be important in the etiology of prostatitis. It is generally not worthwhile to perform a workup for prostatitis in men with PRNGU because the urethral inflammation in PRNGU can complicate the evaluation and the empiric treatment regimens overlap.

B. URINARY TRACT INFECTION

In men, isolated acute cystitis is uncommon, and the majority of cases are due to anatomic or functional abnormalities, including prostatic hypertrophy or genitourinary instrumentation. Men with cystitis present with dysuria, frequency, and suprapubic pain. PRNGU can usually be distinguished from cystitis by the symptom profile and objective evidence of urethritis.

C. OTHER CONDITIONS

Associations with urethritis have been found with urethral strictures, periurethral abscesses, intraurethral condylomata acuminata, and foreign bodies. The etiologies of urethral strictures include trauma, inflammation (including postinfectious causes), and congenital abnormalities. Patients should be asked about possible urethral trauma, as well as insertion of devices or medications into the urethra. Anatomic abnormalities can be definitively diagnosed by endoscopic evaluation, but only a small minority of patients with PRNGU is found to have anatomic abnormalities. Patients with an anatomic cause of urethritis frequently complain of urinary outflow obstruction. In general, however, if a patient has normal urinary flow as measured by a uroflow study, he is unlikely to have a clinically important anatomic abnormality that would benefit from endoscopic evaluation.

Complications

Patients with PRNGU and their partners have not been demonstrated to have any significant morbidity. Specifically, there are no data to suggest an association between PRNGU and infertility or upper genital tract disease in patientsí female partners.

Treatment

The management of patients with PRNGU is largely empiric. Urethritis should be documented in all patients presenting with persistent or recurrent symptoms. If no objective evidence of NGU is found, patients should be reassured (ie, that there is no inflammation suggestive of persistent infection) and reexamined at a later date if symptoms persist. If there is objective evidence of NGU, management strategies are as follows. If the patient was not adherent with therapy or was not abstinent from sexual contact until symptoms had resolved and treatment of both patient and partners was completed (or 7 days after single-dose azithromycin therapy), the patient (and partners) should be retreated with the original regimen. If the patient and his partners were adherent with recommended therapy, the clinician should reevaluate for gonorrhea and chlamydia. Some authorities recommend performing culture (or PCR) for trichomonas prior to empiric treatment, but as mentioned previously, these tests are not routinely available, and wet mount has poor sensitivity for trichomonas in men. Evaluation for HSV is low yield and generally not recommended.

Optimal treatment of PRNGU has not been defined, and different regimens have not been compared prospectively. It is our recommendation that at the first visit for PRNGU the patient be treated with 1 g of azithromycin orally as a single dose (or a 7-day course of erythromycin, 500 mg orally four times daily) and 2 g of metronidazole orally once. If the patient returns with PRNGU and no new exposures are identified, we do not recommend further evaluation for gonorrhea and chlamydia. In such men, we recommend a 3-week course of erythromycin, 500 mg orally four times daily. Others recommend doxycycline, 100 mg orally twice daily for 3 weeks, or ofloxacin, 300 mg orally twice daily for 1 week (levofloxacin, 500 mg/d orally, should be as effective). After a prolonged course of antibiotics, it is unlikely that further treatment with antimicrobials will be beneficial. However, consideration should be given to chronic prostatitis as a cause of PRNGU, and some practitioners recommend a longer empiric course of antibiotics (eg, a 4- to 6-week course of fluoroquinolones) for patients who continue to have symptomatic urethritis.

The only randomized, controlled study of treatment of PRNGU compared a 3-week course of erythromycin, 500 mg orally four times daily, with placebo and demonstrated improvement in signs and symptoms with treatment. However, many men in this study had been exposed to multiple antibiotic courses prior to enrollment in the study.

No data are available to support further evaluation or treatment of previously treated asymptomatic partners of patients with PRNGU unless the cause of the PRNGU was documented to be chlamydia or trichomonas.

Hooton TM, Wong ES, Barnes RC, et al. Erythromycin for persistent or recurrent nongonococcal urethritis. *Ann Intern Med* 1990;113:21–26. [PMID: 2190516] (This trial, the only randomized, controlled trial of persistent or recurrent urethritis, demonstrated an improvement in pyuria in the erythromycin group. The article suggests the prostate may be an important focus of infection for PRNGU.)

When to Refer to a Specialist

Following the initial antimicrobial course for NGU, retreatment with a macrolide antibiotic and metronidazole, and an extended course of erythromycin, the clinician should consider referring patients with PRNGU to a urologist for further evaluation. However, as detailed previously, the urologic evaluation rarely identifies an anatomic cause for urethritis.

Prognosis

Most patients with PRNGU improve following initial retreatment with a macrolide antibiotic and metronidazole, and many of the remaining cases resolve after an extended course of erythromycin therapy. In many of those whose disease recurs or does not improve following those treatments, symptoms resolve spontaneously over time. As previously noted, patients can be reassured that there is no documented association between PRNGU and any serious sequelae.

 PRACTICE POINTS

- If no objective evidence of NGU is found, patients should be reassured that there is no inflammation suggestive of persistent infection and reexamined at a later date if symptoms persist.

Relevant Web Sites

[Centers for Disease Control and Prevention 2006 sexually transmitted diseases treatment guidelines:]
http://www.cdc.gov/std/treatment/default.htm
[King County, Washington, 2003 sexually transmitted diseases clinical practice guidelines:]
http://www.metrokc.gov/health/apu/std/std-clinicalguidelines.pdf

Pelvic Inflammatory Disease

8

Craig R. Cohen, MD, MPH

ESSENTIALS OF DIAGNOSIS

- *No set of signs or symptoms is pathognomonic for pelvic inflammatory disease (PID), and most laboratory tests are nonspecific for its diagnosis.*
- *Because clinically mild and subclinical PID causes most cases of postinfectious tubal factor infertility, ectopic pregnancy, and chronic pelvic pain due to pelvic scarring in women, a low threshold should be used to make the diagnosis of PID.*
- *All sexually active young women and other women at risk for sexually transmitted diseases (STDs) who complain of acute lower abdominal or pelvic pain; demonstrate uterine, adnexal, or cervical motion tenderness on examination; and have no other causes for these symptoms, should be diagnosed and treated for PID.*

General Considerations

PID is the most common serious infection acquired by sexually active women in the United States. Between 750,000 and one million women develop PID annually, with a 1.5% annual incidence among adolescents and higher rates among nonwhite populations. Since the early 1990s, the numbers of hospitalizations and initial visits to outpatient facilities including physicians' offices for PID has steadily declined. Nevertheless, PID led to 123,000 initial visits to physicians' offices in 2003, a figure that underestimates the true number of new outpatient PID cases in the United States because the nature of physician office reporting is inherently incomplete, and excludes emergency department visits.

Postinfectious tubal factor infertility is the second most common cause of female infertility in the United States. Yet the majority of women with this condition do not have a clear history of PID, suggesting that many cases of PID are subclinical and therefore go untreated. Several studies have shown that upon in-depth questioning, 70–80% of patients with tubal factor infertility have a history of lower abdominal pain. Demographic and microbiologic factors associated with acute and subclinical PID are similar, supporting the hypothesis that they share the same pathophysiologic mechanisms. Therefore, until improved tests are available to diagnose subclinical disease, clinicians should use a low threshold in making the diagnosis of PID, and women at risk of an STD should be educated to recognize the symptoms of PID and to seek immediate care and treatment.

Pathogenesis

Neisseria gonorrhoeae and *Chlamydia trachomatis* are common causes of PID. In a recent US multicenter study of women with mild to moderate PID, these pathogens accounted for 20% and 21% of cases, respectively; coinfection with *N gonorrhoeae* and *C trachomatis* was found in 6% of cases. These bacteria initially cause an endocervical infection; however, as a result of poorly defined anatomic, pathologic, and immunologic changes, between 10% and 20% of primary endocervical gonococcal and chlamydial infections will lead to an ascending infection of the endometrium and fallopian tubes. Over the past two decades, the proportion PID cases caused by *N gonorrhoeae* and *C trachomatis* has declined in parallel with the overall reduction of these STDs in the US population.

In many studies, neither gonorrhea nor chlamydia is detected in 60% or more of women with PID. Anaerobic and facultative bacteria have frequently been isolated from the tube, cul-de-sac, and endometrium of women with PID. The highest prevalence of such organisms was seen in studies using culdocentesis, raising the question of transvaginal contamination. Lower prevalences of anaerobic bacteria have generally been discovered in laparoscopically collected specimens. Many of the anaerobic bacteria isolated from the upper genital tract are also commonly found in low concentrations in normal vaginal flora, and at far greater concentrations among women with bacterial vaginosis. In fact, the presence of bacterial vaginosis has been associated with a twofold or greater increased risk of PID.

Prevotella bivius, Bacteroides species, *Peptostreptococcus* species, staphylococci, group B–D streptococci, *Gardnerella vaginalis, Escherichia coli,* and more recently, using molecular techniques, novel bacteria including *Leptotrichia* species and *Atopobium vaginae* have been isolated from the upper genital tract of women with salpingitis and pelvic abscesses. These organisms have also been isolated from women with gonococcal and chlamydial PID, supporting the hypothesis that *N gonorrhoeae* and *C trachomatis* may cause primary infection of the upper genital tract that is followed by secondary infection of the endometrium and fallopian tubes by vaginal organisms such as those associated with bacterial vaginosis. However, anaerobic bacteria are isolated less commonly in women with milder disease. Because of the data just cited, some anaerobic coverage is included in all the inpatient and most outpatient antibiotic regimens recommended for the treatment of PID by the Centers for Disease Control and Prevention (CDC; see Tables 8–3 and 8–4).

Hebb JK, Cohen CR, Astete SG, et al. Detection of novel organisms associated with salpingitis, by use of 16S rDNA polymerase chain reaction. *J Infect Dis* 2004;190:2109–2120. [PMID: 15551209] (The finding of novel phylotypes associated with salpingitis has important implications for the etiology, pathogenesis, and treatment of PID.)

Prevention

Primary measures to identify and treat asymptomatic genital tract infections such as *C trachomatis* have decreased the frequency of PID. Although condom use is associated with a decreased risk of PID, increased numbers of recent sex partners and history of a prior STD are associated with an increased risk. Therefore, women at risk of an STD, specifically adolescents, HIV-infected women, and women who report high-risk sexual behaviors, should be counseled on the need to reduce their sexual exposure. Hormonal contraception, including combined oral contraceptives and depomedroxyprogesterone, do not appear to affect the risk of PID. Although controversy remains, most experts agree that currently marketed intrauterine devices (IUDs) do not increase risk of PID except at the time of insertion; however, women require screening for *N gonorrhoeae* and *C trachomatis* prior to IUD insertion.

Secondary measures to prevent the sequelae of PID include early identification and treatment of upper genital tract infection. Not surprisingly, antibiotic treatment helps prevent tubal damage. Infertility after PID occurs in 12% of women given antibiotics compared with 55–75% of women in the preantibiotic era. Although early antibiotic treatment appears to prevent tubal factor infertility, current antibiotic regimens do not sufficiently prevent other sequelae of PID.

Scholes D, Stergachis A, Heidrich FE, et al. Prevention of pelvic inflammatory disease by screening for cervical chlamydial infection. *N Engl J Med* 1996;334:1362–1366. [PMID: 8614421] (Reports on a strategy of identifying, testing, and treating women at increased risk for cervical chlamydial infection to reduce the incidence of PID.)

Clinical Findings

A. SYMPTOMS AND SIGNS

Early diagnosis of PID is important for effective treatment and prevention of sequelae. However, due to the complexity and lack of objective clinical criteria to diagnose PID, many women with mild PID may go undiagnosed, and those with severe disease may be misdiagnosed with gastrointestinal or noninfectious gynecologic conditions. No set of signs or symptoms is pathognomonic for PID. In other words, no set of signs and symptoms is sufficiently sensitive and specific; the addition of factors to increase specificity leads to an unacceptable decline in sensitivity. Compared with laparoscopic diagnosis, the clinical diagnosis of PID has a positive predictive value of 65–90%. Although laparoscopy and endometrial biopsy provide objective evidence for the diagnosis of PID, waiting to make the diagnosis on the basis of these tests can lead to a delay in treatment. The benefit of early antibiotic treatment outweighs the risk of overdiagnosis and overtreatment in most cases.

In 2002, the CDC changed its guidelines for PID diagnosis, in essence making the clinical criteria for PID more sensitive at the loss of specificity. The 2006 guidelines continue to suggest that a clinical diagnosis of PID should be made in sexually active young women and other women at risk for STDs who complain of acute (usually defined at 30 days or less) lower abdominal or pelvic pain and uterine, adnexal, or cervical motion tenderness, and in whom no other cause for the illness can be identified.

More detailed diagnostic evaluation often is needed, because incorrect diagnosis and management may lead to delays in treatment of other causes of abdominal or pelvic pain. The additional criteria listed in Table 8–1 may be used to enhance the specificity of the minimum criteria.

B. LABORATORY FINDINGS

Most laboratory tests are nonspecific for diagnosis of PID. A human chorionic gonadotropin (hCG) test of urine should be performed in any reproductive-aged woman who presents with acute abdominal or pelvic pain to rule out an ectopic or other pregnancy complication. The finding of an elevated erythrocyte sedimentation rate ($\geq$15 mm/h) has a sensitivity ranging from 76% to 81% and a specificity ranging from 25% to 57%; an elevated C-reactive protein level has a sensitivity of

Table 8–1. Centers for Disease Control and Prevention criteria for the clinical diagnosis of pelvic inflammatory disease.

Minimum criteria[a]

Acute lower abdominal or pelvic pain, *plus* at least one of the following on examination:
  • Uterine tenderness
  • Adnexal tenderness
  • Cervical motion tenderness

Additional criteria[b]

Oral temperature ≥38.3C
Abnormal cervical or vaginal mucopurulent discharge
Vaginal fluid neutrophils on saline microscopy ≥1 per 400 × field)
Elevated C-reactive protein
Elevated erythrocyte sedimentation rate
Cervical *Neisseria gonorrhoeae* or *Chlamydia trachomatis* infection

---

[a]Empiric treatment should be started in women with a mild to moderately severe clinical presentation if they meet the minimum criteria, are at risk for a sexually transmitted disease, and have no other cause for illness identified.
[b]Additional criteria can be used to more accurately diagnose PID and should be reserved for women with severe presentations to help rule out other serious diagnoses. Further evaluation of women with uncertain diagnoses can be made histologically, laparoscopically, and sonographically.
Based on Centers for Disease Control and Prevention; Workowski KA, Berman SM. Sexually transmitted diseases treatment guidelines, 2006. *MMWR Recomm Rep* 2006;55 (RR-11):1–94. [PMID: 16888612]

74–93% and a specificity of 50–90%. An elevated white blood cell count (≥10,000 cells/mm³) has a relatively poor positive and negative predictive value but may be useful to help identify other causes of acute abdominal or pelvic pain such as appendicitis. Finally, although fewer than 40% of PID cases are caused by *N gonorrhoeae* and *C trachomatis*, in women with appropriate clinical findings a positive test for either pathogen is highly suggestive of PID and may influence the treatment of sexual contacts and help motivate the patient to reduce sexual risk behaviors, thus decreasing the likelihood of recurrent infection.

In a recent study, the presence of vaginal neutrophils diagnosed by microscopic evaluation of a saline wet mount preparation of vaginal fluid (≥1 per 400 × field) had a high sensitivity (91%) and negative predictive value (95%), but low specificity (26%) and positive predictive value (17%) for the diagnosis of upper genital tract infection. In other words, a normal vaginal discharge without the presence of white blood cells on saline wet mount makes the diagnosis of PID unlikely, and

alternative diagnoses should be entertained. This simple diagnostic test should be considered for use in the clinical evaluation of a patient with suspected PID.

C. IMAGING STUDIES

Ultrasound provides a noninvasive test to help diagnose PID. It may also be used to follow the course of patients with a tubo-ovarian abscess or pyosalpinx, and may help rule out other causes of acute pelvic pain. In one study, the sensitivity of pelvic ultrasonography was 94% for severe PID, 80% for moderate PID, and 64% for mild PID. In another study, transvaginal ultrasonography appeared to improve the sensitivity for ultrasonographic diagnosis of mild PID. In general, thickening or dilation of the fallopian tubes (sensitivity 32%, specificity 97%), fluid in the cul-de-sac (sensitivity 37%, specificity 58%), multicystic ovary (sensitivity 42%, specificity 86%), or tubo-ovarian abscess (sensitivity 32%, specificity 97%) can be used to help confirm the clinical diagnosis of PID. Pelvic ultrasound is available in most clinical settings; however, because of its low sensitivity, routine use of transvaginal ultrasonography to confirm the diagnosis of PID has limited clinical utility and should be reserved for patients with an acute abdomen or suspected pelvic masses, or when otherwise clinically indicated.

D. SPECIAL TESTS

Endometrial biopsy specimens can be easily obtained using an endometrial suction curette or similar instrument. Histologic evidence of endometritis includes polymorphonuclear lymphocytes in the endometrial epithelium (≥5 per 400 × field), and plasma cell infiltrate in the endometrial stroma (≥1 per 120 × field). Demonstration of both polymorphonuclear lymphocytes and plasma cells has a sensitivity of 92% and a specificity of 87% when compared with the laparoscopic diagnosis of salpingitis. Gentle technique should be used when performing this procedure, especially when sampling an infected uterus, to avoid uterine perforation. In comparison with the other diagnostic procedures, endometrial biopsy is less costly than laparoscopy and probably more sensitive than ultrasound for diagnosis of mild PID. However, it has limited use in most clinical settings and may delay the initiation of treatment.

Boardman LA, Peipert JF, Brody JM, et al. Endovaginal sonography for the diagnosis of upper genital tract infection. *Obstet Gynecol* 1997;90:54–57. [PMID: 9207813] (Endovaginal sonography has limited clinical utility in the diagnosis of upper genital tract infection due to its low sensitivity.)

Yudin MH, Hillier SL, Wiesenfeld HC, et al. Vaginal polymorphonuclear leukocytes and bacterial vaginosis as markers for histologic endometritis among women without symptoms of pelvic inflammatory disease. *Am J Obstet Gynecol* 2003; 188:318–323. [PMID: 12592233] (This prospective study demonstrates the demographic and microbiologic similarities of acute and subclinical PID.)

Table 8–2. Differential diagnosis of pelvic inflammatory disease.

Ectopic pregnancy
Septic abortion
Rupture, torsion, hemorrhage of an ovarian cyst
Endometriosis
Acute appendicitis
Inflammatory bowel disease
Urinary tract infection
Nephrolithiasis

Differential Diagnosis

The differential diagnosis of PID includes other gynecologic, urologic, and gastrointestinal disorders (see Table 8–2). Ectopic pregnancy, appendicitis, and adnexal torsion are the most serious conditions to exclude. Most of those severe conditions can be ruled out clinically (ie, by use of a urine pregnancy test, and, if needed, through diagnostic imaging to rule out adnexal torsion and other gynecologic conditions).

Complications

Although most women with PID recover completely from acute infection, serious irreversible reproductive organ damage can occur. Tissue fibrosis can cause fallopian tube obstruction and pelvic adhesions that lead to sequelae such as tubal factor infertility, ectopic pregnancy, and chronic pelvic pain. As previously noted, following PID, infertility occurs in 12% of women; in addition, the risk of ectopic pregnancy is increased 7- to 10-fold, and approximately 20% of women develop chronic pelvic pain. HIV-1–infected women have a two- to threefold increased risk of severe PID, including tubo-ovarian abscess.

Treatment

A. Antimicrobial Therapy

Broad-spectrum antimicrobial therapy is required to treat acute bacterial PID. Early antibiotic therapy within 3 days of symptom onset has been associated with reduced risk for sequelae and therefore is strongly recommended. Although single-agent regimens have been used successfully to treat PID, two- and three-drug regimens that cover gonorrhea, chlamydia, and common aerobic and anaerobic isolates are recommended by the CDC. Treatment should be empiric and not based on lower genital tract cultures that are costly, may delay onset of treatment, and often do not predict pathogens in the upper genital tract.

A multicenter, randomized, controlled treatment trial of women with clinical symptoms and signs of mild to moderate PID compared inpatient intravenous cefoxitin and doxycycline treatment with outpatient treatment consisting of a single intramuscular injection of cefoxitin and oral doxycycline. In this trial, rates of short-term clinical and microbiologic improvement were similar between the two groups, and subsequent 3-year pregnancy rates were equal (42% in both arms). Furthermore, there were no statistically significant differences between inpatient and outpatient groups in time to subsequent pregnancy or in the proportion of women with PID recurrence, chronic pelvic pain, or ectopic pregnancy. Based on these findings, inpatient treatment and hospitalization should be reserved for patients with an unclear diagnosis (particularly if a serious surgical diagnosis cannot be excluded), patients with abscesses, or those who have failed oral antibiotic therapy or are unable to tolerate oral medication. Although it is reported to be associated with more severe disease, HIV-1 infection, unless associated with severe immunodeficiency (CD4 T-cell count <200µL), is not an absolute indication for parenteral antibiotics. In cases requiring hospitalization, parenteral therapy should continue until the patient is afebrile for 48 hours or more with a significant reduction (usually ≥50%) in abdominal and pelvic tenderness, and, if present at admission, a greater than 50% decrease in the diameter of tubo-ovarian masses. After discontinuation of parenteral therapy, broad-spectrum oral therapy (eg, doxycycline, 100 mg orally twice daily for uncomplicated PID; or doxycycline, 100 mg, with metronidazole, 500 mg, twice daily orally, in cases of pyosalpinx and tubo-ovarian abscess) is continued to complete a full 2-week antibiotic course.

The addition of metronidazole to outpatient treatment regimens remains controversial, and owing to gastrointestinal and other side effects may reduce overall treatment adherence. Although more data are required, metronidazole should be used in patients with PID and concomitant bacterial vaginosis but may be withheld in those with clinically mild to moderate PID who do not have bacterial vaginosis.

Outpatient and inpatient PID treatment regimens recommended by the CDC are outlined in Tables 8–3 and 8–4.

B. Surgical Drainage of a Pelvic Abscess

The use of broad-spectrum antibiotic regimens that include anaerobic coverage has led to a decrease of extirpative surgery during the acute phase of PID. Surgical drainage of pelvic abscesses is reserved for ruptured pelvic abscess, masses that persist after antibiotic treatment, abscesses larger than 4–6 cm as observed by ultrasound, and fluctuant pelvic masses attached to the cul-de-sac in the midline that can easily be drained through the vagina.

Table 8–3. Recommended oral treatment regimens for pelvic inflammatory disease.

Regimen A
  Ofloxacin, 400 mg PO twice daily for 14 d, or
  levofloxacin, 500 mg PO once daily for 14 d
    with or without
  Metronidazole, 500 mg PO twice daily for 14 d.[a]

Regimen B
  Ceftriaxone, 250 mg IM as a single dose
    Or
  Cefoxitin, 2 g IM, plus probenecid, 1 g orally in a single dose concurrently once
    Or
  Other parenteral third-generation cephalosporin (eg, ceftizoxime or cefotaxime)
    Plus
  Doxycycline, 100 mg PO twice daily for 14 d
    with or without
  Metronidazole, 500 mg PO twice daily for 14 d[b]

---

[a]Metronidazole is added to provide anaerobic coverage.
[b]Many authorities recommend the addition of metronidazole, 500 mg PO twice daily, to this regimen for additional anaerobic coverage and the treatment of bacterial vaginosis.
Based on Centers for Disease Control and Prevention; Workowski KA, Berman SM. Sexually transmitted diseases treatment guidelines, 2006. *MMWR Recomm Rep* 2006; 55(RR-11):1–94.

C. POSTERIOR COLPOTOMY

A posterior colpotomy can be performed if three conditions are met: (1) the abscess is midline, (2) it is adherent to the cul-de-sac, and (3) it dissects the rectovaginal septum. Adequate anesthesia is administered, and the patient is placed in the dorsal lithotomy position and examined under general anesthesia. The posterior portion of the cervix is grasped, and the posterior vaginal fornix is incised sharply and extended 1–2 cm. The peritoneum and abscess cavity are punctured using either a long clamp or a suction canula. Insertion of the index finger or a suction canula will aid in exploration of the abscess cavity and gentle breaking of fibrous adhesions to allow complete drainage. A Penrose or similar drain is left in place until drainage has decreased to less than 25 mL per 24 hours. If an abscess is not midline and attached to the cul-de-sac, damage to bowel may occur during the procedure. Ultrasound may assist the clinician in determining the position of the inflammatory mass, although laparoscopy is probably superior at determining the location of the bowel and abscess.

D. TRANSABDOMINAL DRAINAGE

Transabdominal drainage under laparoscopic guidance is used to drain persistent pelvic abscesses that are not

Table 8–4. Recommended parenteral treatment regimens for pelvic inflammatory disease.

Regimen A[a]
  Cefotetan, 2 g IV q 12 h
    Or
  Cefoxitin, 2 g IV q 6 h
    Plus
  Doxycycline, 100 mg IV or orally q 12 h

Regimen B[b]
  Clindamycin, 900 mg IV q 8 h
    Plus
  Gentamicin, loading dose IV or IM (2 mg/kg of body weight), followed by maintenance dose (1.5 mg/kg) q 8 h. Single daily dosing may be substituted.

Alternative parenteral regimens[c]
  Ofloxacin, 400 mg IV q 12 h, or levofloxacin, 500 mg IV once daily
    with or without
  Metronidazole, 500 mg IV q 8 h
    Or
  Ampicillin plus sulbactam, 3 g IV q 6 h
    Plus
  Doxycycline, 100 mg IV or PO q 12 h

---

[a]Parenteral therapy may be discontinued 24 h after patient improves clinically, and oral therapy with doxycycline (100 mg twice daily) should continue for a total of 14 d.
[b]Parental therapy may be discontinued 24 h after patient improves clinically, and oral therapy with doxycycline (100 mg twice daily) or clindamycin (450 mg orally 4 times daily) should continue for a total of 14 d.
[c]Because of concerns regarding the anaerobic coverage of quinolones, metronidazole should be included for this regimen.
Based on Centers for Disease Control and Prevention; Workowski KA, Berman SM. Sexually transmitted diseases treatment guidelines, 2006. *MMWR Recomm Rep* 2006;55 (RR-11):1–94.

suitable for colpotomy drainage. Ultrasound and computed tomography (CT)–guided placement of percutaneous catheters is also possible. About 90% of large abscesses can be cured with percutaneous drainage. Under laparoscopic guidance, percutaneous catheters are inserted into the pelvic abscess. Suction and irrigation of the cavity is performed, and the drain is left in place postoperatively until drainage is less than 25 mL per 24 hours. Loops of bowel may obscure the pelvic abscess, making insertion of transabdominal drains difficult. Laparoscopic guidance is associated with a decreased likelihood of bowel injury compared with use of ultrasound or CT to guide drain placement. Care should be taken to identify and drain multiloculated abscesses.

E. COUNSELING

Although the proportion of cases of PID caused by gonorrhea and chlamydia has been declining over the past 20 years, based on a continued strong association between PID and increased sexual exposure and the growing understanding of newly discovered sexually transmitted organisms that may cause PID (eg, *Mycoplasma genitalium*) consensus opinion remains that most cases of PID are sexually transmitted. Therefore, counseling efforts should focus on decreasing a patient's sexual exposure (eg, reduction of number of partners, condom use, etc). Often a women's risk of exposure to STDs is related to the sexual risk of her male sex partner. Therefore, in addition to counseling the patient, clinicians need to direct STD prevention messages toward the patient's male partner. Ideally, all sex partners for the past 3 months should receive empiric therapy consisting of an oral agent active against *N gonorrhoeae* (eg, cefpodoxime, 400 mg orally given once), and either doxycycline, 100 mg twice daily orally for 1 week, or azithromycin, 1 g given as a single oral dose. Although sexual behaviors of homosexual women are associated with a reduced risk of most STDs, female partners of women with PID should also receive appropriate treatment and counseling.

To provide motivation for women to reduce their sexual exposure, counseling may also include messages concerning the increased risk of infertility and other sequelae associated with subsequent episodes of PID (infertility risk increases with the number of PID episodes: 12% with one episode, 21% with two episodes, and 40% with three or more episodes).

HIV-1 testing and counseling should be offered. Among hospitalized patients with PID, the risk of HIV-1 infection has been demonstrated to be two to seven times greater than in similarly aged women receiving prenatal care in the same community.

Ness RB, Soper DE, Holley RL, et al. Effectiveness of inpatient and outpatient treatment strategies for women with pelvic inflammatory disease: Results from the Pelvic Inflammatory Disease Evaluation and Clinical Health (PEACH) Randomized Trial. *Am J Obstet Gynecol* 2002;186:929–937. [PMID: 12015517] (The results of this hallmark study found that among women with mild to moderate PID, there is no difference in reproductive outcomes between women randomized to intravenous cefoxitin and doxycycline versus outpatient treatment that consisted of a single intramuscular injection of cefoxitin and oral doxycycline.)

When to Refer to a Specialist

In most cases, PID can be managed by a primary care clinician. However, when another significant gynecologic disorder (eg, adnexal torsion) cannot be ruled out or there is lack of clinical improvement after 3 or more days of antibiotic therapy, or diagnosis of a pelvic mass, the patient should be referred to a gynecologist for evaluation and clinical management. Surgical referral should be made when appendicitis cannot be excluded.

Prognosis

The clinical cure rate following early use of the suggested antibiotic regimens ranges from 90% to 97%. Mortality from PID is rare in industrialized countries and usually occurs secondary to rupture of an abscess and the sepsis that follows. In addition to symptom resolution, the avoidance of sequelae should serve as important markers of the success of various treatment strategies—an approach that has only been investigated once in a randomized clinical trial of PID treatment. Nevertheless even with timely and appropriate treatment, tubal infertility, chronic pelvic pain, and increased risk for ectopic pregnancy are increased in women after PID treatment. Repeat episodes of PID further increase those risks. STD prevention and a low threshold for treatment are important means to reduce those adverse outcomes.

 PRACTICE POINTS

- A normal vaginal discharge without the presence of white blood cells on saline wet mount makes the diagnosis of PID unlikely, and alternative diagnoses should be considered.

Relevant Web Sites

[Centers for Disease Control and Prevention fact sheet on pelvic inflammatory disease:]

http://www.cdc.gov/std/PID/STDFact-PID.htm

Proctitis & Proctocolitis

Anne M. Rompalo, MD

PROCTITIS & OTHER SEXUALLY TRANSMITTED INTESTINAL SYNDROMES

ESSENTIALS OF DIAGNOSIS

- A thorough sexual history, including information about the practice of rectal sex (receptive or insertive) or oral-anal sex, with or without condoms.
- Screening for rectal pathogens based on sexual risk history.
- Anoscopy in patients with symptoms of anorectal pain, tenesmus, or discharge.
- Collection of specimens for gonorrhea, chlamydia, and serologic tests for syphilis and HIV, and stool specimens for culture and ova and parasite examinations in patients with symptoms of proctocolitis.

General Considerations

Proctitis is an inflammatory condition of the rectum that usually occurs secondary to infection introduced during sexual activity. A more extensive condition—proctocolitis—may occur after oral ingestion of a pathogen that produces colorectal inflammation. Both conditions are noted more frequently in men who have sex with men (MSM). Proctitis is commonly caused by gonorrhea, chlamydia, and herpes simplex virus (HSV) infections, and proctocolitis by enteric bacteria or parasites.

The incidence of acute, sexually transmitted proctitis and proctocolitis, which decreased dramatically during the 1980s and early 1990s, began increasing again in the mid-1990s. As a consequence of successful antiretroviral therapy for HIV infection and AIDS, declining concern about HIV and AIDS, and renewed physical health, many HIV-infected men in the United States have increasingly been engaging in sexual risk behaviors associated with the spread of STDs. Consistent condom use between HIV-infected sex partners in some cities has also declined, resulting in substantial increases in rates of syphilis and rectal STDs.

A. PATHOGENESIS

Sexually transmitted intestinal infections may be transmitted by direct rectal inoculation or indirectly in the course of oral-anal contact. Conventional sexually transmitted diseases (STDs) most often cause rectal infections through direct inoculation by anal intercourse, although perineal contamination by cervicovaginal secretions among women has been described. *Chlamydia trachomatis* and *Neisseria gonorrhoeae* infect columnar epithelium and infect the anorectal mucosa via oral-genital and rectal insertive intercourse. HSV, human papillomavirus, and *Treponema pallidum* infect stratified squamous epithelium and can be transmitted similarly to the anorectal region. Although not considered "classical" STDs, enteric pathogens, parasites, and hepatitis A and B can be transmitted during direct oral-anal contact, (anilingus) or during oral-genital contact after rectal intercourse. Exposure to as few as 10–100 organisms of *Shigella*, *Entamoeba histolytica* cysts, or *Giardia lamblia* cysts may precipitate infection.

B. RISK FACTORS

Multiple partners, anonymous partners, and individual sexual practices that increase the risk of acquiring specific diseases are associated with increased risk of acquiring any STD. Individuals who engage in receptive anal intercourse or anilingus are at high risk for acquiring sexually transmitted proctitis and enteritis.

Anal intercourse continues as a prevalent sexual practice in both homosexual and heterosexual populations. Studies report that up to 43% of adult women have participated in anal intercourse. Teen definitions of sexual activity may not include oral or anal sex, and the prevalence of anal sex among teens engaging in abstinence-only programs is unknown. Clinicians, social workers, and disease intervention specialists must develop a tactful approach for eliciting information regarding anorectal sexual exposure and other high-risk behaviors, because this information may result in more rapid disease detection, treatment, and control.

Centers for Disease Control and Prevention (CDC). Lymphogranuloma venereum among men who have sex with men—Netherlands, 2003–2004. *MMWR Morb Mortal Wkly Rep* 2004;53:985–988. [PMID: 15514580] (Recent report of the introduction and the spread of an unusual subtype of *C trachomatis* [L2b] presenting as proctitis in European MSM.)

Halkitis PN, Parsons JT, Wilton L. Barebacking among gay and bisexual men in New York City: Explanations for the emergence of intentional unsafe behavior. *Arch Sex Behav* 2003;32:351–357. [PMID: 12856896] (Study describing various reasons for increases in sexual risk behavior, in particular, behavior that might transmit HIV infection.)

Kent CK, Chaw JK, Wong W, et al. Prevalence of rectal, urethral, and pharyngeal chlamydia and gonorrhea detected in 2 clinical settings among men who have sex with men: San Francisco, California, 2003. *Clin Infect Dis* 2005;41:67–74. [PMID: 15937765] (Clinical epidemiologic study describing the prevalence and correlates of rectal gonorrhea and chlamydia in clinics in San Francisco.)

Klausner JD, Kohn R, Kent C. Etiology of clinical proctitis among men who have sex with men. *Clin Infect Dis* 2004;38:300–302. [PMID: 14699467] (Retrospective review of the infectious causes of proctitis in MSM seen at the San Francisco municipal STD clinic.)

Quinn TC, Stamm WE, Goodell SE, et al. The polymicrobial origin of intestinal infections in homosexual men. *N Engl J Med* 1983;309:576–582. [PMID: 6308444] (Classic early description of the different causes of proctitis and proctocolitis.)

Prevention

Because the incidence of acute sexually transmitted rectal and gastrointestinal syndromes is increasing, the diligence of clinicians in counseling patients regarding safer sex practices should not lessen. All patients, regardless of their sexual preferences, should have a careful history to elicit information about gender of sex partners, specific sexual practices, and the method and frequency of condom or other barrier use. This will provide important clues to direct proper evaluation, specimen collection, therapeutic choices, and counseling regardless of patients' presenting symptoms. Consistent condom use and handwashing using soap and water have been recommended to reduce the transmission of gastrointestinal infections. Although latex barriers are also recommended during oral-anal sex, few persons in practice use that barrier method. Vaccination against hepatitis A is an effective preventive measure, particularly in persons who engage in anal or oral-anal sex. Sexually active persons should be informed about these measures, evaluated to determine the need for hepatitis A vaccination, and offered vaccination, if deemed susceptible.

Clinical Findings

Several pathogens are associated with sexually transmitted intestinal syndromes (see Table 9–1). Symptoms and clinical manifestations vary, depending on the pathogen involved and the location of the infection. The latter half of this chapter discusses symptoms and signs, laboratory findings, and treatment for common pathogens that can cause proctitis and proctocolitis.

Polymicrobial infection often occurs and can cause upper intestinal and perianal symptoms. Nonetheless, asymptomatic infections are prevalent, and the clinician should routinely inquire about rectal exposure regardless of the patient's sexual preferences, so as to perform screening tests or anoscopic evaluation when appropriate.

Table 9–1. Clinical findings in common sexually transmitted gastrointestinal syndromes.

	Proctitis	Proctocolitis
Symptoms	Rectal pain, discharge, tenesmus	Symptoms of proctitis, along with cramps and diarrhea
Pathogen	*Neisseria gonorrhoeae* *Chlamydia trachomatis* *Treponema pallidum* herpes simplex virus	*Entamoeba histolytica* *Shigella flexneri* *C trachomatis* (lymphogranuloma venereum) *Giardia lamblia* *Salmonella* spp
Mode of acquisition	Receptive anal intercourse	Direct or indirect fecal-oral contact
Anoscopic findings	Rectal exudate ± friability	Rectal exudate, friability that may extend into sigmoid colon

A. PROCTITIS

Inflammation involving the rectal mucosa is termed *proctitis*. The perianal area up to the anal verge is composed of keratinized, stratified squamous dermal epithelium. Lesions caused by syphilis, HSV, or condylomata acuminata, therefore, generally have the same appearance as they do in other genital areas. The stratified squamous epithelium gradually changes to stratified cuboidal epithelium from the anal verge up to the anorectal (pectinate or dentate) line. Infection in this area with an extensive network of sensory nerve endings may be painful, sometimes resulting in constipation or tenesmus as a result of anal sphincter muscle spasm. Above the anorectal line, the rectum is lined by columnar epithelium, and infections of this region that spare the anus are relatively painless. Anorectal sexually transmitted infections, therefore, may be asymptomatic. Symptoms of proctitis, however, include anorectal pain, mucopurulent or bloody rectal discharge, tenesmus, and constipation.

B. PROCTOCOLITIS

Infections that involve the rectum and the colon are termed *proctocolitis*. Symptoms may include those of proctitis as well as abdominal pain, bloating, cramping, and sometimes diarrhea and fever.

C. INITIAL EXAMINATION

In order to classify patients into syndromes to direct diagnostic and therapeutic choices, a thorough physical examination is essential. Careful inspection of the perianal region may detect lesions or masses that can be tested for pathogens such as HSV or sampled for dark-field examination. Anoscopy may reveal rectal exudates or rectal bleeding. If the patient has proctitis, sigmoidoscopy often reveals disease limited to the rectum, whereas with proctocolitis, the disease process extends above 15 cm, into the sigmoid colon.

Differential Diagnosis

The differential diagnosis of infectious proctitis includes gonorrhea, chlamydia (including lymphogranuloma venereum subtypes), HSV, and, rarely, syphilis. Further discussion of each of these infectious causes is provided later in this chapter. Noninfectious causes include inflammatory bowel disease and neoplastic disease (anorectal cancer). Infectious proctocolitis may be caused by extension of proctitis or other enteric bacterial pathogens (eg, *Shigella* or *Salmonella* species) or by parasites such as *Entamoeba* and *Giardia lamblia*. Other potential bacterial causes of proctocolitis, such as *Campylobacter, Yersinia,* and the various *E coli* species, are beyond the scope of this chapter.

Complications

Although most infectious causes of sexually transmitted intestinal syndromes respond readily to treatment, untreated proctitis or proctocolitis may persist and lead to abscesses, fistulae, and strictures. In the preantibiotic era, chronic infection sometimes led to rectal strictures and rectal obstruction that required surgical intervention. Rectal infections substantially increase the risk of HIV acquisition, because the inflamed rectal mucosa is rich with immunologic target cells and defects in the epithelial barrier provide an opening for viral entry.

When to Refer to a Specialist

If the diagnosis is uncertain or treatment fails to resolve the patient's symptoms, further evaluation, including sigmoidoscopy or colonoscopy and biopsy, may be required. Radiologic imaging (eg, radiographs, computed tomography scan, and magnetic resonance imaging) has a limited role in the management of proctitis and proctocolitis, except to rule out toxic megacolon, which is usually associated with *Clostridium difficile* colitis.

Prognosis

The Centers for Disease Control and Prevention (CDC) classifies rectal gonococcal and chlamydial infections as "uncomplicated," recommending the same single-dose therapy for rectal infections as for urogenital infections. Rectal infections respond similarly to uncomplicated infections at other anatomic sites, and treatment failure or persistent infection is uncommon (<5% of patients). Some experts recommend that patients with rectal gonorrhea or chlamydia undergo repeat testing at 3 months to rule out reinfection. Rectal herpes infection can be managed episodically with antiviral treatment at the earliest onset of symptoms or with chronic antiviral suppression to reduce the frequency of outbreaks.

PATHOGENS CAUSING PROCTITIS

1. Neisseria Gonorrhoeae

The rectum is a common site for gonococcal infection. In a recent retrospective review of 101 patients who presented to an STD clinic for evaluation of proctitis symptoms, 30% had gonorrhea. Rectal gonorrhea among MSM results from direct inoculation through receptive rectal intercourse. The rectal mucosa may also be infected in 35–50% of women with gonococcal cervicitis and in several studies carried out in the pre-AIDS era was the only site of infection in approximately 5% of women with gonorrhea. Although rectal gonorrhea in women is associated with direct inoculation through rectal intercourse, infections in women may occur without acknowledged rectal sexual contact, are positively correlated with the duration of endocervical infection, and are assumed to result from perineal contamination with infected cervical secretions.

Clinical Findings

A. Symptoms and Signs

Many rectal gonococcal infections are asymptomatic. A recent evaluation of rectal, urethral, and pharyngeal chlamydial and gonococcal infections among MSM attending a municipal STD clinic and a gay men's community health center in San Francisco found a 7% prevalence of rectal gonorrhea, 84% of which was asymptomatic. When present, however, symptoms associated with gonococcal infections may be subtle and missed if not sought. Rectal gonorrhea symptoms may develop 5–7 days after exposure and include mild anorectal pain, scant bleeding, pruritus, and mucopurulent discharge manifested only by a coating of stools with exudate. Occasionally, more severe symptoms may occur; these include tenesmus and constipation. External inspection of the perirectal area and anus may rarely show erythema and discharge. Anoscopic evaluation commonly reveals mucopus in the anal canal, especially around the anal crypts. The rectal mucosa may appear completely normal or erythematous and friable, especially near the anorectal junction.

B. Laboratory Findings

If available, Gram stain of a rectal specimen can be performed as an immediate diagnostic tool. The sensitivity of a "blind" anorectal swab evaluated by Gram stain has been reported in the range of 40–60% compared with culture, although when positive this result is highly specific. In men with symptomatic rectal gonorrhea, Gram stain sensitivity was 79% when obtained via anoscopy compared with 53% when obtained via a "blind" rectal swab. Culture performance, however, is similar regardless of swabbing technique.

Nucleic acid amplification tests (NAATs) are available for gonococcal detection in urethral, rectal and pharyngeal specimens. Although NAATs are not currently cleared by the Food and Drug Administration (FDA) for rectal or pharyngeal specimens, increasingly laboratories are offering such testing for these specimens.

Treatment

Data from the CDC's Gonococcal Isolate Surveillance Project (GISP) 2004 indicate that fluoroquinolone-resistant *N gonorrhoeae* is more common among MSM than among heterosexual men (18% vs 2%). Therefore, fluoroquinolones should not be used for gonorrhea treatment among MSM, regardless of the site of infection.

Current STD treatment guidelines for urogenital gonococcal infection recommend a single 125-mg intramuscular injection of ceftriaxone, which cures 99.1% of uncomplicated urogenital and anorectal infections, or cefixime in a single 400-mg oral dose, which cures 97.1% of uncomplicated infections. If cefixime is not available, single-dose oral cefpodoxime, 400 mg, may be used. Empiric treatment for acute proctitis and proctocolitis syndromes consists of ceftriaxone, 125 mg intramuscularly, plus doxycycline, 100 mg orally twice a day for 7 days. This regimen offers coverage for the most common sexually transmitted pathogens that cause these symptoms (see Table 9–1) and is especially effective against *N gonorrhoeae*, *Chlamydia*, and incubating *T pallidum*.

Centers for Disease Control and Prevention (CDC). Increase in fluoroquinolone-resistant Neisseria gonorrhoeae among men who have sex with men—United States, 2003, and revised recommendations for gonorrhea treatment, 2004. *MMWR Morb Mortal Wkly Rep* 2004;53:335–338. [PMID: 15123985] (The CDC recommends against the use of fluoroquinolones [eg, ciprofloxacin] in the treatment of gonorrhea in MSM and in persons who may have acquired gonorrhea in Hawaii or California.)

Young H, Manavi K, McMillan A. Evaluation of ligase chain reaction for the non-cultural detection of rectal and pharyngeal gonorrhoea in men who have sex with men. *Sex Transm Infect* 2003;79:484–486. [PMID: 14663126] (A study demonstrating the utility of nucleic acid amplification testing in place of culture for the detection of gonorrhea in the pharynx and rectum.)

2. Chlamydia Trachomatis

Chlamydial infection is a cause of acute proctitis in MSM who practice receptive rectal intercourse. In a recent study of the etiology of clinical proctitis among MSM, 19% of 101 patients had chlamydial proctitis.

Clinical Findings

A. Symptoms and Signs

Rectal *C trachomatis* infections are usually asymptomatic or mildly symptomatic when caused by the non-lymphogranuloma venereum (LGV) strains of chlamydia. Non-LGV strains or serovars, usually genital immunotypes D or K, can cause a mild proctitis with symptoms of rectal discharge, tenesmus, or anorectal pain. In a recent prevalence study among MSM attending either an STD clinic or a Gay Men's Health Clinic, 44 of 213 (21%) men with symptoms of proctitis had *Chlamydia* isolated compared with 272 (8%) of 3579 asymptomatic men. Regardless of symptoms, chlamydial infections of the rectum are usually associated with friable rectal mucosa and mucopurulent discharge as seen on anoscopy. Gram stains of rectal specimens show increased polymorphonuclear cells, even in asymptomatic patients. Sigmoidoscopy can be normal or can reveal mild inflammatory changes with small erosions or follicles in the lower 10–15 cm of the rectum.

In contrast, direct rectal inoculation with LGV strains (L1, L2, or L3) of *C trachomatis* may cause severe anorectal pain, a bloody mucopurulent discharge, and tenesmus in women and men who practice unprotected anal intercourse. Recent reports, however, suggest that some rectal LGV infections may be asymptomatic. A complete review of recent diagnostic recommendations for LGV infections can be found in Chapter 17.

B. LABORATORY FINDINGS

C trachomatis rectal infection may be confirmed by culture or by direct immunofluorescent stain. Enzyme immunosorbent assays for detection of chlamydial antigens in rectal samples have high false-positivity rates. NAATs have been used with good reported sensitivity and specificity, but no commercial product is currently FDA cleared for use with rectal specimens. At one time serologic testing was considered useful for the diagnosis of classic urogenital LGV, and a complement-fixation titer greater than 1:64 was considered suggestive of LGV infection, but data are incomplete, leading most experts to recommend against the use of serology in the diagnosis of rectal LGV infection.

Treatment

Doxycycline, 100 mg twice daily for 7–10 days, is effective in the treatment of non-LGV chlamydial proctitis and proctocolitis. Azithromycin, 1 g as a single dose, is effective for chlamydial urethritis and cervicitis and has been recommended for uncomplicated rectal infections. The recommended therapy for LGV infections is doxycycline, 100 mg twice daily for 21 days. Alternative regimens include erythromycin base, 500 mg orally four times daily for 21 days. Although azithromycin given as a 1-g oral dose once a week for 3 weeks may be effective, clinical data are lacking.

3. Treponema Pallidum

Primary and secondary syphilis rates declined steadily in the United States throughout the 1990s. Recently, however, these rates have begun to increase.

Clinical Findings

A. SYMPTOMS AND SIGNS

Primary syphilis can present as an anorectal chancre from 9 to 90 days after inoculation by an infected partner. Classically, the chancre is painless. If located in the perirectal area it may have well-demarcated indurated edges and a clean base. Although the chancre may be asymptomatic, patients may also present with itching, bleeding, rectal discharge, constipation, and tenesmus, and it may be easily misdiagnosed as a rectal fissure. If the primary chancre is located above the anal verge, within the anal canal, its appearance may be atypical. Patients with internal chancres may present with symptoms of pain on defecation or rectal bleeding, which may be mistaken for trauma, hemorrhoids, or neoplasms. Often these chancres go undetected unless digital rectal examinations and anoscopic evaluations are performed.

Therefore, if the patient reports any anorectal symptoms and recent anorectal sexual activity, anoscopy should be included in the physical examination.

Lesions of secondary syphilis may also appear in the perirectal skin and rectal mucosa. Condylomata lata, which are generally smooth, heaped, wartlike lesions, or mucous patches are clinical manifestations associated with the secondary stage of syphilis. Condylomata lata may be easily confused with the more highly keratinized condylomata acuminata, but condylomata lata are usually moist, shiny, and smooth appearing, whereas warts are dry, dull, and rough appearing.

B. LABORATORY FINDINGS

Darkfield examination of fluid collected from any observed lesions in the perianal and anal region may be useful to immediately detect motile treponemes. If one typical treponeme is detected, the diagnosis of primary syphilis can be made. However, because 10^5 treponemes per milliliter are required for visualization, a negative test result does not rule out syphilis. Darkfield examination of rectal lesions is not helpful, as nonpathogenic treponemes can be found in the intestines and are easily confused with *T pallidum*. Because darkfield microscopy is not available to most primary care physicians, most diagnoses of anorectal syphilis are based on the physical examination and the results of serologic tests for syphilis.

C. SPECIAL TESTS

Serologic tests for syphilis include the rapid plasma reagin (RPR) or the Venereal Disease Research Laboratories (VDRL) screening tests, which if positive, are confirmed by more specific tests such as the fluorescent treponemal antibody absorption (FTA-ABS) test or the *T pallidum* particle agglutination (TP-PA) assay. These tests may be nonreactive in 10–25% of patients with primary syphilis, if patients have not been infected long enough to mount a detectable antibody response. Some laboratories have begun to screen blood samples using treponemal EIA tests. Persons with a positive EIA screening test should have a standard nontreponemal test with titer to guide patient management decisions. For further discussion regarding EIA screening test interpretation, see Chapter 19.

Treatment

The drug of choice for primary and secondary syphilis remains 2.4 million units of intramuscular benzathine penicillin. Penicillin-allergic patients with primary or secondary syphilis can be treated with a 2-week course of doxycycline, 100 mg twice daily, regardless of HIV status. For further discussion, see Chapter 19.

4. Herpes Simplex Virus

Anorectal herpes infection is usually acquired by anal intercourse, but oral-anal contact with a partner who has orolabial herpes can also result in transmission. Most anorectal HSV isolates have been type 2 (HSV-2), but HSV type 1 also occurs. In a study of primary HSV proctitis, 70% of cases were caused by HSV-2 and 30% by HSV-1.

Clinical Findings

A. SYMPTOMS AND SIGNS

The clinical presentations of HSV infections are varied and range from asymptomatic to mild, moderate, or severe. The presentation of a primary first-episode infection, in which the patient has no serologic evidence of prior HSV-1 or HSV-2 infection and becomes infected with either type, may be severe. Primary anorectal HSV may involve the perianal skin and anal canal, and may extend to the rectum. Symptoms can include severe pain, with rectal discharge, tenesmus, and constipation. Nerve root S4–S5 dysesthesias, sacral paresthesias, urinary retention, and temporary impotence have been reported in up to 50% of patients with primary first-episode anorectal HSV infections. Patients may also have symptoms consistent with viremia such as fever, chills, malaise, headache, and meningismus. Symptoms and signs associated with recurrent disease tend to be milder, as with other forms of genitourinary HSV infections, and are not typically accompanied by urinary retention or impotence.

On examination of the perianal area, typical herpetic vesicles, pustules, or ulcerations may be seen. In severe cases, perirectal edema and erythema may be confused with a yeast infection. Anoscopic examination may be painful and may reveal an edematous, friable mucosa with ulcerations. In immunocompetent individuals, the infection rarely extends above 15 cm.

B. LABORATORY FINDINGS

Culture or direct immunofluorescent stains confirm the diagnosis. PCR testing may be used for diagnosis of perianal lesions.

Treatment

In a prospective, double-blind, placebo-controlled trial evaluating therapy for primary HSV proctitis, acyclovir, 400 mg orally taken five times daily for 10 days, was clinically efficacious compared with placebo. No other controlled trial has been conducted recently, but some experts believe that acyclovir, 400 mg orally three times daily, valacyclovir, 1 g orally twice daily, and famciclovir, 250 mg orally three times daily—all given for 7–10 days—can be administered according to the same recommended dosing schedules as for other first-episode genitourinary HSV infections.

HIV-infected patients or other immunocompromised patients can present with severe mucocutaneous HSV. These patients should receive 5–10 mg/kg of intravenous acyclovir every 8 hours until clinical improvement is attained. Patients may be placed on oral HSV suppression using acyclovir, 400 mg twice daily. A double-blind, placebo-controlled, crossover trial of famciclovir, 500 mg orally twice daily, versus placebo for 8 weeks reported clinically and statistically significant reductions in the symptoms associated with HSV infection and in the symptomatic and asymptomatic shedding of HSV among HIV-infected persons.

PATHOGENS CAUSING PROCTOCOLITIS

Enteric pathogens cause infections that are associated with the ingestion of fecally contaminated food or water. However, certain sexual practices, especially anilingus, may allow direct exposure to these pathogens. These sexual behaviors can promote transmission of *Campylobacter, Shigella, Salmonella, Entamoeba histolytica, Giardia,* and several other enteric pathogens, which may result in symptoms of proctocolitis or gastroenteritis, or both.

1. Shigella

Shigella is the third most common cause of bacterial gastroenteritis in the United States, with the majority of cases occurring among young children and their caretakers. However, increases in *Shigella* infection among adult men were recently reported, attributable to outbreaks among MSM.

The infective dose for shigellosis is very small (10–100 organisms), and transmission can occur rapidly. An infected individual can be very contagious. Therefore, whenever *Shigella* is detected by a diagnostic laboratory, it is immediately reported to the local public health department and the infected individual is contacted for immediate therapy and interview.

Clinical Findings

Clinically, patients with *Shigella* infections may present with an array of symptoms. Symptoms may be absent or may include abrupt onset of watery or bloody diarrhea with associated nausea, tenesmus, cramping, and fever. Rarely, toxic megacolon has been reported as a complication of infection. Examination of stool shows red blood cells and mucopus, and sigmoidoscopy may reveal an inflamed, friable mucosa extending above 15 cm. Diagnosis is confirmed by stool culture on selective media.

Treatment

Treatment is supportive and consists mainly of hydration. Antimotility agents should not be given. Antibiotics are not recommended to treat shigellosis in otherwise healthy patients, and their use should be reserved to prevent complications in immunocompromised patients. If given, antibiotics should be selected according to regional antibiotic sensitivities because of widespread development of resistance. Ciprofloxacin, 500 mg orally twice daily for 5–7 days, has been reported as effective therapy. In severely ill patients receiving antibiotic therapy, stool and blood cultures should be repeated to monitor therapeutic response, because antibiotic resistance may develop and recurrences are common. Contact tracing to detect asymptomatic carriers is an important public health measure, but the value of treating sexual contacts is unknown.

Centers for Disease Control and Prevention (CDC). *Shigella sonnei* outbreak among men who have sex with men—San Francisco, California, 2000–2001. *MMWR Morb Mortal Wkly Rep* 2001;50:922–926. [PMID: 11699845] (Report documenting an outbreak of shigellosis among MSM in San Francisco. The authors recommend treatment [eg, ciprofloxacin, 500 mg orally twice daily for 5–7 days] to decrease the duration, transmission, and severity of symptoms in those with severe illness or the need to protect close contacts. Antimicrobial resistance to ampicillin, trimethoprim-sulfamethoxazole, and tetracyclines was common [>95% of isolates tested].)

2. Salmonella

Although *Salmonella* has been reported as a cause of proctocolitis and enterocolitis in homosexual men, its impact is most significant among AIDS patients, in whom a 20-fold increased incidence is noted. *Salmonella* bacteremia in an HIV-infected person is diagnostic of AIDS. Infections in immunocompromised individuals, usually due to *Salmonella typhimurium* and *Salmonella enteritidis*, are frequently associated with bacteremia that recurs despite directed therapy.

Diagnosis is made by culture of stool on selective media. Treatment is individualized according to symptom severity and antibiotic sensitivity. In immunocompetent patients with mild illness, supportive therapy without antibiotics is usual. In AIDS patients with *Salmonella* infection, ciprofloxacin, 750 mg twice daily for 2–4 weeks, is generally recommended, and ciprofloxacin, 500 mg, is given indefinitely if relapse occurs.

PARASITIC INFECTIONS

Sexual transmission as a mode of spread for parasitic infections was suggested in 1972. The prevalence of *Giardia lamblia* and *Entamoeba histolytica* has been reported to be as high as 30–40% in selected populations of MSM and correlates better with a history of anilingus than with travel to endemic areas.

1. Giardia Lamblia

G lamblia is usually a waterborne disease but can be sexually transmitted through anal-oral contact. Because it is typically an infection of the small intestine, it can cause symptoms of enteritis. Symptoms include diarrhea, bloating, abdominal cramps, and nausea. Multiple stool examinations are often required to document infection with *G lamblia*. When stool examination findings are negative, sampling of jejunal mucus by the Enterotest or by small bowel biopsy confirms the diagnosis.

Therapeutic choices include metronidazole, 250–500 mg orally three times daily for 7 days, but this regimen is associated with a 10–20% failure rate. Tinidazole, given as a 2-g oral single dose, is recommended for giardiasis, and nitazoxanide, 500 mg orally twice daily for 3 days, is a new thiazolide antiparasitic agent with excellent activity and tolerance. Older regiments include paromomycin, 500 mg orally three times daily, or furazolidone, 100 mg four times daily for 7–10 days.

2. Entamoeba Species

Two distinct species of *Entamoeba*, a pathogenic form (*Entamoeba histolytica*) and a nonpathogenic form (*Entamoeba dispar*), can cause gastrointestinal infection. These forms are morphologically identical.

E histolytica has been found in the stool of both symptomatic and asymptomatic individuals. If symptoms are present, they can vary from mild diarrhea to fulminant bloody amebic dysentery. Amebic proctocolitis and other inflammatory bowel diseases have the same appearance on colonoscopy. Diagnosis is best confirmed by the identification of *E histolytica* cysts or trophozoites on examination of fresh stool specimens, although PCR tests have been developed for both parasites.

E dispar is considered nonpathogenic, and identification of this form is clinically significant because the patient may not need therapy. Until recently, the inability of microscopy to distinguish between the two ameba species, and the time it takes to culture and subsequently differentiate *Entamoeba* by isoenzyme analysis, made specific diagnoses difficult, but the development of highly sensitive and specific PCR techniques has simplified diagnosis.

If *E histolytica* is identified in screening specimens of asymptomatic individuals, therapy is given to prevent continued infection and avoid transmission. Recommended therapy is with the luminal amoebicide, iodoquinol, at a dose of 650 mg orally three times daily for 20 days. Alternative regimens include paromomycin, 25–30 mg/kg/day orally in three doses for 7 days, or diloxanide furoate, 500 mg orally three times daily for 10 days; the latter is only available through the CDC. Metronidazole, 750 mg orally three times daily for 10 days, is the treatment of choice for invasive, symptomatic infection. This regimen, however, does not eradicate organisms in the intestinal lumen and must be followed by a course of iodoquinol in the dose indicated above.

Entamoeba nana, Entamoeba coli, and Entamoeba hartmanni have frequently been identified in the stool of homosexual men. *Iodamoeba butschlii* and *Dientamoeba fragilis* are less commonly identified, and the significance of any of these parasites as potential pathogens has not been established. Several protozoan parasites, which include *Cryptosporidium, Isospora, Cyclospora,* and *Microsporidia,* have been reported among AIDS patients with severe and sometimes unrelenting diarrhea. The epidemiology of these infections is not fully understood, and the role of sexual transmission has not been studied but should be addressed in future research.

Roy S, Kabir M, Mondal D, et al. Real-time-PCR assay for diagnosis of Entamoeba histolytica infection. *J Clin Microbiol* 2005;43:2168–2172. [PMID: 15872237] (Two types of PCR versus stool antigen testing were compared for the detection of *E histolytica;* all were highly specific, with real-time PCR being the most sensitive.)

PRACTICE POINTS

- *If a patient reports any anorectal symptoms and recent anorectal sexual activity, anoscopy should be included in the physical examination.*

Relevant Web Sites

[Centers for Disease Control and Prevention lymphogranuloma venereum project:]
http://www.cdc.gov/std/lgv
[Medical Letter on Drugs and Therapeutics:]
http://www.medletter.com/html/prm.htm#Parasitic

Cervicitis

Jeanne M. Marrazzo, MD, MPH

ESSENTIALS OF DIAGNOSIS

- Inflammatory condition of the cervix defined by the presence of mucopurulent endocervical discharge, easily induced endocervical friability, or edematous cervical ectopy.
- Most often a result of chlamydia, gonorrhea, trichomoniasis, or genital herpes infection.
- Associated with an increased risk of upper genital tract infection, adverse pregnancy outcomes, and HIV acquisition.

General Considerations

Cervicitis is typically the consequence of infection with sexually acquired pathogens, most commonly *Chlamydia trachomatis* or *Neisseria gonorrhoeae* and, occasionally, *Trichomonas vaginalis* or herpes simplex virus (HSV). The diagnosis is made when either mucopurulent discharge or easily induced bleeding (friability) is present at the endocervical os; more subtle signs include edema of the cervical ectropion (edematous ectopy). Recent data suggest that disruption of normal vaginal flora, most often manifesting as bacterial vaginosis, may also promote cervicitis. Although *C trachomatis* is probably the most common cause of cervicitis, and *N gonorrhoeae* is also implicated, the majority of women (80–90%) infected with these pathogens have no signs of cervicitis.

Pathogenesis

The cervix consists of an underlying connective tissue matrix overlaid by two types of distinct epithelium, each of which is vulnerable to infection by distinct pathogens. The endocervical canal and ectropion (cervical ectopy), if present, are lined by columnar epithelial cells. These cells, which line what is commonly called the *endocervix*, provide vulnerable targets for infections with *C trachomatis* and *N gonorrhoeae*. The *ectocervix*, in contrast, is lined by squamous epithelium that is contiguous with the vaginal mucosa. For this reason, the ectocervix is susceptible to *T vaginalis*, an agent more commonly associated with vaginitis.

Estrogen, produced endogenously or administered exogenously, promotes the formation and maintenance of cervical ectopy, which is present in adolescents, pregnant women, and women who take estrogen-containing contraceptives. Estrogen is also needed to maintain adequate thickness of the squamous cervicovaginal epithelium (≥20 cell layers). This promotes sustenance of a healthy population of hydrogen peroxide-producing *Lactobacillus* species, which maintain normal (acidic) vaginal pH. The quality of endocervical mucous is also affected by these hormones. Relatively high levels of estrogen during the follicular phase leading up to ovulation thin the endocervical mucous; this can result in elaboration of so-called physiologic discharge. In the luteal phase of the cycle, progesterone increases the viscosity and reduces the volume of endocervical mucous.

Recently, some investigators have proposed a direct role for these hormones in modulating the balance of cell-mediated (Th1) and humoral (Th2) immune responses, with estrogen predominance promoting Th2 and progesterone augmenting Th1 responses. Because endocervical mucous possesses intrinsic antimicrobial activity by virtue of lactic acid, low pH, and antimicrobial peptides, these hormonal changes are potentially important in mediating susceptibility to and natural history of cervical infection. For example, it is not at all clear why only a subset of women develops inflammatory signs of cervicitis when infected by chlamydia, gonorrhea, or trichomoniasis.

Prevention

Acquisition of the sexually transmitted diseases (STDs) that cause cervicitis—in particular, chlamydia, gonorrhea, trichomoniasis, and genital herpes—is markedly reduced when condoms are used consistently and correctly.

No data speak to the effect of condoms on cervicitis in which no microbiologic etiology is apparent.

Clinical Findings

A. History

A thorough sexual history—including assessment of number and gender of recent partners, specific sexual practices (oral, anal, vaginal sex), whether sex partners are symptomatic or have been recently diagnosed with an STD or STD-related syndrome, recent Papanicolaou (Pap) smear history, and use of condoms or other prevention methods—should be obtained from women who present with cervicitis.

Symptoms referent to the lower genital tract that should be elicited include dysuria, urinary hesitancy or frequency, and abnormal vaginal discharge. Elements of the history that might suggest upper genital tract involvement should be assessed, including lower abdominal or pelvic pain or cramping, right upper quadrant pain, and pain or bleeding with intercourse or other penetrative sex.

Patients should be specifically queried about a history of douching and any use of intravaginal products, including lubricants, over-the-counter therapeutic preparations (especially antifungal products), and so-called feminine deodorants, all of which can cause a chemical or allergic mucosal reaction. Information about these factors can help to narrow the differential diagnosis considerably and direct subsequent management.

B. Symptoms and Signs

Symptoms of cervicitis include abnormal vaginal discharge (increase in amount; change in color [often yellow, green, or brown] or odor [malodorous]), intermenstrual bleeding, and bleeding that occur after intercourse or other penetrative sexual contact. However, most women with cervicitis do not complain of symptoms, and even when symptoms are present, they are nonspecific and may indicate vaginitis without cervical involvement. If endometritis or other pelvic inflammatory disease (PID) accompanies cervicitis, lower abdominal pain or cramping, often exacerbated with intercourse, may be present.

Mucopurulent discharge issuing from the endocervical canal and easily induced bleeding are the most easily recognized signs of endocervicitis. Both may be present simultaneously. Edematous ectopy is a more subtle sign and is characterized by a swollen, irregular mucosal surface to the ectropion. Signs of infection affecting the ectocervix depend on the responsible pathogen. *T vaginalis* can cause an erosive inflammation of the ectocervical epithelium, classically manifest as "strawberry cervix" or *colpitis macularis*. This process may appear as a range of epithelial disruption, from small isolated petechiae to large punctuate hemorrhages with surrounding areas of pale mucosa.

Genital infection with HSV types 1 and 2 can cause cervicitis, particularly in the case of women who experience severe clinical manifestations of primary infection with HSV-2. Although most primary HSV-2 infections are asymptomatic, some women (15–20%) experience a severe primary infection that may include cervicitis. Cervicitis in this setting is characterized by diffuse erosive and hemorrhagic lesions, usually in the ectocervical epithelium, and often accompanied by frank ulceration. Other manifestations of primary HSV-2 genital infection are usually evident, including external herpetic lesions, neurologic manifestations (including aseptic meningitis, urinary retention, and lumbosacral radiculitis), fever, and inguinal lymphadenopathy. Cervicitis may recur with clinical recurrences of genital HSV-2; however, it is typically not severe. Subclinical shedding of HSV-2 does not appear to be directly related to cervicitis. HSV-1 may also cause cervicitis similar to that described for HSV-2; however, the manifestations are typically less severe, and usually occur only during the primary genital infection with HSV-1. As with genital herpes, other causes of genital ulcer disease can cause lesions on the cervix; these include the chancre of primary syphilis and ulcers of chancroid.

Mycoplasma genitalium has recently been implicated as a sexually transmissible cause of cervicitis, but its exact prevalence, incidence, and natural history are not known; prospective studies are underway. Various case reports have attributed cervicitis to infection with certain *Streptococcus* species—most notably, *S agalactiae* (group B streptococcus) and *S pyogenes*—but reliable estimates of how commonly this might occur, if a causal relationship exists, are not available, nor is the approach to treating these agents if they are suspected etiologies of cervicitis clear.

Apart from the previously noted infections, numerous noninfectious and infectious systemic inflammatory processes and local insults can precipitate cervical inflammation that may present clinically as apparent cervicitis. The former group includes Behçet syndrome, sarcoidosis, ligneous conjunctivitis, and tuberculosis. Substances that either erode the endocervical mucous plug or cause an irritant mucositis can also cause signs of cervicitis. Commonly used, commercially available douching and feminine deodorant preparations often include detergents that have surfactant properties, and many include various chemicals such as antihistamines and cornstarch. In one large study in which commercial sex workers were randomized to use vaginal sponges impregnated with 1 g of nonoxynol-9 (N-9), cervical erosions as assessed by colposcopy were seen more commonly among N-9 users, who were also more likely to acquire HIV infection during the course of the study than were nonusers. Because N-9 has shown no benefit in reducing acquisition of HIV and STDs, it is no longer recommended for this purpose.

Even seemingly obvious signs of endocervical inflammation may have variable precision for chlamydia and gonorrhea, because the predictive value of individual cervical findings suggestive of cervicitis may vary with patients' age and other STD-related risk factors. For example, the presence of easily induced endocervical bleeding in a 16-year-old girl who reports recent unprotected sex with a new male partner is highly predictive of chlamydial infection; the predictive value of this sign is much lower for chlamydia in a 35-year-old woman in a long-term, monogamous relationship.

C. LABORATORY FINDINGS

1. Gram stain—Gram stain of a smear of endocervical secretions was used for many years to support a diagnosis of cervicitis; however, its independent value, especially in predicting chlamydial infection, has been variable, and its sensitivity for detection of *N gonorrhoeae* at the cervix is only 50%. If this test is used, clinicians should first use a large cotton-tipped swab to gently remove adherent vaginal secretions from the face of the cervix before inserting a small cotton- or Dacron-tipped swab approximately 2 cm into the endocervical canal, rotating once or twice, then removing and swabbing the material on a fresh glass slide for staining. High-power fields should be examined (at 1000 × magnification, oil immersion), specifically focusing on areas that have abundant endocervical mucous that appears pink under Gram stain.

Most clinic guidelines recommend a threshold level of 10–30 polymorphonuclear (PMN) leukocytes per high-power field, with PMN counts above this level supporting a diagnosis of cervicitis. The sensitivity of this test increases and specificity decreases as this threshold cutoff is decreased.

2. Pap smear—Although inflammatory changes on Pap smear are associated with an increased likelihood of detection of several STDs, including chlamydia, gonorrhea, trichomoniasis, and human papillomavirus, this test is neither specific enough to direct empiric therapy for these pathogens nor practical in delineating immediate etiologies of cervicitis for empiric therapy. Thus, it is not recommended as a means of evaluating women for the presence of cervicitis.

3. Microscopy—A finding of PMNs (>5–10 per high-power field) on saline microscopy of vaginal fluid has been associated with an increased risk of cervical chlamydia and gonorrhea; further data are needed.

D. SPECIAL TESTS

1. Chlamydia tests—Women with cervicitis should be tested for chlamydia and gonorrhea. One of the most sensitive diagnostic assays, a nucleic acid amplification test (NAAT), should be used if at all possible. NAATs include polymerase chain reaction (PCR), transcription-mediated amplification, and strand displacement amplification. Use of these techniques is particularly important for chlamydia, because the sensitivity of NAAT for *C trachomatis* is at least 20% higher than that of unamplified DNA probes, enzyme immunoassay, and direct fluorescent antibody assays. These tests perform equally well in the presence of blood, mucopus, or pregnancy, and exhibit excellent specificity (>98%). Chlamydial infection at the cervix can be detected using any of three patient specimens: cervical swab, first-catch urine, or vaginal fluid.

a. Cervical swab specimen—A swab can be obtained directly from the cervix; this approach may be useful if a pelvic examination is performed for other indications, such as a Pap smear or assessment for PID. However, in general, clinicians need not perform a speculum examination for the sole purpose of obtaining a cervical swab for NAAT, because the sensitivities of NAAT performed on either a urine specimen or a vaginal swab are also excellent.

b. First-catch urine specimen—A first-catch urine specimen (defined as the first 10–15 mL of urine stream) can be obtained. This test not only has the advantage of not requiring a pelvic examination, but also will detect the minority of chlamydial infections that occur in the female urethra and not at the cervix (10–15% of all lower genital tract infections in women). Importantly, women should be instructed not to cleanse or wipe the periurethral area prior to voiding, and not to collect a midstream sample (sometimes familiar to them from previous experience with collection of urine culture for evaluation of cystitis).

c. Vaginal fluid specimen—Swabs of vaginal fluid can be used. These may be collected by the clinician performing the examination or, occasionally, by the patient; however, not all NAATs are currently FDA cleared for patient collection of vaginal swabs.

2. Gonorrhea tests—Although NAATs may be used to diagnose gonococcal infection at the cervix, the sensitivity of traditional culture is relatively close to that of NAATs, which do not offer the same degree of enhanced sensitivity for this pathogen as for *C trachomatis*. Culture is especially appropriate if there are concerns about the possibility of fluoroquinolone-resistant *N gonorrhoeae* (eg, a woman being assessed in Hawaii or California, history of travel outside the United States during the time frame in which the infection may have been acquired, or sexual contact with a bisexual man). Notably, several NAATs offer combination assays for both chlamydia and gonorrhea with the use of a single specimen.

3. Other tests—Examination of vaginal fluid should be performed to look for the presence of bacterial vaginosis, because treatment of concurrent infection might enhance the resolution of cervicitis. The presence of three of the four Amsel criteria establishes the diagnosis of bacterial vaginosis: (1) homogeneous vaginal discharge, (2) vaginal fluid pH higher than 4.5, (3) clue cells comprising more than 20% of total vaginal epithelial cells seen on 100 × magnification on saline microscopy, and (4) an amine (fishy) odor on addition of potassium hydroxide. If microscopy if not available, pH testing of vaginal fluid offers valuable information; abnormally high vaginal pH is the most sensitive of the four Amsel criteria in diagnosing bacterial vaginosis: a normal pH (<4.5) makes bacterial vaginosis highly unlikely. Saline microscopy also offers the opportunity to look for motile trichomonads and for PMNs. Trichomonads may also be identified by newly available rapid antigen–based diagnostic tests for *T vaginalis*.

Further workup should be determined by the specific clinical scenario. For example, if ulcerations are present on the cervix, specific tests for HSV are indicated and may include direct (culture or antigen detection [PCR]) or serologic assays. If the sexual and social history suggests that the woman is at increased risk for syphilis (eg, having sex with a man who reports sex with other men, exchange of sex for drugs or money), serologic screening should be performed and, if available, direct darkfield microscopy of exudate from the lesion. No test for *M genitalium* is commercially available at the present time.

E. Special Examinations

All women with cervicitis require a pelvic examination to rule out PID, because the presence of cervicitis is associated with a considerably increased risk of both silent endometritis and symptomatic PID. PID should be diagnosed if either cervical motion tenderness or uterine or adnexal tenderness is present; if PID is suspected, women should be treated with appropriate antibiotic regimens (see Chapter 8). Importantly, the single-dose antibiotic regimens recommended for the treatment of cervicitis are not adequate in the treatment of PID.

Manhart LE, Critchlow CW, Holmes KK, et al. Mucopurulent cervicitis and Mycoplasma genitalium. *J Infect Dis* 2003;187: 650–657. [PNMID: 12599082] (This study showed a strong, direct association between the presence of *M genitalium* and a clinical diagnosis of cervicitis, as well as individual signs, including mucopurulent endocervical discharge, easily induced endocervical bleeding, and elevated PMN count on Gram stain of endocervical secretions. The associations persisted after the investigators controlled for chlamydia, gonorrhea, age, menstrual cycle, and the presence of ectopy.)

Differential Diagnosis

Because cervicitis is a clinically determined syndrome, the differential diagnosis is based on etiology. As previously described, the cause can be infectious, with an STD predominating, or noninfectious.

Complications

Cervicitis is associated with three major consequences. First, it is a marker for the presence of inflammation, and potential infection, in the upper genital tract. This can occur either as overt PID or as silent inflammation of the uterine lining (endometritis). Second, the presence of cervicitis during pregnancy has been associated with an increased risk of adverse pregnancy outcomes even when no specific pathogen was detected. Third, cervicitis influences the dynamics of HIV transmission. It increases a woman's risk of infection with HIV, probably by recruiting vulnerable lymphocytes to the site of inflammation, and, among women already infected with HIV, increases the amount of HIV shed at the cervix. Concomitantly, treatment of cervicitis in HIV-infected women effects a reduction in the quantity of HIV shed at the cervix. This observation provides an especially compelling rationale for screening and treatment of this condition among HIV-infected women.

Treatment

Tables 10–1 and 10–2 outline the general approach to management of cervicitis, and treatment based on suspected or documented microbial etiology. Presumptive therapy directed at *C trachomatis* should be provided, because the prevalence of this common STD is high among young women in the United States. The approach involving possible infection with *N gonorrhoeae* is less clear. Women with cervicitis who fall into subgroups with high prior likelihood of gonococcal

Table 10–1. General considerations in the management of patients with cervicitis.

Evaluate for a history of genital herpes, vaginitis, or use of irritative intravaginal preparations (spermicides, deodorants, chemical douches).
All women should have diagnostic tests for *Chlamydia trachomatis* and *Neisseria gonorrhoeae* using the most sensitive assays available (ideally, nucleic acid amplification tests).
Provide empiric therapy:
- Most women should be treated for chlamydial infection.
- Consider therapy for gonococcal infection based on age, risk, and local or patient subgroup prevalence.
- Treat concomitant causes of any vaginitis appropriately.
- Eliminate intravaginal use of products that could irritate cervicovaginal mucosa (douches, other).
Evaluate (ideally) and treat (presumptively) sex partners as index patient was treated.

Table 10–2. Suggested treatment for the most common causes of cervicitis.

Etiology	Management	Comments
Chlamydia trachomatis	Azithromycin, 1 g PO (single dose) *or* Doxycycline, 100 mg PO twice daily for 7 d	Minority of infected women have signs of cervicitis Urine NAATs[a] are highly sensitive for diagnosis of cervical infection
Neisseria gonorrhoeae	Single dose of any of following: • Cefixime, 400 mg PO • Ciprofloxacin, 500 mg PO[b] • Levofloxacin, 250 mg PO[b] • Ceftriaxone, 125 mg IM *Alternative:* • Cefpodoxime, 400 mg PO • Cefuroxime axetil, 1 g PO • Spectinomycin, 2 g IM	Availability of oral cefixime has been precarious, leading many experts to advocate use of alternative oral cephalosporins; formal efficacy studies are underway Fluoroquinolone resistance is increasing rapidly in *N gonorrhoeae;* may not be appropriate empiric therapy (see text for discussion) Minority of infected women have signs of cervicitis Urine NAATs are highly sensitive for diagnosis of cervical infection
Trichomonas vaginalis	Metronidazole, 2 g PO (single dose) *or* Tinidazole, 2 g PO (single dose) *or* Metronidazole, 500 mg PO twice daily for 7 d	
Herpes simplex virus (HSV)	Any of the following given orally for 7–10 d: • Acyclovir, 400 mg 3 times daily • Famciclovir, 250 mg 3 times daily • Valacyclovir, 1 g twice daily	Primary infection with HSV-2 may cause an especially erosive, hemorrhagic cervicitis

[a]NAAT, nucleic acid amplification test; includes polymerase chain reaction, transcription-mediated amplification, and strand displacement assay.
[b]Fluoroquinolones are not recommended for use in patients in California and Hawaii, or in men who have sex with men, due to increased incidences of fluoroquinolone-resistant *N gonorrhoeae* in these populations.

infection should be empirically treated; these subgroups include adolescents in many inner-city areas of the United States. Presumptive therapy for gonorrhea should also be considered if the likelihood of a woman's return for treatment based on a diagnostic test that turns out to be positive is judged to be low. Other considerations that should weigh toward empiric therapy include report of an STD-related risk behavior (especially report of new or multiple sex partners in the prior 60 days) and recent history of STD (especially chlamydial or gonococcal infection in the prior year). Recurrent infection with *C trachomatis* is very common among women, ranging from 8% to 25% in several studies, and probably relates predominantly to resumption

of unprotected sex with untreated partners. Recurrence of gonorrhea is likely to be equally common. For this reason, it is imperative to treat sex partners of women for whatever infection was either detected or presumptively treated in the woman (typically, chlamydia and sometimes gonorrhea).

Appropriate treatment of cervicitis—especially if it is caused by *C trachomatis* or *N gonorrhoeae*—is especially important among HIV-infected women, because at least one small study demonstrated a decline in the amount of HIV-1 shed from the cervical mucosa after empiric treatment of cervicitis aimed at chlamydial and gonococcal infection. This is likely to reduce these women's risk of transmitting HIV-1 to sex partners.

M genitalium appears to be more sensitive to macrolide than tetracycline antibiotics, but further study is required to confirm the efficacy of these agents in curing lower genital tract infection with this organism. *M genitalium* is difficult to culture and, to date, clinical studies have relied on PCR assays to detect it. The implication of this for determining microbiologic cure in such studies is not yet clear.

The approach to treating cervicitis in which no identifiable STD is detected is unclear. Scant evidence suggests that women should be evaluated for bacterial vaginosis at the time they present with cervicitis, and the concurrent condition should be treated if present. Among 51 women with cervicitis and bacterial vaginosis who received doxycycline and ofloxacin as empiric treatment for chlamydia and gonorrhea and were then randomized to receive either intravaginal metronidazole or placebo, those who received metronidazole had a higher rate of resolution of cervicitis at 2 and 4 weeks post-treatment. Women whose bacterial vaginosis resolved were more likely to have resolution of cervicitis at 2 weeks, regardless of which regimen they received.

Further management of cervicitis for which neither an identifiable STD nor bacterial vaginosis plays a role is empiric, and substantiated by little rigorous evidence, because no published data have addressed this issue. Certainly, intravaginal use of products that could potentially damage cervicovaginal mucosa, including douches, spermicides, lubricants, and other products, should be discouraged. Therapeutic approaches used and anecdotally successful include more extended courses of broadspectrum antibiotics or ablative therapy, but neither can be recommended on the basis of available evidence.

Marrazzo JM, Handsfield HH, Whittington WL. Predicting chlamydial and gonococcal cervical infection: Implications for management of cervicitis. *Obstet Gynecol* 2002;100:579–584. [PMID: 12220782] (Among 6230 women for whom chlamydia and gonorrhea test results were available, the positive predictive value of any cervical sign was low (<19%) for these infections among women 25 years of age or older and quite high among adolescents (40%), prompting the authors to suggest that empiric treatment for cervicitis should take age into consideration.)

Nyirjesy P. Nongonococcal and nonchlamydial cervicitis. *Curr Infect Dis Rep* 2001;3:540–545. [PMID: 11722812] (An excellent overview of the challenging clinical scenario in which no etiologic agent is identified as a cause of cervicitis, a condition for which little or no data are available.)

When to Refer to a Specialist

The vast majority of cervicitis cases are uncomplicated; the major concern in most clinical situations is assessing the affected patient for PID. However, a subset of women has cervicitis that persists after treatment aimed at chlamydia, gonorrhea, trichomoniasis, and bacterial vaginosis. Although data on this condition are very limited, an identifiable cause is usually not evident, and prolonged therapy with antibiotics are not indicated. When endocervical discharge is copious and women suffer consequent symptoms, some gynecologists have used cryotherapy for ablation of the affected area, especially if ectopy is present. Referral to a gynecologist in such cases should be considered.

Prognosis

Cervicitis associated with STD-related infections typically resolves completely when antibiotic therapy aimed at causative pathogens is provided. However, relatively few studies of the natural history of this condition are available, and persistent cervicitis occurs in a minority of affected women. The incidence of persistent cervicitis is unknown, but anecdotally, is probably 5% or less.

PRACTICE POINTS

• Clinicians need not perform a speculum examination for the sole purpose of obtaining a cervical swab for NAAT, because the sensitivities of NAAT performed on either a urine or a vaginal swab are also excellent.

Bacterial Vaginosis

11

Jane R. Schwebke, MD

ESSENTIALS OF DIAGNOSIS

- *Grayish-white vaginal discharge.*
- *Presence of vaginal epithelial clue cells.*
- *Vaginal pH higher than 4.5.*
- *Positive "whiff" test.*
- *Decreased numbers of lactobacilli.*
- *Increased bacteria count, consisting mainly of short rods observed on wet mount.*

General Considerations

Bacterial vaginosis is the most frequent cause of vaginal discharge in the United States. Symptoms include vaginal discharge and odor, but half of women with bacterial vaginosis are asymptomatic. Previously given little attention and called nonspecific vaginitis or *Gardnerella* vaginitis, bacterial vaginosis is now known to be significantly associated with complications of pregnancy, including preterm rupture of membranes, preterm delivery, and low birth weight. Additionally, it has been associated with gynecologic complications such as postabortal endometritis, posthysterectomy vaginal cuff cellulitis, pelvic inflammatory diseases (PID), and urinary tract infections. It also appears to be a risk factor for acquisition of sexually transmitted diseases (STDs), including HIV.

Pathogenesis

The pathogenesis of bacterial vaginosis remains obscure, but the bulk of the epidemiologic data suggests that the disease is sexually transmitted. However, understanding of transmission is limited because the causative agent remains unknown and there is no clinical correlate of infection or disease in men. In terms of the microbiologic findings in bacterial vaginosis, lactobacilli, especially

hydrogen peroxide—producing strains, are greatly diminished and are replaced with large numbers of *Gardnerella vaginalis* as well as multiple types of anaerobic bacteria and mycoplasmas. The decline in lactobacilli, which produce lactic acid, a key component in the maintenance of the normally low vaginal pH, results in increased vaginal pH. That increase in pH allows for the overgrowth of anaerobic bacteria, which apparently coat epithelial cells ("clue cells") and produce a grayish-white vaginal discharge. The metabolites from anaerobic bacteria are rich in amines responsible for the characteristic fishy odor.

Larsson PG, Forsum U. Bacterial vaginosis—a disturbed bacterial flora and treatment enigma. *APMIS* 2005;113:305–316. [PMID: 16011656.]

Hillier SL. The complexity of microbial diversity in bacterial vaginosis. *N Engl J Med* 2005;353:1886–1887. [PMID: 16267319]

Prevention

The use of condoms appears to be protective against acquisition of bacterial vaginosis. Although bacterial vaginosis may be an STD, antimicrobial therapy directed at anaerobic bacteria (eg, metronidazole) of the male partner has yet to be proved effective. Among women who have sex with women, examination and treatment of the sex partner is likely to be of benefit in preventing recurrence in the index case, because studies have found high concordance rates of bacterial vaginosis among sex partners in this setting. Twice-weekly prophylactic use of intravaginal metronidazole has proven to be efficacious in preventing recurrences.

Clinical Findings

A. SYMPTOMS AND SIGNS

Symptomatic bacterial vaginosis causes vaginal discharge or odor, or both. The odor is usually described as fishy and may be more noticeable after unprotected intercourse or during menses. Half of women with bacterial vaginosis complain of no symptoms. On examination, a homogenous, milky discharge adherent to the walls of the vagina may be present.

B. LABORATORY FINDINGS

Because a single etiologic agent has not been identified, clinical criteria (Amsel criteria) are used to make the diagnosis. According to these criteria, bacterial vaginosis is present if three of the following findings are present: (1) elevated vaginal pH (>4.5), (2) positive amine odor when vaginal fluid is mixed with 10% potassium hydroxide (KOH)—the so-called "whiff" test, (3) presence of clue cells (squamous epithelial cells covered with adherent bacteria) in a saline (wet mount) preparation of the vaginal fluid, and (4) homogenous vaginal discharge.

When examining vaginal fluid under the microscope, the morphotypes of the bacteria should also be noted. For example, if only *Lactobacillus* morphotypes are present (moderately long rods) it is unlikely that the patient has bacterial vaginosis. On the other hand, motile curved rods that represent *Mobiluncus* are highly suggestive of bacterial vaginosis. White blood cells usually are not present in the vaginal fluid of a patient infected only with bacterial vaginosis; their presence in the vaginal fluid should alert the clinician to the possibility of coinfection in either the vagina or the cervix.

Amsel R, Totten PA, Spiegel CA, et al. Non-specific vaginitis: Diagnostic and microbial and epidemiological associations. *Am J Med* 1983;74:14–22. [PMID: 6600371] (Discussion of the clinical criteria for diagnosis of bacterial vaginosis.)

C. SPECIAL TESTS

1. Gram stain—Gram stain is a reliable means of diagnosing bacterial vaginosis and has the advantage of being a permanent record that can be reviewed. Standardized criteria have been developed that facilitate interpretation, resulting in good intra- and interobserver reproducibility. In a multicenter study comparing the vaginal Gram stain with the Amsel criteria, the sensitivity and specificity of the Gram stain were found to be 89% and 83%, respectively. With Gram stain considered as the "gold standard," the sensitivity and specificity of the Amsel criteria were 70% and 94%, respectively, suggesting that the use of the Amsel criteria may lead to underdiagnosis of bacterial vaginosis. Although the vaginal Gram stain is generally used in research settings, it is also offered in some clinical laboratories.

2. Other diagnostic tests—The following point-of-care tests for bacterial vaginosis are also available: (1) a rapid card test for detection of pH and amines; (2) detection of proline aminopeptidase in the vaginal fluid; (3) a rapid colorimetric test for sialidase, an enzyme that is elevated in bacterial vaginosis; and (4) an oligonucleotide probe technique based on high concentrations of *G vaginalis* (see Table 11–1). The first three tests are useful for initial screening but will not rule out mixed infections.

Bradshaw CS, Morton AN, Garland SM, et al. Evaluation of a point-of-care test, BVBlue, and clinical and laboratory criteria for diagnosis of bacterial vaginosis. *J Clin Microbiol* 2005;43: 1304–1308. [PMID: 15750100]

Differential Diagnosis

Other causes of vaginal complaints include yeast vaginitis, trichomoniasis, atrophic vaginitis, and other miscellaneous conditions. Vaginal complaints should never be diagnosed without analyzing objective laboratory data except, perhaps, in the case of recurrent infections that have been previously documented.

Complications

Bacterial vaginosis is associated with obstetric and gynecologic complications. In cross-sectional studies, bacterial vaginosis is a risk factor for preterm birth and low birth

Table 11–1. Commercially available tests for bacterial vaginosis.

Test Name	Principle of Test	Manufacturer	Comment
Quickvue Advance pH and Amine Test Card	Detects elevated vaginal pH and amines	Quidel Corporation (San Diego, CA)	90% sensitivity versus multiple comparisons
Quickvue Advance *Gardnerella vaginalis* Test	Detects proline and aminopeptidase	Quidel Corporation (San Diego, CA)	91% sensitive compared with Amsel criteria or Gram stain
Osom BV Blue	Detects sialidase	Genzyme Corporation (Cambridge, MA)	85% sensitive compared with Amsel criteria
BD Affirm VPIII	DNA probe for elevated levels of *G vaginalis*	Becton-Dickinson (Franklin Lakes, NJ)	84–98% sensitive compared with wet mount, culture, Amsel criteria, or Gram stain

weight. However, prospective treatment studies have yielded inconsistent results as to the benefit of screening and treating for bacterial vaginosis in pregnancy. Gynecologic complications include postoperative infections following gynecologic surgery; acquisition of STDs, including PID; acquisition and transmission of HIV; and recurrent urinary tract infections. Screening and treating for bacterial vaginosis prior to elective gynecologic procedures is recommended. The leading hypothesis for the association of bacterial vaginosis with STDs and HIV is that the absence of protective hydrogen peroxide–producing lactobacilli found in patients with bacterial vaginosis precedes and facilitates the acquisition of these infections. Women with bacterial vaginosis should be screened for STDs at appropriate intervals. Screening for bacterial vaginosis in asymptomatic women is not generally recommended. Some experts recommend screening in pregnant women with a history of adverse pregnancy outcomes, but the data supporting the benefit of screening and treatment in that population are limited.

Treatment

Options for treatment include both oral and topical metronidazole and clindamycin. Oral metronidazole should be administered at a dose of 500 mg twice daily for 7 days. The 2-g one-time-only dose used for trichomoniasis is not efficacious for bacterial vaginosis. Metronidazole may be used in the first trimester of pregnancy. Meta-analyses have failed to document any adverse events associated with its use during pregnancy. Oral clindamycin is an additional option at a dose of 300 mg twice daily for 7 days.

Intravaginal medications are as efficacious for treating bacterial vaginosis as oral agents and do not produce systemic side effects, although local side effects such as vaginal yeast infections may occur. Options include metronidazole gel at bedtime for 5 nights, clindamycin cream at bedtime for 7 nights, clindamycin ovules for 3 days, and sustained-release clindamycin as a single dose. There is concern that topical agents may not be adequate therapy for pregnant patients, in whom upper tract colonization with bacterial vaginosis–associated bacteria may have occurred; however, no studies have addressed this issue specifically

Reconstitution of the vaginal flora with exogenous lactobacilli has been suggested as an adjunct to antibiotic therapy; however, this requires use of a human-derived strain for effective colonization and is not commercially available. Therapy with yogurt, lactobacilli suppositories, or acidifying agents has not been found to be useful.

The treatment of asymptomatic bacterial vaginosis is controversial and is currently not recommended, with the exception of screening and treating for the condition prior to elective gynecologic procedures as a means of decreasing postoperative infections.

Recurrent episodes of bacterial vaginosis are common, and up to 50% of cases may recur in 6 months. Some data are available on the prophylactic use of intravaginal metronidazole gel twice weekly at bedtime to prevent recurrent episodes. The consistent use of condoms also appears to be protective against recurrent bacterial vaginosis.

Sobel JD, Ferris D, Schwebke J, et al. Suppressive antibacterial therapy with 0.75% metronidazole vaginal gel to prevent recurrent bacterial vaginosis. *Am J Obstet Gynecol* 2006;194:1283–1289. [PMID: 16647911]

When to Refer to a Specialist

Women with recurrent bacterial vaginosis may be referred to a gynecologist or infectious disease specialist for additional management.

Prognosis

Cure rates with any of the recommended therapies are 70–80%, and recurrence rates are high. Many women have frequent recurrences.

PRACTICE POINTS

- The treatment of asymptomatic bacterial vaginosis is controversial and is currently not recommended, with the exception of screening and treating for the condition prior to elective gynecologic procedures as a means of decreasing postoperative infections.

Relevant Web Sites

[American Social Health Association STD information page:]
http://www.ashastd.org
[Centers for Disease Control and Prevention fact sheet on bacterial vaginosis:]
http://www.cdc.gov/std/bv/STDFact-Bacterial-Vaginosis.htm

SECTION II
Infections

Chancroid

12

Stephanie N. Taylor, MD, & David H. Martin, MD

ESSENTIALS OF DIAGNOSIS

- *Tender papule develops into a pustule after an incubation period of 4–7 days; the pustule ruptures within a few days to produce a nonindurated, painful ulcer with a purulent base and undermined or ragged borders.*
- *Unilateral tender inguinal adenopathy may progress to a bubo (fluctuant lymph node mass) that spontaneously ruptures or requires drainage.*
- *Isolation of the causative organism,* Haemophilus ducreyi, *by special culture media.*

General Considerations

Chancroid is a sexually transmitted genital ulcer disease caused by *Haemophilus ducreyi*, a small, fastidious, gram-negative rod. Worldwide, chancroid incidence exceeds that of syphilis in many developing countries. In 1997, the World Health Organization estimated that there were six million new cases of chancroid. Based on polymerase chain reaction (PCR) assays, chancroid prevalence has been shown to range from 23% to 56% in endemic areas (Africa, Asia, and the Caribbean). In the United States and western Europe outbreaks are episodic. The infection is also up to 25 times more prevalent in men than in women, a difference recognized in both naturally occurring and experimental disease in humans and macaques. In fact, although controversial,

it has been suggested that women may be asymptomatic carriers or reservoirs of the infection.

Although chancroid is uncommon in North America, outbreaks occur in the inner cities of the United States. The most recent of these began in the late 1980s in an outbreak attributed to sexual behavior associated with crack cocaine use and sex in exchange for drugs or money. The number of cases peaked in 1988, when 5001 cases were reported. Since then, the number of cases has sharply declined to an all-time low of 30 cases reported in 2004. Currently chancroid is rare in the United States and Canada.

The reasons for the decline in reported chancroid cases are multifactorial and not completely understood. There did not appear to have been a decline in sexual risk behavior or crack cocaine use in the at-risk populations. Improved provider education and awareness, condom promotion, partner notification and treatment programs, and the addition of chancroid treatment to the syndromic management of genital ulcers all may have played a role. Previous localized chancroid outbreaks appear to have been controlled by identifying and treating reservoir core groups such as commercial sex workers.

A major constraint to understanding chancroid epidemiology has been the lack of sensitive and specific diagnostic tests. The organism is fastidious and difficult to culture. When diagnosis is based on clinical criteria alone, the infection is likely to be grossly over-reported in some circumstances and under-reported in others. The development of sensitive and specific PCR assays for *H ducreyi*, it is hoped, will correct the problem of misdiagnosis in the future.

Chancroid has been shown to facilitate HIV transmission by providing both a portal of entry and an exit for the virus. In other words, chancroid increases both the transmissibility and the susceptibility of HIV and may do so by two mechanisms. First, increased viral shedding occurs in the ulcer exudates in HIV-infected patients with chancroid, thus making the virus available for transmission during sexual intercourse. Studies have shown that the mere presence of lesions does not always prevent chancroid patients from having sex. Second, recruitment of CD4 cells, the primary targets of the virus, to chancroidal ulcers serves to increase susceptibility of HIV-infected individuals to HIV acquisition. Finally, there are challenges in chancroid treatment among HIV coinfected patients as prolonged duration of ulceration and more frequent treatment failures have been reported.

Pathogenesis

H ducreyi enters the skin through microabrasions that occur during sexual intercourse. A local tissue reaction leads to development of an erythematous papule that progresses to a pustule. The lesion then undergoes central necrosis to ulcerate. Histologic evaluation of these lesions reveals a deep necrotic ulcer surrounded by an infiltrate of neutrophils, macrophages, Langerhans cells, and CD4 and CD8 cells. Viable *H ducreyi* are demonstrable in lesions, but very few organisms have been found within phagocytes. This finding, combined with a lack of interaction noted between the organisms and surrounding cells, suggests that *H ducreyi* is primarily an extracellular organism with the ability to resist cellular uptake and phagocytosis through mechanisms that have not yet been completely elucidated.

H ducreyi pathogenesis has been studied in tissue culture, animal models, and a human challenge model. Virulence factors identified include the presence of a pilus, lipooligosaccharide, a cytolethal distending toxin, a hemolysin, a hemoglobin-binding outer membrane protein, a copper-zinc superoxide dismutase, a zinc-binding periplasmic protein, and a filamentous hemagglutinin-like protein. These potential virulence factors and isogenic mutants of *H ducreyi* developed to facilitate examination of these factors have been studied extensively in tissue culture, animal models, and human challenge models. *H ducreyi* virulence is no doubt multifactorial, as is the case for many other organisms.

Al-Tawfiq A, Spinola S. *Haemophilus ducreyi*: Clinical disease and pathogenesis. *Curr Opin Infect Dis* 2002;15:43–47. [PMID: 11964905] (This article focuses on recent advances in pathogenesis and clinical management of chancroid.)

Lewis DA. Chancroid: From clinical practice to basic science. *AIDS Patient Care STDs* 2000;14:19–36. [PMID: 12240879] (Comprehensive review of chancroid, including research models that have been used for the identification of virulence factors and potential antigens for vaccine development.)

Prevention

Prevention and control of chancroid is important for several reasons. Foremost among these is the association of

chancroid with HIV transmission in parts of the world where both infections are endemic. Because chancroid lesions are often painful, patients often seek and receive treatment early, making it possible for partners to be notified and treated in a timely manner. Chancroid thrives in populations with high sexual activity, especially where many men are having sex with relatively fewer women, usually sex workers. If these factors can be reduced significantly, transmission will slow or even cease and chancroid prevalence will markedly diminish.

Successful chancroid control has been carried out in Thailand and other countries where multifaceted interventions have been implemented. Promotion of condom use, syndromic management of genital ulcers, treatment of patients who have reactive syphilis serology, contact tracing and treatment, education, and monthly presumptive treatment with azithromycin have contributed to reductions in chancroid and genital ulcer disease in Thailand and South Africa. Treatment of core groups in Canadian epidemics also has had a dramatic effect on the number of cases of chancroid.

Additional insights regarding chancroid prevention were provided by an *H ducreyi* human challenge model in which azithromycin not only successfully treated infection, but also blocked experimental reinfections for up to 2 months. Based on these observations it is now thought that the success of the South African intervention trial may have been due not only to azithromycin treatment efficacy, but also to the drug's prophylactic effect.

Clinical Findings

A. Symptoms and Signs

Chancroid begins as a papule that evolves into a pustule after an incubation period of 4–7 days. The pustule then erodes into the classic nonindurated, painful ulcer with a purulent base and ragged, undermined borders (see Figure 12–1). The

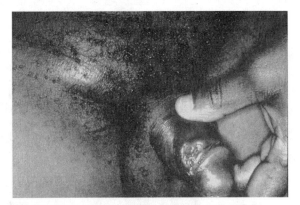

Figure 12–1. Classic appearance of chancroid ulcer. (Reproduced from Martin DH, Mroczkowski TF. Dermatologic manefestations of STD's other than HIV. Infect Dis Clinics North Amer 1994;8:550, with permission from Elsevier)

ulcers can be single or multiple and usually remain confined to the genital area (see Figure 12–2). Vesicle formation is not a feature of chancroid. In some cases mild constitutional symptoms have been associated with infection.

In men ulcers are most likely to be found on the internal or external surface of the prepuce, coronal sulcus, or frenulum. The shaft of the penis, prepucial orifice, urethral meatus, and glans penis may also be involved. In women most lesions are found at the vaginal entrance, including the labia majora and minora, fourchette, vestibule, and clitoris. About 50% of male patients present with a single ulcer, but a study of women with chancroid reported a mean number of 4.5 discrete ulcers. Smaller ulcers may also coalesce or merge to form a single giant ulcer or serpiginous ulcers. Other clinical variants of chancroid have been recognized and are outlined in Table 12–1. Ulcers have been rarely reported at extragenital sites such as the thighs, anus, breasts, hands, mouth, abdomen, and feet, but these lesions are secondary to local contact or autoinoculation and do not represent hematogenous dissemination from the primary genital lesion(s).

In HIV-infected patients multiple ulcers are more common, duration of ulceration is longer, and treatment failure is more often a problem. Interestingly, no cases of opportunistic, systemic, or disseminated chancroid have been reported in patients coinfected with HIV.

Unilateral tender inguinal lymphadenopathy is also a characteristic finding in up to 50% of patients with chancroid. This may progress to development of buboes or fluctuant lymph nodes, which can rupture spontaneously or require drainage. *H ducreyi* has been isolated

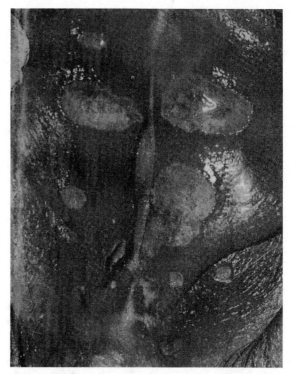

Figure 12–2. Multiple chancroid ulcers on the vulva. (Reproduced, with permission, from Wolff K, Johnson RA, Summond D. *Fitzpatrick's Color Atlas & Synopsis of Clinical Dermatology,* 5th ed. McGraw-Hill, 2005.)

Table 12–1. Clinical variants of chancroid.

Variant	Clinical Features
Dwarf chancroid	Small, superficial, relatively painless ulcer
Giant chancroid	Large granulomatous ulcer at the site of a ruptured inguinal bubo, extending beyond its margins
Follicular chancroid	Seen in women in association with hair follicles of the labia majora and pubis; initial follicular pustule evolves into a classic ulcer at the site
Transient chancroid	Superficial ulcers that may heal rapidly, followed by a typical inguinal bubo
Serpiginous chancroid	Multiple ulcers that coalesce to form a serpiginous pattern
Mixed chancroid	Nonindurated tender ulcers of chancroid appearing together with an indurated nontender ulcer of syphilis having an incubation period of 10–90 d
Phagedenic chancroid	Ulceration that causes extensive destruction of genitalia following secondary or superinfection by anaerobes such as *Fusobacterium* spp or *Bacteroides* spp (Vincent organisms)
Chancroidal ulcer	Most often a tender, nonindurated, single large ulcer caused by organisms other than *Haemophilus ducreyi;* lymphadenopathy is conspicuous by its absence

Adapted, with permission, from Sehgal VN, Srivastava G. Chancroid: Contemporary appraisal. *Int J Dermatol* 2003;42:185.

from pus removed from these buboes. Lymphadenitis and subsequent bubo formation have been noted less frequently in women.

B. LABORATORY FINDINGS

Laboratory diagnosis of chancroid depends on identification of *H ducreyi* in genital ulcer secretions or bubo pus. Gram stain of these secretions can reveal gram-negative, pleomorphic coccobacilli in a "schools of fish," "railroad," or "fingerprint" pattern, but this test lacks both sensitivity and specificity. Stains are misleading due primarily to the polymicrobial contamination of the ulcer bases. Therefore, direct microscopy is not recommended for the routine diagnosis of chancroid.

For many years culture was considered the "gold standard" for chancroid diagnosis and for the evaluation of new diagnostic tests. Unfortunately, culture of *H ducreyi* is difficult due to the fastidious nature of the organism. It is optimal for clinical samples to be plated directly onto special culture media in the clinic setting or be rapidly transported to the laboratory because there is no widely available, proven transport media. Even under ideal clinical conditions and with the cultures performed in highly experienced laboratories, the sensitivity of culture is still only about 75%.

PCR-based methods with improved sensitivity have been developed and now should probably be considered the new "gold standard" for *H ducreyi* identification. A genital ulcer disease multiplex PCR assay (M-PCR), which simultaneously amplifies gene targets for *H ducreyi*, *Treponema pallidum*, and herpes simplex virus types 1 and 2, is available for research purposes at the Centers for Disease Control and Prevention (CDC). Specimens can be transported to the laboratory and stored at −70°C for batch testing using this method. Unfortunately, PCR assays are not commercially available. However, they continue to be valuable tools for outbreak and epidemiologic investigations.

Antigen detection methods using monoclonal antibodies to detect *H ducreyi* in ulcer secretions have been developed and are simple, rapid, sensitive, and inexpensive, but also not available commercially.

Serologic methods to detect antibody to *H ducreyi* also have been described using both outer membrane protein and lipooligosaccharide. Although these methods are not able to distinguish recent from past infections, they provide useful screening tools for community-level epidemiologic studies.

Lewis DA. Diagnostic tests for chancroid. *Sex Trans Inf* 2000;76:137–141. [PMID: 10858718] (Excellent review of methods used for the identification *H ducreyi* and diagnosis of chancroid.)

Morse SA. New tests for bacterial sexually transmitted diseases. *Curr Opin Infect Dis* 2001;14:45–51. [PMID: 11979115] (Excellent review of recent advances in diagnostic methods and DNA amplification tests for chancroid and other STDs.)

Patterson K, Olsen B, Thomas C, et al. Development of a rapid immunodiagnostic test for *Haemophilus ducreyi*. *J Clin Microbiol* 2002;40:3694–3702. [PMID: 12354868] (Describes the development of a 15-minute diagnostic method that with further work could be a valuable beside tool in areas where chancroid is endemic.)

Differential Diagnosis

Because definitive laboratory diagnosis of chancroid is rarely available in most clinical settings, health care providers must usually rely on clinical diagnosis. Unfortunately, the clinical diagnosis of chancroid based on physical examination alone has low sensitivity and specificity, even in the hands of experienced STD experts. Although the suggestive combination of painful ulcer and tender adenopathy occurs in 33% of patients, the accuracy is only 30–50% based solely on clinical features. The CDC recommends that a probable diagnosis of chancroid be made if the following criteria are present: (1) the patient has one or more painful ulcers; (2) the patient has no evidence of syphilis by darkfield examination of ulcer exudate or by serologic testing performed at least 7 days after onset of ulcers; (3) the clinical presentation, appearance of genital ulcers, and, if present, regional lymphadenopathy are typical for chancroid; and (4) the result of a test for herpes simplex virus performed on the ulcer exudate is negative.

Despite many distinguishing features, there is considerable overlap between the clinical appearance of chancroid, primary syphilis, and herpes simplex virus. Thus, these genital ulcer diseases are often confused with one another. Table 12–2 outlines the classic differences in clinical presentation of these three diseases.

The classic chancroid triad of painful ulcer, purulent base, and undermined edges occurs in less than 50% of patients. In addition, it is estimated that 10% of patients with chancroid are coinfected with syphilis or herpes. For this reason a syndromic approach to genital ulcer disease management—empirically treating prevalent infections—is recommended when both chancroid and syphilis are present in the community. The syndromic management approach results in patients receiving treatment for both chancroid and syphilis at the time of initial presentation. Although genital herpes is the most common cause of genital ulceration worldwide, empiric antiviral treatment for this disease is generally not recommended.

Lewis DA. Chancroid: Clinical manifestations, diagnosis, and management. *Sex Trans Inf* 2003;79:68–71. [PMID: 12576620] (Thorough review of chancroid, including information on syndromic and other management issues related to genital ulcer disease.)

Complications

Some patients with bubo formation secondary to chancroid develop extensive adenitis and large inguinal

Table 12–2. Differential diagnosis of chancroid.

Disease	Characteristics of Lesion	Other Clinical Findings
Chancroid	Painful nonindurated ulcer with irregular undermined borders and a purulent exudative base	Associated with tender, suppurative lymphadenopathy in up to 50% of patients
Primary syphilis	Painless, clean-based, indurated ulcer or chancre	—[a]
Genital herpes	Crops of small vesicles or blisters on an erythematous base that rapidly evolve into tiny, shallow ulcers; these may coalesce to form larger ulcers	Fever in primary cases Dysuria, urethritis, and (rarely) urinary retention

[a]Rash and other symptoms of secondary syphilis develop after resolution of the initial lesion.

abscesses. To avoid spontaneous rupture and a possible draining sinus or giant ulcer formation, buboes larger than 5 cm should be either aspirated or incised and drained. In the past it was thought that aspiration was preferable because of the potential for sinus tract formation subsequent to incision and drainage. This concern has not been substantiated. Although needle aspiration is an easier procedure, a recent study demonstrated that incision and drainage, when combined with appropriate antibiotic therapy, was an effective strategy and had the advantage of avoiding the need for frequent reaspiration.

Another complication of chancroid is development of superinfected ulcers due to organisms such as *Fusobacterium, Bacteroides* species, and other mixed aerobic and anaerobic flora. These ulcers may become very large and are extremely destructive to genital tissues. Such superinfected lesions may require debridement. In addition, these lesions and other large chancroid ulcers may result in disfiguring scars.

Phimosis, a late complication of chancroid, results from thickening and scarring of the foreskin and may require referral for therapeutic circumcision.

Treatment

A. PHARMACOTHERAPY

Control of chancroid requires treatment of index cases and exposed partners with effective antibiotics (see Table 12–3). Although *H ducreyi* has acquired resistance to several antibiotics through both plasmid- and chromosomally mediated mechanisms, several regimens are available for cure, resolution of clinical symptoms, and prophylaxis.

Plasmid-mediated resistance has been documented for sulfonamides, tetracyclines, penicillins, chloramphenicol, and aminoglycosides. Chromosomally mediated resistance is reported for penicillin, ciprofloxacin, ofloxacin, and trimethoprim. For many years, trimethoprim-sulfonamide

Table 12–3. Recommended treatment regimens for chancroid.[a]

Azithromycin, 1 g PO in a single dose
or
Ceftriaxone, 250 mg IM in a single dose
or
Ciprofloxacin, 500 mg PO twice daily for 3 d
or
Erythromycin base, 500 mg PO 3 times daily for 7 d

[a]Ciprofloxacin is contraindicated in pregnant and lactating women. Azithromycin and ceftriaxone offer the advantage of single–dose therapy.
Based on Centers for Disease Control and Prevention; Workowski KA, Berman SM. Sexually transmitted diseases treatment guidelines, 2006. *MMWR Recomm Rep* 2006;55 (RR-11):1–94.

regimens were the therapy of choice, but rapid and widespread resistance now precludes use of this combination. In addition, several isolates with intermediate resistance to ciprofloxacin and erythromycin have been reported, reminding clinicians of the need to maintain surveillance for *H ducreyi* antibiotic susceptibility in endemic areas.

B. FOLLOW-UP

Patients should be reexamined 3–7 days after initiation of treatment, at which time subjective improvement should occur. Objective improvement should be noted within 7 days. If there is no improvement several factors should be considered, including whether the diagnosis was correct, compliance with therapy, coinfection with another STD or HIV, and the possibility of antibiotic resistance. Resolution of symptoms also depends on ulcer size and whether or not patients are circumcised. Healing is slowed for ulcers located under the foreskin in uncircumcised men, and large ulcers may require 2 weeks or longer to heal. Slow clinical resolution of fluctuant lymphadenopathy can also be expected and usually requires needle aspiration or incision and drainage.

Patients coinfected with chancroid and HIV require special follow-up and monitoring because of the increased likelihood of treatment failure and slow-healing ulcers. HIV-infected patients require longer courses of therapy, and treatment failure can occur with any regimen. Of particular interest is the 30% failure rate of single-dose ceftriaxone reported in an African treatment trial. Because of this trial and limited data from other reports concerning the therapeutic efficacy of single-dose ceftriaxone and azithromycin regimens in HIV-infected patients, these regimens should be used only if close follow-up can be ensured. Some experts prefer to use the 7-day regimen of erythromycin in treating HIV-infected persons.

Follow-up should also be provided for all persons who have had sexual contact with chancroid patients during the 10 days preceding the onset of the patient's symptoms. These partners should be examined and treated for chancroid regardless of whether symptoms of the disease are present.

It is also recommended that all chancroid patients be tested for HIV and syphilis at the time of diagnosis and 3 months later if initial test results were negative.

Centers for Disease Control and Prevention; Workowski KA, Berman SM. Sexually transmitted diseases treatment guidelines, 2006. *MMWR Recomm Rep* 2006;55(RR-11):1–94. [PMID: 16888612] (Compiled by the leading experts in the field; contains the most recent STD treatment guideline recommendations.)

Sehgal VN, Srivastava G. Chancroid: Contemporary appraisal. *Int J Dermatol* 2003;42:182–190. [PMID 12653911] (A contemporary update and appraisal of chancroid epidemiology, clinical presentations, diagnosis, and treatment.)

Wu JJ, Huang DB, Pang KR, Tyring SK. Selected sexually transmitted diseases and their relationship to HIV. *Clin Dermatol* 2004;22:499–508. [PMID: 15596321] (A review for the practicing clinician of the epidemiology, clinical manifestations, diagnostic methods, and treatment of chancroid and four other cutaneous STDs in HIV-infected patients.)

When to Refer to a Specialist

In the developed nations where chancroid is seldom seen, all patients suspected of having this disease should be referred to a clinician experienced in STD management. Such individuals generally know if there are local clinical or public health laboratories available with the expertise to identify the organism. State health departments can send properly collected ulcer swab specimens for *H ducreyi*–specific PCR or M-PCR to the CDC's reference laboratory for testing. The importance of such referrals is that if chancroid is documented to have been acquired domestically rather than in an endemic area of the world, it may represent the onset of a new chancroid epidemic with important public health implications, as previously discussed.

Prognosis

Effective antibiotic therapy exists for chancroid cure, resolution of clinical symptoms, and interruption of transmission. The prognosis is excellent in this regard, but because patients are capable of being reinfected, it is essential that sex partners be contacted and treated with effective therapy, even in the absence of symptoms.

Providers should also maintain heightened awareness of the potential for sporadic chancroid outbreaks as well

PRACTICE POINTS

- *Vesicle formation is not a feature of chancroid.*
- *A syndromic approach to genital ulcer disease management—empirically treating prevalent infections—is recommended when both chancroid and syphilis are present in the community.*

as for development of antibiotic resistance in endemic settings. Finally, because of the association of chancroid with HIV transmission and the challenges of definitive diagnosis, it is critical that syndromic assessment and treatment of genital ulcers be implemented at the appropriate time and that patients receive treatment for both chancroid and syphilis when necessary.

Relevant Web Sites

[Centers for Disease Control and Prevention case definition of chancroid:]
http://www.cdc.gov/epo/dphsi/casedef/chancroid_current.htm
[Sexually Transmitted Diseases Resource on chancroid:]
http://herpes-coldsores.com/std/chancroid.htm
[American Social Health Association patient information on chancroid:]
http://www.ashastd.org/learn/learn_chancroid.cfm
[CDC sexually transmitted diseases treatment guidelines 2006:
http://www.cdc.gov/std/treatment
[CDC clinical slide file of STDs]
http://www2a.cdc.gov/stdclinic/

Genital Chlamydial Infections

13

William M. Geisler, MD, MPH, & Walter E. Stamm, MD

ESSENTIALS OF DIAGNOSIS

- *Clinical diagnosis is difficult because most genital chlamydial infections are asymptomatic and even when symptoms or signs are present, they are nonspecific.*
- *Diagnosis relies on tests that detect the causative organism, Chlamydia trachomatis.*
- *Nucleic acid amplification tests (NAATs) have the greatest sensitivity and can be performed on noninvasively collected specimens (eg, urine or self-collected vaginal swabs).*

General Considerations

Chlamydia trachomatis is responsible for a wide spectrum of clinical disease, particularly in the genital tract (see Table 13–1). Despite the availability of effective antimicrobial therapy and improved preventive efforts, genital chlamydial infections remain a worldwide public health concern, and the World Health Organization estimates that 90 million new cases occur worldwide each year. Genital chlamydial infection remains the most commonly reported bacterial sexually transmitted disease (STD) in the United States, producing an estimated four million new infections each year, according to the Centers for Disease Control and Prevention (CDC).

From the time genital chlamydial infections first became a reportable disease in the United States in 1986, a greater number of cases have been reported in women versus men, a finding that has been attributed to emphasis on chlamydial screening in women. Chlamydia causes significant morbidity, especially in women, who can develop upper genital tract infection (pelvic inflammatory disease [PID]), which can lead to chronic pelvic pain, tubal abscesses, ectopic pregnancy, and infertility;

chlamydia is the leading preventable cause of infertility worldwide. Genital chlamydia can also increase the risk of acquisition and transmission of HIV.

Among the many risk factors for genital chlamydial infection (see Table 13–2), age is the strongest risk factor, with CDC surveillance studies demonstrating the highest chlamydial prevalence occurring in men and women younger than 25 years of age. A history of prior chlamydial infection is another strong predictor for current chlamydial infection. The majority of chlamydial infections in men and women are asymptomatic; therefore, the diagnosis of infection relies on identification of the organism through diagnostic testing. The availability of highly sensitive nucleic acid amplification tests (NAATs) should help to facilitate both improved rates of diagnosis and more widespread chlamydial screening, because such tests can be performed on noninvasively collected specimens (eg, urine and self-collected vaginal swabs). However, many barriers to screening exist, including lack of patient access to health care providers and lack of routine chlamydial testing in many medical settings.

Current management of genital chlamydial infection relies on effective antimicrobial therapy for infected patients and their sex partners, and routine rescreening 3 months after treatment. Although antimicrobial resistance in chlamydial infections has not been a major concern to date, evidence is building that suggests this may be a future problem. Recurrence of chlamydial infection in women is common, and the CDC recommends retesting at approximately 3 months following therapy. Development of an effective chlamydial vaccine is one of the priorities for the prevention and control of chlamydia, but efforts to date have been hindered by an incomplete understanding of the human host immune response to *C trachomatis*.

Miller WC, Ford CA, Morris M, et al. Prevalence of chlamydial and gonococcal infections among young adults in the United States. *JAMA* 2004;291:2229–2236. [PMID: 15138245] (Reveals the prevalence of chlamydial infection and associated substantial racial and ethnic disparities in a nationally representative sample of young adults living in the United States.)

Table 13–1. Clinical syndromes caused by *Chlamydia trachomatis*.

Urethritis (men or women)
Epididymitis
Prostatitis[a]
Cervicitis
Pelvic inflammatory disease
    Endometritis
    Salpingitis
    Perihepatitis (ie, Fitz-Hugh-Curtis syndrome)
Bartholinitis
Proctitis and proctocolitis (men or women)
Conjunctivitis (men, women, or neonates)
Pharyngitis (men, women, or neonates)
Respiratory tract infection (neonates or
    immunosuppressed adults)
    Upper: Rhinitis or bronchitis
    Lower: Pneumonitis or pneumonia
Reiter syndrome (men or women)
Culture-negative endocarditis (men or women)[a]

---

[a]Although *C trachomatis* is associated with these syndromes, there is limited evidence establishing the organism as an etiologic agent of these syndromes.

Pathogenesis

Chlamydiae are obligate intracellular bacteria that are energy parasites of infected host cells. In the genital tract, *C trachomatis* primarily infects columnar and transitional epithelial cells but not squamous epithelial cells, explaining in part why chlamydial infection in the female genital tract occurs in the endocervix and upper genital tract, but not the vagina. *C trachomatis* can be classified through molecular typing into strains causing ocular infections (trachoma), strains causing lymphogranuloma venereum (LGV) infection, and strains causing the characteristic lower genital tract and other mucosal infections outlined in Table 13–1.

All chlamydiae undergo a unique intracellular developmental cycle (see Figure 13–1) that is completed in 48–72 hours when infected cells release newly replicated

Table 13–2. Risk factors for genital chlamydial infection.

Adolescence and young adulthood
History of prior genital chlamydial infection
New or multiple sex partners
Nonwhite race or ethnicity
Lower socioeconomic status
Bacterial vaginosis
Oral contraceptive use (cervical ectopy)

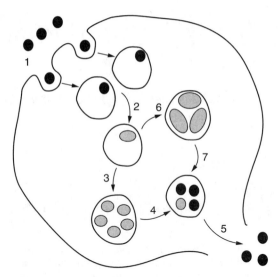

Figure 13–1. The unique intracellular developmental cycle of *Chlamydia trachomatis*. The organism exists primarily in two forms: an elementary body (EB; black circles), which is the infective form that is metabolically inactive, and a reticulate body (RB, light-colored ovals), which is the reproductive form that is metabolically active. The numbered stages in the figure correspond to the following events of the cycle: (1) *Endocytosis* of the EB into an inclusion; (2) *differentiation* of the EB into an RB; (3) *replication* (several rounds) of the RB by binary fission; (4) *redifferentiation of RBs* into EBs; (5) *exocytosis* of EBs, which can go on to infect other cells; (6) under environmental stress (eg, immune mediators, nutrient deprivation, etc), RBs can differentiate into larger aberrant forms that are noninfectious and nonreplicating (ie, *persistence*); (7) upon removal of environmental stress, there is *redifferentiation of aberrant forms* into EBs.

chlamydial organisms; as a result, the incubation time in genital chlamydial infection ranges from 7 to 21 days (compared with as few as 24–48 hours in gonococcal infection). Diagnostic assays, especially those other than NAATs, that are performed within the first few days after exposure to chlamydia may yield a false-negative result due to low organism burden at that point.

The natural history of chlamydial infection is not yet fully understood, but Geisler and others have recently found that approximately 20% of individuals with genital chlamydial infection detected by screening have spontaneous resolution of their infection prior to returning for therapy, suggesting the host immune response, at least under some circumstances, eradicated the organism from the lower genital tract. In the majority of individuals, if not treated, infection tends to persist for weeks to months, and perhaps over a year in a small proportion of individuals.

Stamm WE. *Chlamydia trachomatis*—the persistent pathogen: Thomas Parran Award Lecture. *Sex Transm Dis* 2001;28: 684–689. [PMID: 11625221] (Reviews chlamydial epidemiology, pathogenesis, and approaches to prevention over the past 25 years.)

Clinical Findings

Symptoms, physical examination findings, and immediate laboratory findings (eg, results of urethral or endocervical Gram stains) in lower genital tract chlamydial infection are nonspecific and do not reliably distinguish chlamydia from other infections causing the same genital tract syndromes. Diagnostic assays to detect *C trachomatis* are essential to confirm the diagnosis of chlamydia. Imaging studies are not usually needed in uncomplicated genital chlamydial infection and will not be discussed further.

Clinical findings in upper genital tract chlamydial infection (see Chapter 8) and anorectal infection (see Chapter 9) in men and women are discussed elsewhere in this book. Conjunctivitis caused by *C trachomatis*, usually resulting from autoinoculation from the genital tract, is rare. *C trachomatis* has been detected in the pharynx by culture and NAAT, yet it remains unclear whether clinically evident pharyngitis occurs and whether the organism is transmissible from the pharynx. The discussion that follows focuses on clinical findings in chlamydial infection of the *lower* genital tract.

A. SYMPTOMS AND SIGNS

1. Men—Over 50% of men with urethral chlamydial infection are asymptomatic. Symptoms of chlamydial infection may include painful urination, urinary frequency, meatal itching or discomfort, and urethral discharge. If the patient has not voided recently, a urethral discharge may be apparent on examination and typically is clear or cloudy, often with mucus strands; accompanying the discharge may be meatal erythema or swelling, or both. However, it is important to recognize that asymptomatic urethral chlamydial infection without discharge occurs commonly. If no spontaneous discharge is noted, the urethra should be stripped ("milked") from the base of the penis to the urethral meatus and examined again. Unlike the LGV chlamydial strains, the non-LGV strains do not cause genital ulcers or significant lymph node swelling.

2. Women—At least 75% of women with endocervical chlamydial infection are asymptomatic, and even when symptoms are present, they are nonspecific and often overlap with symptoms found in other vaginal or endocervical infections. Symptoms may include new or increased vaginal discharge, intermenstrual bleeding, lower abdominal pain, or pain during intercourse. Up to 50% or more of women with endocervical chlamydial infection have concomitant urethral infection and may present with painful urination or urinary frequency, or both. Many women also have asymptomatic rectal infection. Symptoms and signs of proctitis are rare with such non-LGV chlamydial strains.

Even in the absence of symptoms, older studies using chlamydia culture have demonstrated up to one third of chlamydia-infected women have signs of infection on pelvic examination (Geisler and colleagues, utilizing NAATs, found fewer than 10% of asymptomatic women had signs of infection.) Mucopurulent endocervical discharge, easily induced endocervical bleeding ("friability"), and edematous ectopy are the signs most suggestive of chlamydial infection, yet all are nonspecific and may be seen in other sexually transmitted endocervical infections. Abnormal vaginal discharge (originating from the endocervix) may also be present.

Although cervical ectopy may predispose to chlamydial infection (through increased exposure to susceptible columnar epithelial cells), ectopy *without edema or congestion* may be present in up to 60–80% of sexually active female adolescents and young adults, especially those using oral contraceptives, and is not indicative of chlamydial infection.

Concomitant chlamydial infection of the Bartholin ducts may occur, manifesting as ductal erythema and swelling, often with purulent ductal exudate.

B. LABORATORY FINDINGS

In chlamydial urethral infection, a Gram-stained smear made from an endourethral swab specimen often indicates the presence of urethritis (≥5 polymorphonuclear leukocytes [PMNs] per high-power field). However, Geisler and colleagues found that almost 20% of patients with chlamydial urethritis detected by NAAT had fewer than 5 or no PMNs visualized on a Gram-stained endourethral smear, suggesting that chlamydial infections may often mount a minimal inflammatory response or it may attenuate over time. Although an endourethral Gram stain can establish with a high degree of certainty whether gonorrhea is present in symptomatic urethritis, it does not exclude chlamydial infection, because *C trachomatis* cannot be visualized on a Gram stain.

If microscopy is not available, then urinalysis can be performed on a first-voided urine specimen (ie, the first 10–15 mL of urine voided), and in younger men, the finding of a positive leukocyte esterase test or microscopic pyuria (>10 white blood cells in spun urine sediment per high-power field) is consistent with urethritis due *C trachomatis* or another sexually transmitted pathogen. A positive leukocyte esterase test or pyuria in older men might represent a urinary tract infection or sexually transmitted urethritis, and diagnostic testing should address both.

In chlamydial endocervical infection, a Gram-stained smear of an endocervical swab specimen in a nonmenstruating woman often indicates the presence of cervicitis

(≥30 white blood cells per high-power field). However, analogous to urethritis, in some patients with endocervical chlamydial infections, fewer than 30 white blood cells per high-power field are visualized, and some studies have suggested that a cutoff of more than 10 white blood cells per high-power field correlates better with cervicitis. Geisler and other researchers have also investigated the relationship of vaginal leukocyte counts (based on viewing a vaginal specimen wet mount at 400 × power) to endocervical chlamydial infection. In a recent study by Geisler and colleagues (performed in women with bacterial vaginosis), the presence of >5 white blood cells in at least one high power field predicted chlamydial infection, yet did not exclude the presence of other organisms.

C. Diagnostic Tests

Because symptoms, examination findings, and microscopy do not reliably distinguish chlamydial infection from other organisms causing the same syndromes, patients suspected of having genital chlamydial infection should have specific diagnostic testing for *C trachomatis*. Confirmation of chlamydial infection is important for purposes of patient treatment, patient education, sex partner treatment, and for communicable disease reporting (to monitor the prevalence of chlamydia). Many different diagnostic assays are available for detection of *C trachomatis* (see Table 13–3). These vary in terms of test sensitivity, cost, and patient convenience.

Table 13–3. Diagnostic assays for detection of *Chlamydia trachomatis*.

Assay	Sensitivity[a] (%)
Nucleic acid amplification tests (NAATs)[b]	80–95
Polymerase chain reaction	
Strand displacement amplification	
Transcription-mediated amplification	
Direct fluorescent antibody	70–85
Tissue culture	70–85
Nucleic acid hybridization (DNA probe)	60–80
Enzyme immunoassay	50–75

[a]Estimated range of sensitivity, which may differ by gender, specimen type, or clinical presentation of infection.
[b]In contrast to most assays for chlamydia detection, which are performed only on genital swab specimens, NAATs can also be performed on urine or vaginal swabs (provider- or patient-collected).

1. Screening recommendations—Populations with the greatest risk for genital chlamydial infection, yet who have unrecognized chlamydial infection, should also undergo chlamydial screening. The CDC and the US Preventive Services Task Force each currently recommends annual chlamydial screening for all sexually active women 25 years of age and younger, as well as for older at-risk women (eg, with new or multiple sex partners). The importance of annual chlamydial screening for young women is further emphasized by the inclusion of such screening as an element of the Health Plan Employer Data and Information Set (HEDIS) measures widely used to compare the quality of health care provision. The benefits of chlamydial screening have been demonstrated in parts of the United States where screening and treatment programs for women have reduced both the prevalence of infection and PID rates. Although no guidelines have been provided for chlamydial screening in men, consideration should be given for screening men 25 years of age and younger or those at higher risk if resources permit, especially in clinical populations with a high prevalence of disease.

2. Nonculture tests—Chlamydia culture has been the reference standard against which all other tests have been compared. However, nonculture tests are now far more commonly used because they are less technically demanding and may be less expensive and or more sensitive than chlamydia culture.

The earliest nonculture screening tests for *C trachomatis* were based on detection of chlamydial antigen, rather than growth of the organism, and included enzyme immunoassays and direct fluorescent antibody tests. Nucleic acid hybridization tests (ie, DNA probes) then became available. These nonculture tests were less expensive and less technically demanding than culture; however, they also had lower test sensitivities and therefore failed to detect infections more often than culture, with the exception of direct fluorescent antibody testing, the sensitivity of which was similar to culture. Serologic assays for chlamydia have also been available yet are not widely used in the diagnosis of urogenital chlamydial infection because they do not distinguish past from current *C trachomatis* infection; cross-reacting antibody can occur with infections caused by other chlamydial species (eg, *C pneumoniae*); they may be negative in early or acute chlamydial infection, especially in men presenting with symptomatic nongonococcal urethritis (NGU); and titers are often low with superficial mucosal infections.

NAATs became available for routine clinical use in the mid 1990s and are the preferred and recommended means for detecting *C trachomatis* infection. These tests offer two distinct advantages over culture or earlier nonculture-based chlamydia tests: (1) higher test sensitivity (approximately 15–20% higher than former tests), resulting from the amplification of nucleic acids, thereby improving the likelihood of detecting the organism (especially when the bacterial burden is low); and (2) greater patient convenience or satisfaction by using non-invasively collected specimens, including urine, tampons, or self-collected vaginal swabs. Hence, NAATs can facilitate chlamydia screening outside of conventional clinical settings. One disadvantage of NAATs is their higher cost. However, the higher test sensitivity may still allow NAATs to be more cost-effective than other chlamydia tests as their use may decrease the prevalence of genital chlamydia or PID.

3. Additional tests for coinfection—Most individuals undergoing testing for chlamydia should also receive testing for gonorrhea, because coinfection with both organisms is common and their recommended treatments differ.

Gaydos CA. Nucleic acid amplification tests for gonorrhea and chlamydia: Practice and applications. *Infect Dis Clin North Am* 2005;19:367–386. [PMID: 15963877] (Reviews the NAATs currently available for diagnosing chlamydia and their application to clinical care.)

Geisler WM, Yu S, Hook EW III. Chlamydial and gonococcal infection in men without polymorphonuclear leukocytes on Gram stain: Implications for diagnostic approach and management. *Sex Transm Dis* 2005;32:630–634. [PMID: 16205305] (Gram stain evidence of urethral inflammation was absent in 12% of chlamydial and 5% of gonococcal infections, and symptoms and discharge may be absent in chlamydial infection detected by NAAT. Thus, without testing, many infections would go untreated, furthering the possibility of complications or partner transmission.)

Geisler WM, Yu S, Venglarek M, Schwebke JR. Vaginal leucocyte counts in women with bacterial vaginosis: Relation to vaginal and cervical infections. *Sex Transm Infect* 2004;80:401–405. [PMID: 15459411] (An elevated vaginal leucocyte count in women with bacterial vaginosis was a strong predictor of vaginal or cervical infections. Vaginal leucocyte quantification may provide an alternative approach to assessing the need for empiric therapy for chlamydia and gonorrhoea, particularly in resource-limited high STD risk settings that provide syndromic management.)

Differential Diagnosis

A. Men

The differential diagnosis of genital chlamydial infection in men includes infection with *Neisseria gonorrhoeae* as well as other organisms causing NGU (see Chapter 3), primarily *Trichomonas vaginalis*, herpes simplex virus, genital *Mycoplasma* species (*M genitalium)*, and possibly genital *Ureaplasma* species. All of these organisms can manifest as urethritis, with clinical findings similar to those in chlamydial infection.

Although men presenting with symptomatic **gonorrhea** may have a more purulent urethral discharge and usually have gonococcal-like organisms on the urethral Gram stain, approximately 5% of men with symptomatic gonococcal urethritis have no evidence on Gram stain of gonococcal-like organisms, which emphasizes the importance of testing for gonorrhea even in individuals diagnosed with NGU.

Genital herpes is a recognized cause of recurrent NGU, although the epidemiology, clinical findings, and treatment outcomes in NGU resulting from herpes infection have not been well characterized.

T vaginalis is a protozoa causing NGU, which can be prevalent in high-risk populations (in an STD clinic in Birmingham, Alabama, the prevalence of **trichomoniasis** in men with NGU is approximately 15–20%). Trichomoniasis is not routinely tested for in men with NGU, in part due to limited sensitivity of currently available assays when used in men. However, this etiology should always be considered in men with recurrent or persistent NGU and appropriate empiric therapy included in this clinical setting.

Genital **Mycoplasma** species, especially *M genitalium*, are now recognized as legitimate etiologic agents of NGU. However, commercial testing is not routinely available for this organism; research studies have employed culture and polymerase chain reaction techniques. Fortunately, the antimicrobial agents recommended for treatment of chlamydia also have the best activity against *Mycoplasma* urethritis, although tetracycline- or macrolide-resistant isolates of *Mycoplasma* have been reported.

Ureaplasma species have been postulated as an etiology of NGU, but current evidence does not strongly support such an association. Analogous to genital *Mycoplasma* species, commercial testing is not routinely employed to test for genital *Ureaplasma* species, and the treatment employs the same antimicrobials used to treat chlamydia.

B. Women

The differential diagnosis of genital chlamydial infection in women includes *N gonorrhoeae* as well as other organisms causing mucopurulent cervicitis (see Chapter 10); these include herpes simplex virus, bacterial species associated with bacterial vaginosis (eg, *Gardnerella vaginalis*), genital *Mycoplasma* species (*M genitalium)*, and possibly genital *Ureaplasma* species.

Approximately half of all cases of mucopurulent cervicitis are caused by chlamydia or **gonorrhea,** the two infections for which routine testing is performed in patients with cervicitis and for which empiric therapy is given.

Bacterial vaginosis is a common disorder of the genital tract in women characterized by an alteration of the normal acidic, lactobacilli-predominant vaginal ecosystem to a vaginal environment dominated by organisms such as *G vaginalis*, *Mobiluncus* species, and anaerobes, with an accompanying increase in vaginal pH (see Chapter 11). Bacterial vaginosis has been associated with mucopurulent cervicitis, and some experts recommend treating bacterial vaginosis in women with cervicitis, especially if chlamydia and gonorrhea test results are negative.

Genital herpes is a recognized cause of recurrent mucopurulent cervicitis, although the epidemiology, clinical findings, and treatment outcomes in cervicitis resulting from herpes infection have not been well characterized.

Genital *Mycoplasma* **species** (*M genitalium*) and possibly genital *Ureaplasma* **species** may cause mucopurulent cervicitis, but as with urethritis, they are not routinely tested for and would already be empirically treated by the same treatment regimens used for chlamydia.

Complications

A. Upper Genital Tract Infection

A major complication of lower genital tract chlamydial infection is spread of chlamydial infection to the upper genital tract. In men, this can cause acute epididymitis (see Chapter 6), which can lead to other complications, including testicular abscess (and possibly infarction), chronic testicular pain, chronic epididymitis, and infertility. In women, infection of the upper genital tract causes PID (see Chapter 8), which can lead to other complications, including ovarian abscess (and possibly infarction), infertility, chronic pelvic pain, and ectopic pregnancy. These complications are discussed in detail in the previously noted chapters.

B. Reiter Syndrome

Concurrent or preceding genital chlamydial infection has been associated with Reiter syndrome, an aseptic inflammatory polyarthritis, the classic clinical manifestations of which include a trigger infection (STD: urethritis or cervicitis; non-STD: enteritis), associated with conjunctivitis, rheumatoid factor–negative asymmetric polyarthritis, and mucocutaneous lesions. Cardiac and neurologic manifestations can also occur but are rare. Reiter syndrome occurs more commonly in men and those with the HLA-B27 haplotype, the latter also having a more severe clinical course. It is believed that either whole chlamydial organisms or chlamydial nucleic acids or antigens disseminate beyond the genital tract to the synovium of joints and other structures in these patients. To date, viable *C trachomatis* organisms (other than non-LGV strains) have not been isolated outside the genital tract in these patients. Reiter syndrome associated with chlamydial infection is treated with antibiotics and anti-inflammatory agents (eg, indomethacin, nonsteroidal anti-inflammatory agents, etc).

C. Other Complications

Chlamydial proctitis (see Chapter 9) can be complicated by strictures and fistulas; however, this is primarily limited to infections cause by LGV chlamydial strains and is further discussed in the previously noted chapter. *C trachomatis* has also been associated with culture-negative endocarditis, yet this reported association has been based primarily on diagnosis of chlamydia by serologic testing, which lacks specificity. Culture-negative endocarditis attributed to *C trachomatis* is a poorly characterized entity, and currently it remains unclear whether *C trachomatis* causes endocarditis.

Treatment

A. Antimicrobial Therapy

Antimicrobial agents represent the cornerstone of therapy for chlamydial infections. The antimicrobial agents with the greatest in vitro activity against *C trachomatis* and which are clinically most efficacious for uncomplicated chlamydial infection include the tetracyclines, macrolides, azalides (ie, azithromycin), and select fluoroquinolones. All of these agents achieve sufficient intracellular concentrations to treat this obligate intracellular pathogen. The current CDC recommendations for treatment of uncomplicated genital chlamydial infection are summarized in Table 13–4.

1. Recommended regimens—The recommended antibiotic regimens for uncomplicated genital chlamydial infection in nonpregnant individuals are azithromycin, 1 g orally given as a single dose, or doxycycline, 100 mg twice daily orally for 7 days. Despite the convenience and the improved compliance of the single-dose azithromycin regimen, no significant differences have been demonstrated in the clinical efficacy or frequency of adverse reactions for azithromycin versus doxycycline. The major considerations in choosing azithromycin versus doxycycline in nonpregnant patients are cost, convenience, and drug allergies. Azithromycin is more convenient because of single-dose administration, which can be directly observed, but it costs more. Doxycycline is less expensive, yet less convenient because 14 capsules are taken over 7 days and complete treatment is not directly observed in most settings.

2. Alternative regimens—Ofloxacin, 400 mg orally twice daily for 7 days, or levofloxacin, 500 mg orally daily for 7 days, are recommended by the CDC for nonpregnant persons with chlamydial infection as alternatives to the azithromycin or doxycycline regimens previously described. Given the high cost of fluoroquinolones (compared with azithromycin or doxycycline), their longer duration of therapy (compared with azithromycin), and their contraindication in pregnancy (compared with azithromycin), for most patients these agents provide no significant advantage over the recommended doxycycline or azithromycin regimens. One of the previously listed fluoroquinolones may be considered for uncomplicated genital chlamydial infection

Table 13–4. Antimicrobial therapy for uncomplicated genital chlamydial infection.

	Recommended Regimen	Alternative Regimen
Nonpregnant patients	Azithromycin, 1 g PO in a single dose *or* Doxycycline, 100 mg PO twice daily for 7 d	Ofloxacin, 300 mg PO twice daily for 7 d *or* Levofloxacin, 500 mg PO once daily for 7 d *or* Erythromycin base, 500 mg PO 4 times daily for 7 d *or* Erythromycin ethylsuccinate, 800 mg PO 4 times daily for 7 d
Pregnant patients	Azithromycin, 1 g PO in a single dose[a] *or* Amoxicillin, 500 mg PO 3 times daily for 7 d	Erythromycin ethylsuccinate, 800 mg PO 4 times daily for 7 d *or* Erythromycin ethylsuccinate, 400 mg PO 4 times daily for 14 d *or* Erythromycin base, 250 mg PO 4 times daily for 14 d *or* Erythromycin base, 500 mg PO 4 times daily for 7 d

[a]Recent literature supports the efficacy and safety of this regimen, and anecdotal experience suggests it is used far more widely than either erythromycin or amoxicillin for chlamydia-infected pregnant women.
Based on Centers for Disease Control and Prevention; Workowski KA, Berman SM. Sexually transmitted diseases treatment guidelines, 2006. *MMWR Recomm Rep* 2006;55(RR-11):1–94.

when a patient is already being treated with this agent for a different clinical syndrome (eg, urinary tract infection), if a patient has an allergy to tetracyclines and azalides or macrolides, or if the patient presents with PID, in which ofloxacin or levofloxacin regimens (for 14 days) are recommended in the CDC's current STD treatment guidelines (see Chapter 8).

Table 13–4 also lists erythromycin regimens that are considered as alternative therapy. Although erythromycin is inexpensive, the high rate of gastrointestinal side effects (especially diarrhea) limits compliance with the full treatment course and, as a result, may lead to lower clinical cure rates with these regimens. Thus, we do not recommend their use. Other macrolides, such as clarithromycin, do not offer advantages over azithromycin for treatment of genital chlamydial infection.

3. Antimicrobial considerations in special populations—

a. Pregnant women—Doxycycline, ofloxacin, and levofloxacin are contraindicated in pregnant women. The 2006 CDC treatment guidelines recommend either amoxicillin, 500 mg orally three times daily for 7 days, or azithromycin, 1g single dose orally, in this patient population (see Table 13–4). Erythromycin, previously a first-line agent in the 2002 CDC treatment guidelines, is

now listed as a alternative agent in the 2006 guidelines (see Table 13-4). Azithromycin was moved to a first-line agent in the 2006 guidelines because: 1) recent clinical trials of azithromycin versus comparator regimens (erythromycin or amoxicillin) in chlamydia-infected pregnant women have demonstrated azithromycin to be safe and just as or more efficacious as the comparator regimens, 2) anecdotal experience and discussion with experts suggested azithromycin was far more widely used than erythromycin or amoxicillin in these patients, and 3) erythromycin is poorly tolerated in pregnant women, which leads to greater noncompliance and lower efficacy. All three antibiotics are pregnancy category B drugs.

b. Adolescents—Although there is some evidence for development of bone and joint disease in juvenile animals treated with fluoroquinolones, there is sufficient clinical experience in human adolescents (especially those >45 kg) to support use of the alternatively recommended fluoroquinolone regimens for chlamydia if doxycycline or azithromycin cannot be used.

c. HIV-infected individuals—There are no data to suggest that the efficacy of recommended antimicrobial regimens for chlamydia are altered in HIV-infected individuals, and the CDC recommends the same regimens in these patients.

B. Other Management Considerations

1. Sexual activity—To prevent transmission to uninfected individuals, it is recommended that chlamydia-infected patients be instructed to abstain from sexual activity until completion of a recommended treatment regimen (ie, 7 days after receiving single-dose azithromycin or after finishing a 7-day course of doxycycline). For those persons unlikely to abstain during this period, strict compliance with condom use should be reinforced to prevent further transmission. Patients should also use these prevention measures until their sex partners have completed therapy.

2. Management of sex partners—Treatment of sex partners of chlamydia-infected patients is important, both to prevent reinfection of the patient and to prevent further transmission to other susceptible individuals. Traditionally, chlamydia-infected patients have been instructed by providers to notify their partners that they have been exposed to chlamydia and should themselves be seen by a provider for testing and treatment. However, high rates of chlamydia reinfection suggest such partner notification practices often do not lead to treatment of the sex partner.

Recent studies have explored the feasibility and efficacy (in preventing recurrence of chlamydia) of patients or providers delivering medication or a prescription directly to the sex partner (ie, expedited partner therapy [EPT]). Although further studies are needed, it appears that EPT is feasible and may decrease rates of chlamydia recurrence. There are, however, some concerns with EPT. One concern is the risk for an allergic reaction to the EPT in the sex partner, but serious drug reactions to doxycycline or azithromycin are very rare. There is some concern about the legality of EPT, as this issue is not clearly addressed in most states. However, anecdotal evidence and discussion with other experts suggests EPT is already a widespread clinical practice. An additional concern centers on the delivery of medication by male patients to female sex partners who have subclinical PID; providing EPT to these partners might deter them from seeking evaluation by a health care provider, thus leading to treatment for PID that may be insufficient. However, many of these female partners might not have sought provider evaluation anyway, and EPT may provide some benefit. Finally, another potential concern with EPT is reduced opportunities to screen partners for other STDs, including HIV infection, and to provide risk reduction education. Clinicians who use EPT are encouraged to provide educational materials for the partners and encourage them to seek evaluation, which will allow examination for clinical evidence of complications and testing for other STDs.

3. Follow-up and "test of cure"—Nonpregnant patients with uncomplicated genital chlamydial infection do not need repeat clinical or diagnostic evaluation after completion of therapy unless symptoms or signs of infection persist or recur. However, test of cure following treatment of uncomplicated genital chlamydial infections—usually more than 3 weeks after treatment—is recommended for pregnant women, a population in which treatment failures could lead to both maternal and neonatal complications.

4. Approach to treatment failure—Chlamydia-infected patients with symptoms or signs of infection that persist or recur within a short time period (<4 weeks) after treatment are often labeled as "treatment failures." The first step in managing such patients is to repeat the clinical and diagnostic evaluation. This is done to confirm the presence of *C trachomatis* and to rule out other STDs. It is recommended that patients with clinical findings suggestive of chlamydial infection (urethritis, cervicitis, etc) receive empiric treatment with one of the CDC-recommended treatment regimens. Most cases of "treatment failure" are a result of reinfection of the patient by an untreated partner. Therefore, the next step is to ensure that sex partners receive treatment and both the patient and partner abstain until treatment is complete.

No studies have definitely proved that treatment failure in the absence of reexposure to an infected partner occurs following recommended chlamydia treatment regimens, but there is indirect evidence suggesting it may. There is also no strong evidence to support that treatment failure is due to resistant *C trachomatis* isolates. Antibiotic resistance can be induced in vitro in *C trachomatis*, but wild-type resistance does not appear to be common in clinical isolates or to result in sustained transmission.

5. "Repeat testing" to identify chlamydia recurrence—Recurrence of chlamydial infection is common in women, occurring in 10–20% within 6 months of a prior chlamydial infection. The rate of recurrence in men is unclear, but our clinical experience suggests it is common. Recurrence of chlamydial infection can lead to upper genital tract complications in men and women, and may serve as a reservoir for repeated chlamydial infections.

The current CDC treatment guidelines advise that all women with chlamydial infections be retested for chlamydial infection in about 3 months after treatment to rule out reinfection, and we believe that strong consideration should also be given to rescreening high-risk men following chlamydial infection if resources permit. Clinicians should have a system in place to recall patients treated for chlamydial infection for retesting in about 3 months. Some researchers are evaluating the feasibility of having patients repeat chlamydial testing by home self-collection and then mail in specimens (urine in men and vaginal swabs or urine in women).

Centers for DiseccControl and Prevention; Workowski KA, Berman SM. Sexually transmitted diseases treatment guidelines, 2006. *MMWR Recomm Rep* 2006;55(RR-11):1–94. [PMID: 16888612] (These widely accepted guidelines, developed in consultation with professionals knowledgeable in the field of STDs, provides recommendations for management of chlamydial infections).

Geisler WM. Approaches to the management of uncomplicated genital *Chlamydia trachomatis* infections. *Exp Rev Anti Infect Ther* 2004;2:771–785. [PMID: 15482239] (Reviews current and future approaches to management of chlamydia).

Golden MR. Expedited partner therapy for sexually transmitted diseases. *Clin Infect Dis* 2005;41:630–633. [PMID: 16080085] (Informative editorial that includes a summary of the randomized, controlled trials of EPT for chlamydial infection.)

Suchland RJ, Geisler WM, Stamm WE. Methodologies and cell lines used for antimicrobial susceptibility testing of *Chlamydia* spp. *Antimicrob Agents Chemother* 2003;47:636–642. [PMID: 12543671] (This article provides a basis for standardizing the methodologic approach and interpretation of antimicrobial testing of *Chlamydia*, and is one of the few studies to date assessing correlation of clinical outcomes in chlamydial infections with results of susceptibility testing).

When to Refer to a Specialist

Patients who present with recurrent *C trachomatis* infections and who deny reexposure to an untreated sex partner may benefit from referral to a specialist. Chlamydia genotyping is a tool we and other researchers have utilized to determine with a reasonable certainty whether the chlamydia strains in such patients with recurrent chlamydia are the same or a different genotype (the latter likely representing new infection). In those presenting with recurrent infection with the same chlamydial genotype, antimicrobial susceptibility testing may also be considered. However, such testing currently lacks a standardized methodology and is performed by us and only a few other researchers. Finally, referral to a urologist or gynecologist may also be of benefit in evaluating whether an upper genital tract infection (in men, prostatitis or epididymitis; in women, PID) may be present and serving as a nidus for reinfecting the lower genital tract.

Prognosis

Initiation of appropriate antimicrobial therapy leads to improvement and eventual resolution of symptoms and signs of uncomplicated genital chlamydial infection within the first few days of therapy and to clinical and microbiologic cure after the completion of therapy in most patients. The key to prevention of recurrent chlamydial infection is ensuring patient compliance with treatment, achieving treatment of sex partners, providing STD education, and reenforcing the use of barrier precautions. With the availability of highly sensitive diagnostic tests for chlamydia (ie, NAATs), continued efforts toward sex partner treatment, rescreening chlamydia-infected women in a few months, and routine yearly chlamydia screening in women, we anticipate further decline in the prevalence of chlamydial infection and its associated complications in the United States.

PRACTICE POINTS

- *Up to 50% or more of women with endocervical chlamydial infection have concomitant urethral infection and may present with painful urination or urinary frequency, or both.*
- *NAATs are the preferred and recommended means for detecting* C trachomatis *infection.*
- *Clinicians should have a system in place to recall patients treated for chlamydial infection for retesting in about 3 months.*

Relevant Web Sites

[Centers for Disease Control and Prevention fact sheet on chlamydia:] http://www.cdc.gov/std/chlamydia/STDFact-Chlamydia.htm

Genital Herpes

Peter Leone, MD

ESSENTIALS OF DIAGNOSIS

- *Most individuals with genital herpes are unaware of the infection but are able to transmit it to others.*
- *Type-specific serology allows reliable differentiation of chronic type 1 from type 2 infection.*
- *Clinical diagnosis should be confirmed by diagnostic testing of the genital lesion (culture or polymerase chain reaction [PCR]) or a type-specific serologic assay.*

General Considerations

Herpes simplex virus (HSV) infections are endemic in the United States and are a cause of recurrent genital and oral ulcerative disease. Genital herpes infection can be caused by type 2 virus (HSV-2), or less frequently by type 1 (HSV-1). Although most infections are asymptomatic, genital HSV infection, whether type 1 or 2, can cause vesicular and ulcerative disease in adults and severe systemic disease in neonates and immunocompromised individuals. Genital HSV infection increases the risk of HIV acquisition in infected persons.

HSV-2 transmission is almost always sexual, whereas HSV-1 is usually transmitted through nonsexual skin-to-skin contact. Current estimates place the incidence of HSV-2 infection at more than 1.5 million cases annually. In the general population, HSV-2 seroprevalence is low for persons younger than 12 years of age, rises sharply following onset of sexual activity, and peaks by the early 40s. HSV-2 seroprevalence in the United States rose 30% between 1978 and 1991 to 21.7%. The overwhelming majority of individuals with genital HSV infection have undiagnosed initial infections and unrecognized recurrences. Orolabial HSV-2 infection is rare and is almost always associated with genital infection.

HSV-1 infection frequently occurs as orolabial infection in childhood, and approximately 20% of children younger than 5 years of age are seropositive. The seroprevalence of HSV-1 rises almost linearly with increasing age to approximately 70%. In the general population over the past decade, HSV-1 has become an increasingly common cause of genital infection, with an estimated 50% of newly acquired genital herpes attributable to it in some populations.

Fleming DT, McQuillan GM, Johnson RE, et al. Herpes simplex virus type 2 in the United States, 1976 to 1994. *N Engl J Med* 1997;337:1105–1111. [PMID: 9329932] (Classic article.)

Pathogenesis

Primary HSV infection occurs at mucosal sites of inoculation (see Figure 14–1), with retrograde infection propagating to sensory nerve ganglia. Following resolution of primary infection, HSV enters a latent state in sensory nerve ganglia from which reactivation may occur to cause active infection at any mucosal sites innervated by the nerve ganglia.

During primary HSV infection, natural killer cells are important effectors of immunity. Their activation depends on the production of several cytokines in response to the infection. These cytokines also have direct and indirect effects that are important for limiting replication of the virus. As the immune response matures, HSV clearance from infected tissues is T-cell mediated, involving cytokine-mediated effector mechanisms and direct cytolysis of virus-infected cells. In mice and humans, both CD4 and CD8 T cells are important in resolution of infection. Antibody may play a limited role in controlling HSV infection as well.

The efficiency of the immune response appears to influence the quantity of virus establishing latency in the ganglia. Although the elements contributing to this control are incompletely known, interferon-γ (IFN-γ) is likely to be important. IFN-γ activates antiviral genes that inhibit HSV replication and may be required for early decrease in local HSV viral titers. However, it appears from murine models that both IFN-γ and T-cell

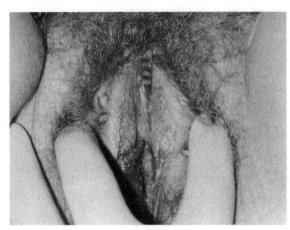

Figure 14–1. Primary genital herpes of the vulva. (Reproduced, with permission, from Holmes KK, et al. *Sexually Transmitted Diseases,* 3rd ed. McGraw-Hill, 1999, Figure 28.)

response can maintain viral latency and clear peripheral infections.

Prevention

There are multiple proven ways to prevent the acquisition and transmission of genital herpes. There are no "right" answers for prevention, and each patient must determine those best suited for his or her lifestyle. All patients diagnosed with genital herpes should be educated to recognize genital herpes outbreaks and given the option of daily suppressive therapy as a means to reduce genital herpes transmission. Measures for reducing transmission and acquisition of genital herpes include:

1. Disclosure of genital herpes infection to new partners. Although it may be difficult at first for patients to inform new partners that they have genital herpes, medical providers should encourage this important and necessary step to allow sex partners to make informed choices and, if appropriate, modify sexual practices to reduce the risk of transmission.

2. Abstinence during outbreaks. Once educated about the typically mild signs and symptoms of outbreaks, most patients are able to recognize symptomatic outbreaks.

3. Correct and consistent condom use. Male latex condom use can reduce transmission, especially during the first 6–12 months after initial infection.

4. Selection of partners with similar HSV serologic status or a history of genital herpes.

5. Chronic suppressive therapy. A recent major study demonstrated a 70% reduction in HSV transmission by infected patients using daily suppressive therapy. The reduction in disease and infection transmission may be attributable to both reduction of genital herpes recurrences and reduction of subclinical shedding.

Clinical Findings

A. SYMPTOMS AND SIGNS

Genital infection with HSV can be differentiated into five categories: first recognized episode, primary first episode, nonprimary first episode, recurrent episode, and subclinical shedding. Symptoms and signs characteristic of each are described below.

1. First recognized episode—The clinical diagnosis of a first episode versus recurrent episodes is unreliable. For the patient, the first recognized episode is an "initial" infection, whether it is a first episode or recurrent infection. The only way to classify a first episode with certainty is to document serologic conversion, but such classification usually serves little clinical purpose. All first recognized episodes can be safely managed as a newly acquired infection given the safety profile of currently recommended oral antiviral medications for HSV. Although both increased frequency of outbreaks and viral shedding are more likely with recent acquisition of infection, recommendations for daily suppressive therapy are based on the patient's desire to control disease (ie, outbreaks) or reduce the risk of transmission, or both.

2. Primary first episode—This refers to infection with either HSV-1 or HSV-2 in an individual who has never had infection with a herpes simplex virus. In immunocompetent hosts, this event often goes unrecognized.

After an incubation period of several days (average, 4 days; range, 1–14 days), a small papule appears that quickly evolves into a vesicle within 24 hours. Vesicles can be clear or pustular, are multiple, and rapidly evolve into shallow, nonindurated, painful ulcers (see Figure 14–2). The appearance of lesions can be associated with dysuria, inguinal lymphadenitis, vaginal discharge, and cervicitis. In primary infection, systemic symptoms including myalgias, malaise, fever, and other "flu-like" symptoms may be associated with the appearance of genital lesions. In the typical presentation, signs or symptoms are minimal and usually are not recognized as primary genital herpes.

Crops of lesions may occur over 1–2 weeks, and crusting and healing of lesions requires an additional 1–2 weeks (see Figure 14–3).

3. Nonprimary first episode—This refers to infection in individuals who have had a previous infection with either HSV type. The typical scenario is an individual

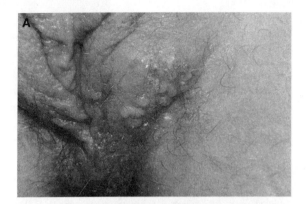

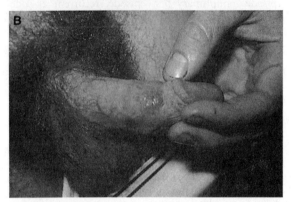

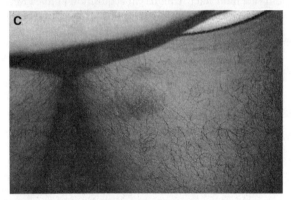

Figure 14–2. A: Vesicular lesions of genital herpes simplex virus (HSV) infection of the vulva. **B:** Genital ulceration resulting from HSV infection of the penile shaft. **C:** HSV infection of the posterior thigh.

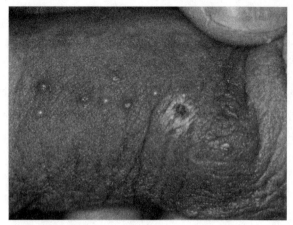

Figure 14–3. Primary HSV infection showing intact vesicles and pustules with surrounding erythema together with an earlier lesion, which is crusted and healing. (Reproduced, with permission, from Holmes KK, et al. *Sexually Transmitted Diseases,* 3rd ed. McGraw-Hill, 1999, Figure 26.)

with prior HSV-1 orolabial infection who subsequently acquires new genital HSV-2 infection. Typically, the first genital herpes outbreak tends to be less severe clinically than a true primary episode due to an existing, partial humoral and cellular immunity. Fewer lesions appear, pain and systemic symptoms are less, and lesion resolution is more rapid than with a primary first episode. The first episode usually resolves within 5–7 days. Nonprimary first episodes are clinically similar to recurrent disease and are often mistaken for recurrent genital herpes, if they are recognized at all.

4. Recurrent episode—Recurrent genital herpes refers to the second or subsequent episodes of genital herpes with the same virus type. HSV-2 is much more likely to recur then HSV-1 and accounts for more than 90% of recurrent genital herpes. The median number of recurrences is four per year, but up to 38% of individuals have six or more recurrences per year. Recurrences are, in general, clinically fairly mild and are often unrecognized. The outbreak usually is not associated with systemic symptoms but may be preceded by a prodrome of local paresthesia or dysesthesia.

Recurrent genital herpes may occur as a cluster of localized vesiculopustular or ulcerative lesions. Lesions tend to lateralize to one side of the midline. "Atypical" lesions are common and may be mistaken for excoriation or irritation. The predominant locations of lesions are on the glans penis or penile shaft in men (see Figure 14–4), the vaginal introitus or labia in women, and the buttocks and anal area in both sexes. A neuropathic prodrome characterized by pain or a burning sensation may occur 6–24 hours prior to the appearance of lesions.

5. Subclinical shedding—Subclinical shedding refers to the detection of virus in the absence of visible lesions. Our understanding of the natural history of genital herpes has shifted from that of intermittent outbreaks to one of low-grade frequent shedding of virus that can be

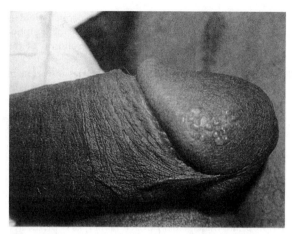

Figure 14–4. Recurrent HSV infection, showing grouped vesicles of the glans penis. (Reproduced, with permission, from Holmes KK, et al. *Sexually Transmitted Diseases,* 3rd ed. McGraw-Hill, 1999, Figure 27.)

detected by viral antigen detection methods (culture or PCR) of the genital tract on 5–20% of days. Subclinical shedding is most common during the first 6–12 months following acquisition of infection, approaching 40% of days. Subclinical shedding of HSV-2 occurs in almost all infected individuals, is of equivalent frequency in both women and men, and tends to diminish in frequency over time. About 50% of shedding episodes are temporarily associated around clinically recognized outbreaks, with virus detected one to several days proceeding or following resolution of lesions. Conversely, and of particular import, 50% of subclinical shedding events are more than 7 days removed from outbreaks. Patients who are counseled about the mild signs and symptoms of recurrent outbreaks may be able to recognize some of those periods when they are at greater risk of transmitting HSV to partners. HSV-1 subclinical shedding is much less common then HSV-2, occurring on 3–5% of days.

B. Diagnostic Tests

Until recently, **viral culture** was the "gold standard" for herpes diagnosis. Culture allows definitive diagnosis and permits distinction of HSV-1 from HSV-2, which is important for prognosis and counseling. Cultures are most sensitive while lesions are in the vesicular-pustular stage. Sensitivity rapidly declines as lesions ulcerate and crust.

PCR is three to five times more sensitive than viral culture, is offered by most reference laboratories, and is quickly replacing viral culture as the "gold standard." It is important to note that a negative culture for HSV does not rule out genital herpes.

Type-specific antibody testing based on HSV glycoprotein G is the most important and reliable diagnostic tool for chronic HSV infection. Antibody tests based on complement fixation, indirect immunofluorescence, or neutralization technologies do not reliably distinguish antibodies to HSV-1 from those to HSV-2. A negative result on an antibody test can be reassuring in that it excludes the diagnosis in a patient who has symptoms suggestive of long-standing or recurrent herpes. A positive result on a test that is not HSV glycoprotein G based is of little diagnostic value, because these serologic assays do not reliably distinguish between type 1 and type 2 infections. Because more then half of US adults are seropositive for HSV-1 as a result of herpes labialis infection, a positive test for HSV-1 antibody does not provide useful diagnostic information for the evaluation of genital ulcer disease. IgM antibody is often present during recurrent HSV outbreaks and does not indicate recent infection.

The newer **type-specific serologic assays** have specificities of more than 98% for the detection of HSV-2 antibody and sensitivities of more than 90%. One assay is a rapid, office-based test that can be run on serum or a whole blood specimen collected by a fingerstick and can provide results in less then 10 minutes. It is imperative to specify and request a glycoprotein G–based test when ordering an HSV serologic test. The following type-specific assays have been cleared by the Food and Drug Administration (FDA): Western immunoblot, HerpeSelect HSV-1 and HSV-2 ELISA (Focus Diagnostics, Cypress, CA), HerpeSelect HSV-1 and HSV-2 immunoblot (Focus Diagnostics, Cypress, CA), BioKit HSV-2 Rapid Assay (Biokit USA, Lexington, MA), and Captia HSV-1 and HSV-2 (Trinity Biotech, Wicklow, Ireland).

Other diagnostic tests for possible herpetic lesions include the following:

1. Direct immunofluorescent antibody testing for HSV antigen. Although more rapid (4–6 hours) than culture, this test may not differentiate HSV-1 and HSV-2.

2. Enzyme-linked immunosorbent assay (ELISA) testing for HSV antigens in clinical specimens. This test offers a rapid alternative to culture (results are available in 3–4 hours), but its use is generally confined to large reference laboratories and teaching institutions.

3. Microscopy of Papanicolaou smears or Giemsa staining (Tzanck test). These tests, although inexpensive, are insensitive, nonspecific, and not recommended.

Ashley RL. Performance and use of HSV type-specific serology test kits. *Herpes* 2002;9:38–45. [PMID: 12106510]

Guerry SL, Bauer HM, Klausner JD, et al. Recommendations for the selective use of herpes simplex virus type 2 serological tests. *Clin Infect Dis* 2005;40:38–45. [PMID: 15614690]

Differential Diagnosis

Discreet genital or anal ulcers in sexually active young adults have a relatively narrow differential diagnosis.

A complete differential diagnosis of genital herpes should include the following infectious etiologies: syphilis, primary HIV, chancroid, lymphogranuloma venereum, and donovanosis. Chancroid is currently rare in the United States and syphilis had been, until recently, at an historic low and is highly concentrated in geographic areas and certain groups. Thus, most genital ulcers (>90%) are caused by HSV.

The chancre of primary syphilis is classically nontender, indurated, and nonpurulent. Those findings can distinguish a syphilitic chancre from other infectious genital ulceration with some certainty. Other ulcer characteristics are less helpful in distinguishing infectious etiologies, but given the far greater prevalence of herpes, most genital ulcer disease is likely due to herpes. Thus, it is critical that diagnostic testing for HSV be performed on all genital lesions whenever possible to prevent missing a diagnosis for other treatable causes of genital ulcer disease, such as syphilis.

In general, genital lesions should always be evaluated by obtaining a "swab" test. This generally means obtaining a specimen for darkfield examination for *Treponema pallidum* and obtaining a specimen for HSV culture or PCR. Serologic screening for syphilis should accompany the diagnostic evaluation for genital lesions. HIV testing is encouraged for all individuals presenting with a genital lesion.

Complications

A primary first episode infection can be severe (see Figure 14–5) and may be associated with symptoms and

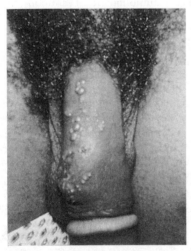

Figure 14–5. Severe primary HSV infection with extensive vesicles, ulcerations, and penile edema. (Reproduced, with permission, from Holmes KK, et al. *Sexually Transmitted Diseases,* 3rd ed. McGraw-Hill, 1999, Figure 25.)

signs of meningitis. On analysis, cerebrospinal fluid is aseptic and usually shows a predominance of lymphocytes. Antiviral therapy will speed the resolution of the clinical illness.

Long-term sequelae from genital herpes infection in adults are rare. Reactivation of HSV-1 infection, usually orolabial infection, in adults can cause keratitis or encephalitis. Genital herpes infection can increase the risk of HIV transmission and possibly the acquisition of other viral infections (eg, hepatitis C). In newborns, herpes infection can be devastating, resulting in permanent neurologic disability or death.

Treatment

Appropriate management of genital herpes is predicated on addressing the following critical areas: accurate etiologic diagnosis (see Clinical Findings, earlier), treatment of disease, reduction of transmission risk, and emotional counseling. The latter is all too often ignored by providers or, if acknowledged, is trivialized. There is an undeserved stigma attached to genital herpes, and most patients require reassurance concerning their sexual well-being, reproductive health, and ability to reduce the risk of transmission of disease and infection to partners. Patients should be encouraged to inform sex partners of their infection but may need help in learning how to disclose their status to partners.

A. PHARMACOTHERAPY

Table 14–1 outlines pharmacologic treatment, based on the 2006 guidelines from the Centers for Disease Control and Prevention (CDC).

Antiviral therapy for initial genital herpes prevents new lesion formation and rapidly reduces viral shedding, infectivity, and the risk of autoinfection. However, it has no effect on the frequency of subsequent recurrences. Episodic treatment shortens the duration of recurrences by 20–30%. Taken daily, antiviral therapy effectively suppresses HSV recurrences and reduces subclinical shedding. Episodic therapy is most effective when started immediately upon the earliest sign or symptom of an outbreak. Self-initiation of therapy is an important element of episodic therapy to prevent delays. Patients, therefore, should be given a prescription for medication to be-filled and kept easily accessible.

All currently recommended oral regimens for genital herpes therapy are well tolerated and associated with few adverse effects. Dosing frequency is the main difference among the current therapies. It should be noted that acyclovir can be given three times daily. Limited clinical trial data exist for this dosing schedule, but considerable clinical experience justifies administering the drug in this manner. All three oral agents are renally excreted and thus can accumulate when renal function is impaired (requiring a reduction in dosage). Acyclovir, valacyclovir,

Table 14–1. Recommended treatment regimens for genital herpes based on type of infection.

Indication	Regimen
Initial infection	Acyclovir, 400 mg PO 3 times daily for 7–10 d *or* Valacyclovir, 1 g PO twice daily for 7–10 d *or* Famciclovir, 250 mg PO 3 times daily for 7–10 d
Recurrent infection	Acyclovir, 400 mg PO 3 times daily for 5 d *or* Acyclovir, 800 mg PO 3 times daily for 2 d *or* Acyclovir, 800 mg PO twice daily for 5 d *or* Valacyclovir, 500 mg PO twice daily for 3 d[a] *or* Valacyclovir, 1 g PO daily for 5 d *or* Famciclovir, 125 mg PO twice daily for 5 d *or* Famciclovir, 1000 mg PO twice daily for 1 d
Suppressive therapy	Acyclovir, 400 mg PO twice daily *or* Valacyclovir, 500 mg PO daily (increased to 1.0 g daily in patients with >9 outbreaks per year) *or* Famciclovir, 250 mg PO twice daily.

[a]Clinicians can order the 1-g dose and order it scored or split, at a cost (for 3-day supply) that is less than or comparable to acyclovir (5-day supply).
Based on Centers for Disease Control and Prevention; Workowski KA, Berman SM. Sexually transmitted diseases treatment guidelines, 2006. *MMWR Recomm Rep* 2006;55(RR-11):1–94.

and famciclovir are not approved for the use in pregnancy but are FDA category B drugs and are probably safe for pregnant women and fetuses. Some experts recommend the use of suppressive acyclovir therapy during the last month of pregnancy for women with a history of recurrent genital herpes. Suppressive therapy has been shown to reduce the likelihood of genital herpes recurrences at term and, thus, the need for cesarean delivery.

Daily suppressive therapy reduces the frequency of recurrences and viral shedding. Suppressive therapy should be offered to all patients with frequent recurrences, those with psychological distress related to genital herpes, and those wishing to reduce the risk of transmission. A recent study involving heterosexual monogamous couples discordant for HSV-2 evaluated use of daily suppressive therapy to reduce risk of transmission. The study demonstrated a 48% reduction of transmission of infection and a 75% reduction in development of clinical genital herpes in susceptible partners. Consideration of suppressive therapy is equally justified to control recurrences as well as to reduce the risk of transmission. Ultimately, patents must decide what their goals for treatment are and make decisions about episodic versus suppressive therapy.

Topical lidocaine jelly 2% is sometimes a useful adjunct to oral antiviral agents for managing severe first episodes in women. It should be applied frequently, and especially before voiding, but for no longer than 24–36 hours. There is a theoretical risk of sensitization, but this is very rarely seen in practice.

Corey L, Wald A, Patel R, et al. Once-daily valacyclovir to reduce the risk of transmission of genital herpes. *N Engl J Med* 2004;350:11–20. [PMID: 14702423]

B. OTHER TREATMENT MEASURES

There is no evidence that salt baths, topical antiseptics, lysine, vitamins, or the multitude of over-the-counter herpes remedies are any more effective than placebo in the treatment or prevention of genital herpes.

C. Optimal Evaluation and Treatment

1. First episodes—Specimens from clinical lesions should be obtained for diagnosis, depending on tests available and stage of presentation of the patient. Viral culture or PCR testing permits distinction of HSV-1 from HSV-2 and allows a definitive etiologic diagnosis for the genital ulcer. Culture yield diminishes quickly as lesions begin to heal, with the highest yield being at the vesiculopustular stage. The need for further immediate tests should be assessed if there is risk behavior or clinical suspicion of syphilis, chancroid, primary HIV, or other sexually transmitted disease. Such tests include darkfield examination, rapid plasma reagin evaluation of serum, Venereal Disease Research Laboratory (VDRL), *T pallidum* particle agglutination (TP-PA) tests, and HIV RNA or HIV antibody testing. Type-specific serologic assays for HSV-1 and HSV-2 can be used as part of the initial evaluation for HSV culture- or PCR-negative lesions. Seroconversion for newly acquired HSV infection may take 8–12 weeks with the use of the current type-specific serologic assays.

An oral antiviral agent should be prescribed for 7–10 days. The patient can expect symptoms to resolve in 3–4 days. If symptoms do not resolve, the patient should be reexamined and the possibility of secondary infection or an alternative diagnosis considered. Persistence of lesions for more then 14 days should prompt consideration of HIV coinfection.

All patients with genital ulcer disease should be reevaluated at 1 week. The clinician should consider repeat serologic testing for syphilis and examination for other genital infections. If the results of initial HSV virologic tests were negative, HSV type-specific serology can be obtained at least 6 weeks and preferably 3 months after presentation. All patients should be counseled about treatment options, with the purpose of obtaining desired outcomes such as controlling disease and reducing transmission of HSV.

2. Recurrent episodes—Virologic specimens should be obtained from active lesions, if the diagnosis has not been confirmed earlier. Consideration should be given to obtaining type-specific serology in patients with atypical-appearing lesions, negative results on virologic tests, or lesions that cannot be tested for the presence of HSV.

HIV testing should be strongly encouraged for patients in whom HIV status has not recently been obtained.

Episodic treatment with an oral antiviral agent should be offered. All patients should be counseled about full treatment options (ie, continued episodic therapy that may be started at the first signs or symptoms of an outbreak or suppressive therapy to prevent recurrences and reduce the risk of transmission).

D. Counseling

Firstly, and most importantly, the medical provider must give accurate information about all aspects of the disease. Newly diagnosed genital herpes can be an emotionally traumatic event for some patients, making comprehension and retention of information difficult at the time of diagnosis. Important information to be discussed at the first visit is listed in Table 14–2.

Time should be offered at a follow-up visit to address the patientís concerns and to provide appropriate counseling. Patients may be given written information and referred to Internet web sites (see listing at end of chapter) and telephone hotlines (eg, the American Social Health Association national herpes hotline, at 919-361-8488, or the CDC national STD hotline, at 800-227-8922 or 800-342-2427 [English] and 800-344-7432 [Spanish]).

When to Refer to a Specialist

Although acyclovir-resistant genital herpes infection is rare, it has occurred in immunocompromised patients whose adherence to antiviral therapy was intermittent. If resistant infection is suspected, consultation with an infectious disease specialist is warranted to confirm the diagnosis and obtain appropriate antiviral therapy.

Prognosis

An outbreak of genital herpes will resolve on its own; however, the frequency of recurrent outbreaks is quite

---

Table 14–2. Recommended counseling messages for persons newly diagnosed with genital herpes.

Many sexually active adults (> 20%) have genital herpes infection, and most (90%) are unaware of the infection.
Effective therapy is available for initial episodes and recurrences, as well as for suppression.
Daily suppressive therapy can prevent transmission.
Recurrent episodes tend to be milder than the initial episode.
Transmission of herpes usually occurs from a partner who was not aware of the infection or did not believe he or she was infectious when exposure occurred.
Genital herpes simplex virus type 2 (HSV-2) infection is associated with an increased risk of HIV acquisition, and with an increased risk of HIV transmission in those dually infected with HSV-2 and HIV.
Genital herpes does not affect fertility, but there is a substantial risk of neonatal transmission in women with infections acquired during pregnancy, particularly the third trimester.

variable. Over a prolonged period, recurrences decline but in some patients, episodic outbreaks continue. Fortunately, antiviral treatment is safe and well-tolerated, and clinical outcomes in patients with recurrent disease can be improved with daily suppressive therapy.

PRACTICE POINTS

- *All patients diagnosed with genital herpes should be educated to recognize genital herpes outbreaks and given the option of daily suppressive therapy as a means to reduce genital herpes transmission.*

- *Episodic therapy is most effective when started immediately upon the earliest sign or symptom of an outbreak.*

Relevant Web Sites

[American College of Obstetricians and Gynecologists:]
http://www.accog.com
[American Social Health Association:]
http://www.ashastd.org
[CDC Division of Sexually Transmitted Diseases:]
http://www.cdc.gov/std

External Genital Warts

15

Peter V. Chin-Hong, MD, & Joel M. Palefsky, MD

ESSENTIALS OF DIAGNOSIS

- *Gray or flesh-colored, pedunculated, and moist papules on the penis, urethra, vulva, cervix, anus, or perineal and perianal areas.*
- *One or several grouped lesions may be present, ranging in size from a few millimeters to several centimeters.*
- *Symptoms may include burning, itching, pain, and fullness (urethra, vagina, or anus); however, many patients are asymptomatic.*

General Considerations

Human papillomavirus (HPV) is one of the most common sexually transmitted diseases (STDs) and is the cause of genital warts (condylomata acuminata), anogenital dysplasia, and invasive cancer. Oral warts may also occur as a direct consequence of HPV infection during sexual activity. At least 75% of sexually active men and women acquire one or more genital HPV types at some point in their lifetime. The incubation period from HPV infection to condyloma is usually 3–4 months, with a range of 1 month to 2 years, but many infected persons have subclinical disease or have regression of disease before it becomes clinically apparent. HIV-infected patients have a higher prevalence of genital warts than HIV-uninfected patients. These may proliferate further during immune reconstitution following the initiation of antiretroviral therapy.

There are more than 100 different HPV types; 40 of these can cause anogenital lesions. HPV types 6 and 11 are most commonly associated with genital warts; these types have a low risk of malignant transformation. Other types (eg, 16, 18, 31, 33, and 35) have a strong association with cervical and other anogenital cancers. Thus, genital warts lie on one spectrum of a continuum of HPV-associated

disease, with warts being one variant of low-grade disease that has little risk of malignant potential. High-grade HPV-associated disease such as cervical intraepithelial neoplasia (CIN) types 2 and 3 are likely the direct precursors to invasive cancer and are the target of screening programs that utilize the Papanicolaou (Pap) test.

Chin-Hong PV, Palefsky JM. Natural history and clinical management of anal human papillomavirus disease in men and women infected with human immunodeficiency virus. *Clin Infect Dis* 2002;35:1127–1134. [PMID: 12384848] (Excellent review of anal HPV disease and HIV infection.)

Conley LJ, Ellerbrock TV, Bush TJ, et al. HIV-1 infection and risk of vulvovaginal and perianal condylomata acuminata and intraepithelial neoplasia: A prospective cohort study. *Lancet* 2002; 359:108–113. [PMID: 11809252] (Prospective study showing that HIV-infected women may be 16 times more likely to develop HPV-related anovaginal disease, including invasive vulvar carcinoma, than HIV-uninfected women.)

Massad LS, Silverberg MJ, Springer G, et al. Effect of antiretroviral therapy on the incidence of genital warts and vulvar neoplasia among women with the human immunodeficiency virus. *Am J Obstet Gynecol* 2004;190:1241–1248. [PMID: 15167825] (Multicenter prospective study showing that warts and vulvar intraepithelial neoplasia are common among women with HIV infection, and highly active antiretroviral therapy decreased their incidence.)

Pathogenesis

Most anogenital HPV is believed to be acquired via sexual transmission. Following acquisition of infection, HPV infection is established initially in the basal cells of the anogenital epithelium. As the basal cells differentiate and rise to the epithelial surface, HPV replicates and virions form. A spectrum of disease occurs, depending on the degree of mitotic activity and replacement of the epithelium with immature basaloid cells. In the cervix, this ranges from genital warts or mild dysplasia (CIN 1) to moderate or severe dysplasia (CIN 2 and CIN 3).

Prevention

The most reliable method of preventing HPV acquisition is abstinence from sexual activity, including skin-to-skin contact. However, there is strong evidence that male latex condoms offer some protection against HPV infection, as well as HPV-associated diseases such as genital warts, CIN 2 or 3, and invasive cervical cancer. Although not recommended by the US Centers for Disease Control and Prevention (CDC), partner evaluation may offer an opportunity to screen and provide education on HPV and other STDs.

Preventive vaccines are promising new options. A multivalent vaccine against four HPV subtypes (6, 11, 16, and 18) was approved by the Food and Drug Administration (FDA) for use in women and girls aged 9–26 years in June 2006. These immunizations use components of the major HPV capsid proteins that assemble into viruslike particles that contain no HPV DNA and thus are not infectious. Vaccination with viruslike particles is designed to induce neutralizing antibodies prior to initial HPV exposure by the host. In large, randomized controlled trials, excellent efficacy has been demonstrated against certain HPV types, including 6, 11 (which can cause anogenital warts), and 16 and 18 (which can cause invasive cervical and other anogenital cancers). Future trials will test the efficacy of combined vaccines for additional types.

Bleeker MC, Hogewoning CJ, Voorhorst EJ, et al. Condom use promotes regression of human papillomavirus-associated penile lesions in male sexual partners of women with cervical intraepithelial neoplasia. *Int J Cancer* 2003;107:804–810. [PMID: 14566831] (Randomized trial in 136 couples showing that condom use significantly shortened the median time to regression of flat penile lesions [7.4 months in the condom group vs 13.9 months in the noncondom group].)

Hogewoning CJ, Bleeker MC, van den Brule AJ, et al. Condom use promotes regression of cervical intraepithelial neoplasia and clearance of human papillomavirus: A randomized clinical trial. *Int J Cancer* 2003;107:811–816. [PMID: 14566832] (Randomized trial in 148 women with CIN and their male sex partners showing that condom use promotes regression of CIN lesions and clearance of HPV.)

Villa LL, Costa RL, Petta CA, et al. Prophylactic quadrivalent human papillomavirus (types 6, 11, 16, and 18) L1 virus-like particle vaccine in young women: A randomised double-blind placebo-controlled multicentre phase II efficacy trial. *Lancet Oncol* 2005;6:271–278. [PMID: 15863374] (Randomized trial in 277 women demonstrating that a vaccine targeting HPV types 6, 11, 16, and 18 could substantially reduce the acquisition of infection and clinical disease caused by common HPV types.)

Clinical Findings

A. SYMPTOMS AND SIGNS

Genital warts appear as characteristic well-circumscribed, exophytic papules that may be pedunculated. Some warts may be flat. The adjacent skin usually appears normal. They range in size from a few millimeters to several centimeters, with some warts coalescing to form larger plaques. The median number of warts in an individual patient is seven although there is a large range from patient to patient.

Most genital warts in circumcised men occur in the penile shaft. In uncircumcised men, they occur mainly in the preputial cavity where the penile shaft meets the glans (see Figure 15–1). Other common locations for genital warts in men include the perianal area (see Figure 15–2), particularly among men who have sex with men (MSM), and the urethral meatus. Less frequently, genital warts are seen on the scrotum and perineum. Although not the focus of this chapter, intra-anal

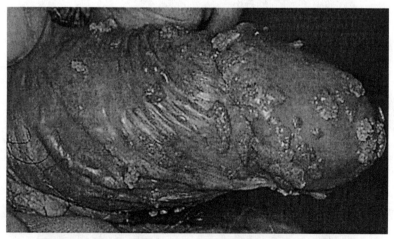

Figure 15–1. Penile warts. Multiple soft papules on the glans penis and the prepuce. (Reproduced, with permission, from Wolff K, Johnson RA, Summond D. *Fitzpatrick's Color Atlas and Synopsis of Clinical Dermatology,* 5th ed. McGraw-Hill, 2005.)

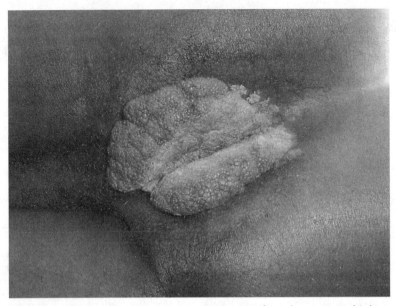

Figure 15–2. Large, circumferential perianal genital warts in an HIV-infected patient. Multiple verrucous papules have coalesced into a large plaque causing obstructive symptoms. (Courtesy of Tina Clark, NP, University of California at San Francisco.)

warts can be very common as well. Among women, most lesions are found in the posterior introitus, the labia majora and minora (see Figure 15–3), and the clitoris. Other less common locations in women are the perineum, vagina, anus, cervix, and urethra.

Patients with genital warts may complain of itching, burning, bleeding, and pain. Patients with large genital warts may have a sensation of fullness and this may interfere with intercourse, vaginal delivery, and defecation. However, many patients have no symptoms.

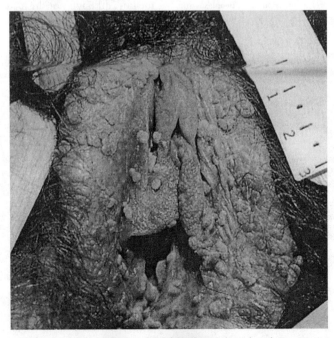

Figure 15–3. Vulvar warts. Multiple soft papules on the labia. (Reproduced, with permission, from Wolff K, Johnson RA, Summond D. *Fitzpatrick's Color Atlas and Synopsis of Clinical Dermatology*, 5th ed. McGraw-Hill, 2005.)

B. Laboratory Findings and Special Examinations

Most genital warts are diagnosed by the characteristic appearance on clinical examination only. If lesions look atypical or have features that may be consistent with malignancy such as induration, ulceration, and pigmentation, biopsy with histologic evaluation should be considered.

1. Colposcopy with acetic acid—Colposcopy uses a powerful light source and binocular lenses to enable providers to identify HPV-associated lesions. Typically colposcopy is used in conjunction with acetic acid to aid in the visualization of affected tissue. Following the application of 3–5% acetic acid for 3–5 minutes, an acetowhite area signifies HPV infected tissue in contrast to normal surrounding tissue. Although originally designed to evaluate the female genital tract, the application of colposcopy has expanded to evaluate other anatomic sites such as the penis and the anus. Cervical colposcopy and high-resolution anoscopy ("colposcopy" of the anal canal) are typically performed after an abnormal cytologic test on cervical and anal cancer screening, respectively. However, this method is occasionally used for the evaluation of genital warts as well.

2. Cytologic tests—The Pap test is the cornerstone of cervical cancer and CIN screening and has been very successful in lowering cervical cancer incidence and mortality where it has been implemented. There is no role for the use of cytologic tests to diagnose genital warts, but women presenting with genital warts should be screened with Pap tests. The CDC recommends that providers perform a cervical Pap test at the time of a pelvic examination for STD screening in women who have not had a Pap test within the preceding 12–36 months. This is because women attending STD clinics have a five times higher prevalence of CIN than women attending family planning clinics, and a history of STDs is a risk factor for invasive cervical cancer. Cervical cancer screening guidelines have been issued by the American Cancer Society, the US Preventative Services Task Force, and the American College of Obstetricians and Gynecologists.

Cervical cytologic findings are classified as abnormal or normal. The abnormal category includes high-grade squamous intraepithelial lesions (HSIL), low-grade squamous intraepithelial lesions (LSIL), atypical squamous cells that may be of undetermined significance (ASC-US), or those that are suspicious for HSIL (ASC-H). (For further discussion of abnormal cervical findings, see Chapter 29.)

Similar to the association between genital warts and CIN, there is a risk of anal intraepithelial neoplasia in men and women with anogenital warts. We believe that certain groups, such as MSM, HIV-infected women and men regardless of sexual orientation, women with a history of vulvar or cervical cancer, and transplant recipients, are at the highest risk of anal intraepithelial neoplasia and anal cancer and should be screened with anal cytology.

Anal cytologic testing every 1–2 years has been projected to be a cost-effective intervention to prevent anal cancer in HIV-infected MSM, with cytologic testing every 2–3 years for HIV-uninfected MSM. To perform anal cytologic testing, we insert a water-moistened Dacron swab in the anal canal, then withdraw the swab slowly while maintaining some pressure against the anal canal. In this way, we obtain exfoliated cells from the lower rectum, squamocolumnar junction, and anal canal. Similar to the system used in cervical cancer and CIN screening, anal cytologic findings are classified as normal, ASC-US, ASC-H, LSIL, and HSIL. Individuals with abnormal findings (ASC-US, ASC-H, LSIL, and HSIL) are referred for high-resolution anoscopy, in which equipment identical to that used in cervical colposcopy is employed to aid in the identification of lesions that have contributed to abnormal cytologic findings.

3. Histologic findings—Histologic examination of genital warts reveals HPV-induced abnormalities in the epidermis, including acanthosis (thickening of the stratum spinosum), parakeratosis (retention of nuclei in the cells of the stratum corneum), and hyperkeratosis (thickening of the stratum corneum), leading to a typical papillomatosis formation. Other characteristic findings on tissue examination of a biopsy specimen are koilocytes (squamous epithelial cells with an abnormal nucleus within a large cytoplasmic halo). Biopsies are not necessary for the diagnosis of genital warts, given their unique clinical appearance. However, we recommend obtaining a biopsy specimen if there are atypical findings such as pigmentation, ulceration, or firm, nodular masses, to rule out high-grade dysplasia or malignant disease.

4. Molecular methods—Techniques using polymerase chain reaction (PCR) and hybrid capture technology are sensitive and specific methods of diagnosing HPV infection. PCR technology uses the action of DNA polymerase on specific primers to amplify target HPV DNA. HPV type-specific PCR assays are available. Hybrid capture employs RNA probes specific for the identification of certain grouped oncogenic (high-risk) or nononcogenic (low-risk) HPV types, but does not give individual type-specific information. PCR and hybrid capture methods can be used to diagnose HPV infection using both exfoliated cells and tissue specimens obtained by biopsy. Although PCR and hybrid capture are commonly used in research settings, only hybrid capture is cleared by the FDA as an adjunct to cervical cytologic screening to detect CIN. PCR and hybrid capture are not routinely used for the diagnosis or management of genital warts.

5. Serologic findings—Enzyme-linked immunoabsorbent assay (ELISA) technology is used to provide IgM and IgG serologic measures of HPV infection by targeting type-specific viruslike particles. Patients with genital warts and other HPV-associated diseases have been found to have type-specific HPV serologic responses to HPV-6 and HPV-11. The significance of HPV sero-logic measures is unclear, and these measures are currently used only in research settings. Antibody responses to HPV may persist for several years or resolve with the resolution of disease, and thus may indicate either current or past infection. There is currently no clinical indication for the use of HPV serology.

Differential Diagnosis

External genital warts should not be confused with manifestations of other STDs such as *condylomata lata* of secondary syphilis. Condylomata lata are characterized by large, white or gray, raised, moist, and flat lesions. In contrast, external genital warts are typically dry and cauliflower-like. If condylomata lata are suspected, serologic tests for syphilis (rapid plasma reagin [RPR], Venereal Disease Research Laboratories [VDRL], with confirmatory treponemal tests such as the *Treponema pallidum* particle agglutination assay [TP-PA]) will be positive, and surface scrapings of the lesion will reveal spirochetes under darkfield microscopy.

The lesions of the poxvirus, *molluscum contagiosum,* are shiny and umbilicated papules that may appear anywhere on the body except the palms and soles. These flesh-colored lesions are 2–5 mm, appear singly or in groups, and may sometimes be difficult to distinguish from genital warts. Unlike genital warts, however, molluscum contagiosum causes smooth and only rarely pedunculated lesions that may express cheesy material. Although most self-resolve in immunocompetent patients, the lesions can be particularly recalcitrant in AIDS patients with low CD4 T-cell counts.

A normal anatomic variant of the corona in men, *pearly penile papules,* can sometimes be mistaken for genital warts. Analogous lesions in women occur in the vulvar introitus. One clue to the diagnosis of these variants of normal anatomy is to look at the base of the lesions. In the normal variants, each normal papilla can be seen to arise from its own base; by contrast, in anogenital warts, multiple papillae typically arise from a single base. (For additional discussion, see Chapter 30.)

Lichen planus, nevi, and *seborrheic keratoses* may also be rarely confused with genital warts.

Complications

Genital warts have little risk of progression to invasive cancer. However, individuals with genital warts usually have shared risk factors for oncogenic HPV types that cause high-grade CIN and anal intraepithelial neoplasia. These are the true precancerous lesions and are the target of Pap screening programs. Genital warts may proliferate and increase in size during pregnancy and can obstruct the pelvic outlet during vaginal delivery. A rare complication in children born to women with genital warts is

recurrent respiratory papillomatosis. Warts develop in the infants' throats, commonly the vocal cords, causing hoarseness or stridor. These warts are frequently removed, usually by laser surgery, to prevent the possibility of respiratory failure. Because the prevalence of recurrent respiratory papillomatosis is so low, cesarean delivery is not usually recommended as a preventive measure in pregnant women with genital warts.

Treatment

Treatment options for genital warts include therapies that are patient applied and those that are clinician administered, based on the size and location of lesions. Some patients elect to forgo treatment, because many lesions regress spontaneously. However, many patients have recurrent disease within 3–6 months after treatment, particularly those who are infected with HIV.

The goals in treatment of external genital warts are to provide symptomatic relief or cosmesis, or to alleviate anxiety. The type of treatment chosen depends on the size and location of the lesion, and the reasons for treatment. Other factors that may influence treatment choices include patient preference, cost, adverse effects of treatment, and provider experience. As noted below, some treatment options are contraindicated in pregnancy, and this needs to be considered. In general, smaller lesions are easier to treat than larger ones. Warts that are smaller than 1 cm^2 at the base are more likely to be successfully treated by topical therapy alone. In contrast, diffuse and large lesions may require surgical intervention. Figure 15–4 outlines a treatment algorithm for genital warts.

We sometimes choose not to treat large, circumferential perianal genital warts if they are not symptomatic. The reason for this is that multiple staged procedures are usually needed for complete treatment, surgery is painful, and lesions are often recurrent. We would only recommend surgery in these cases to remove foci of disease that are causing symptoms, or if the goal is to rule out invasive cancer.

Warts that are located on dry surfaces, are chronic (duration >1 year), or are multiple (>10) are more difficult to treat. Many patients require multiple treatments before successful removal of genital warts, and warts may recur after several months. There is no evidence that one therapeutic modality is superior to another, and the agent chosen may depend on local availability or experience of the clinician in using a particular treatment modality. The impact of treatment on the transmission of genital warts is unknown.

A. Patient-applied Therapies

Imiquimod 5% cream (Aldara) is a topical immune response modifier that induces cytokines locally without a direct antiviral effect. Patients apply 5% cream once daily before bedtime, three times a week for up to 16 weeks. Six to ten hours following the application, the affected

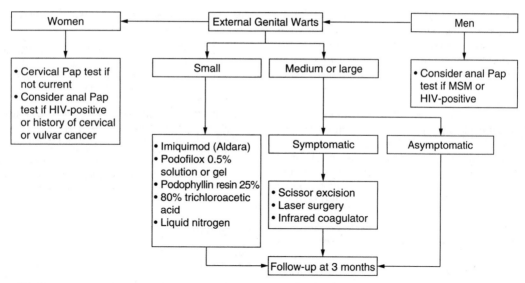

Figure 15–4. Treatment algorithm for external genital warts. MSM = men who have sex with men.

area should be washed off with soap and water. Unlike podophyllotoxin (discussed below), there is no limit to the surface area that can be treated. The major adverse effect is mild to moderate local erythema. The safety of imiquimod in pregnancy has not been established, and it should not be used by pregnant women (category C).

Podofilox 0.5% solution or gel (Condylox Gel) works by arresting the cell cycle in metaphase, leading to cell death. Patients can apply the gel with a finger, or the solution with a cotton swab to palpable warts. Podofilox is used twice daily for 3 days, followed by no therapy for 4 days. Up to four cycles may be performed. A maximum surface area of 10 cm^2 is recommended, and the total daily volume of podofilox should not exceed 0.5 mL. Adverse effects include mild skin irritation, but local ulceration and pain can occur depending on the duration of use. Safety in pregnancy has not been established (category C).

B. Provider-Applied Therapies

Cryotherapy can be performed in the office using liquid nitrogen spray, a liquid nitrogen–soaked swab, or a cryoprobe cooled with nitrous oxide. The freeze-thaw cycle produces cell lysis and destruction of the wart. The freeze margin should extend 2–3 mm beyond the margins of the wart. Cryotherapy can be repeated every 3 weeks. Adverse effects include some pain during and for a variable time after the procedure. Swelling and erythema may also occur. This treatment modality is safe for use during pregnancy.

Podophyllin resin 25% in tincture of benzoin (Podocon-25; Paddock Laboratories, Minneapolis, MN) is similar to podofilox except that it is provider applied.

The liquid is applied to the affected area, allowed to dry, and washed off after 6 hours. Total volume should not exceed 0.5 mL per session. Therapy may be repeated in 1 week. Adverse effects include skin irritation, ulceration, and pain, depending on how much solution is applied. Rarely, polyneuritis, paresthesias, leucopenia, and thrombocytopenia may occur. Safety in pregnancy has not been established (category C).

Trichloroacetic acid (TCA), 80%, destroys affected tissue by protein coagulation. Typically, a small quantity of TCA is applied to the lesion until it appears white or frosted; the acid is then allowed to dry. Care should be taken to ensure that TCA does not run off the lesion to cover areas of normal skin. To provide greater control, we soak the stick end of a cotton swab in a small amount of TCA and apply it by touching the stick end to the lesion. Temporary burning may occur at the time of application to the wart. If too much TCA is applied, or if surrounding tissue is inadvertently treated—resulting in substantial pain—talc, liquid soap, or sodium bicarbonate can be used to neutralize the acid. A barrier of petroleum jelly could also be used to protect areas adjacent to the wart undergoing treatment. As with cryotherapy multiple treatment applications are often necessary. TCA is safe for use during pregnancy.

C. Surgical Options

Use of an *infrared coagulator* (Redfield Corporation, Rochelle Park, NJ) is an FDA-approved option for the treatment of genital warts. The infrared coagulator uses light technology to generate intense heat at the tip of the device, producing coagulative necrosis without a smoke plume. This procedure can be performed in the office using local anesthesia only. The infrared coagulator is particularly useful for larger lesions that would have normally required intraoperative fulguration or laser surgery.

Laser surgery is an option for extensive genital warts, particularly those that have been refractory to other treatment modalities. Trained operators focus the laser on affected tissue. Laser energy is converted into heat, vaporizing the genital wart. The maximum recommended depth of tissue destruction is 1 mm. Adverse effects include pain and scarring, and operators may develop warts by dispersion of virions during the procedure. This procedure is performed in the operating room under anesthesia and is one of the most expensive treatment options for genital warts. It can also be done in the office.

Scissor excision and other excisional procedures are considered first-line therapy by some providers for large warts causing obstructive symptoms. After local anesthesia, the wart is usually excised down to normal tissue or mucosa (using fine scissors or a scalpel), and the roots of the lesion are destroyed by electrocautery, with no further hemostasis required. Suturing is rarely needed. Complications include strictures and scarring, particularly if subcutaneous tissue or submucosal fat is inadvertently cauterized.

D. Other Treatment Options

5-Fluorouracil (5-FU) can be used as a gel with epinephrine and injected intralesionally for the treatment of genital warts. 5-FU acts by blocking the methylation of deoxyuridylic acid, arresting DNA synthesis and causing cell death. Adverse effects—pain and ulceration, with dysuria if used in the urethra—limit the use of this drug. 5-FU is not recommended during pregnancy (category D).

Cidofovir disrupts viral chain elongation by competitively inhibiting the incorporation of deoxycytidine triphosphate (dCTP) into viral DNA. Applied topically as a 1% gel, cidofovir has been demonstrated to be effective in a randomized controlled trial of the treatment of genital warts. This therapy is still experimental.

Interferon alfa can be given systemically, topically (not generally effective), or, as is more often the case, intralesionally. Intralesional interferon is not FDA-cleared for the treatment of genital warts although it is used widely.

Beutner KR, Reitano MV, Richwald GA, Wiley DJ. External genital warts: Report of the American Medical Association Consensus Conference. AMA Expert Panel on External Genital Warts. *Clin Infect Dis* 1998;27:796–806. [PMID: 9798036] (Excellent summary of clinical trials and expert opinion in the management of external genital warts with practice recommendations.)

Centers for Disease Control and Prevention; Workowski KA, Berman SM. Sexually transmitted diseases treatment guidelines, 2006. *MMWR Recomm Rep* 2006;55(RR-11):1–94. [PMID: 16888612]

Metawea B, El-Nashar AR, Kamel I, et al. Application of viable bacille Calmette-Guerin topically as a potential therapeutic modality in condylomata acuminata: A placebo-controlled study. *Urology* 2005;65:247–250. [PMID: 15708031] (Weekly topical application of bacille Calmette-Guérin in the treatment of genital warts attained a high success rate (80–92%) at 6 months compared with the placebo solution, with insignificant side effects and no recurrence.)

Snoeck R, Bossens M, Parent D, et al. Phase II double-blind, placebo-controlled study of the safety and efficacy of cidofovir topical gel for the treatment of patients with human papillomavirus infection. *Clin Infect Dis* 2001;33:597–602. [PMID: 11477525] (Randomized, placebo-controlled trial that found 9 of 19 patients (47%) treated with topical cidofovir gel had a complete response [total healing], compared with none of the patients in the placebo group.)

Prognosis

The natural history of anogenital warts is highly variable. If left untreated, as many as 30% of warts may regress spontaneously within 3 months. If the decision is made to treat, as many as 70% of genital warts may recur within 6 months, depending on the modality of treatment. Recurrence may be a direct result of treatment failure, but the role of reinfection by a sex partner or autoinoculation has not been well elucidated. HIV-infected and other immunocompromised individuals are more likely to have recurrent disease.

PRACTICE POINTS

- One way to differentiate normal anatomic variants such as pearly penile papules from anogenital warts is to look at the base of the lesions. In the normal variants, each normal papilla can be seen to arise from its own base; by contrast, in anogenital warts, multiple papillae typically arise from a single base.

- There is no evidence that one therapeutic modality is superior to another in the treatment of genital warts, and the agent chosen may depend on local availability or experience of the clinician in using a particular treatment modality.

Relevant Web Sites

[CDC fact-sheets, treatment recommendations, and clinician and educational resources regarding HPV-related disease, including genital warts:]

http://www.cdc.gov/std/hpv/default.htm

Gonorrhea

16

Heidi Swygard, MD, MPH, Arlene C. Sena, MD, MPH, Peter Leone, MD, & Myron S. Cohen, MD

ESSENTIALS OF DIAGNOSIS

- In men, findings include urethral discharge, urethral burning with urination, and swelling of the glans penis.
- In women, findings include lower abdominal pain; cervicovaginal discharge, "spotting," and bleeding; and pain with intercourse.
- Disseminated infection produces a rash consisting of papules or pustules with an erythematous border; monoarticular arthritis or tenosynovitis may also be present.
- Definitive diagnosis can be made by Gram stain, culture, molecular probe assay, or nucleic acid amplification testing.

General Considerations

Neisseria gonorrhoeae may cause several adverse health outcomes, including local genitourinary infections, upper reproductive tract disease, and disseminated gonococcal infections. An important impact of *N gonorrhoeae* infection is that it can facilitate acquisition of the human immunodeficiency virus (HIV) and shedding of HIV in semen.

The global incidence of gonorrhea infections remains high, with an estimated 62 million new cases each year. The highest rates occur in sub-Saharan Africa, south and Southeast Asia, the Caribbean, and Latin America. Although the overall prevalence of gonorrhea has declined in the United States since 1975, it remains the second most commonly reported communicable disease. Rates remain high in certain groups, including African-Americans and Hispanics, men who have sex with men (MSM), adolescents, and populations in the southeastern United States. Race in itself is not a risk factor for

gonorrhea but may be a surrogate marker for socioeconomic and behavioral factors that increase the risk for infection.

Screening is an important tool for identifying and treating asymptomatic infection, the most common manifestation of gonorrhea, which serves as a source of ongoing community transmission. In addition to screening efforts directed at women to reduce the complications of untreated disease in this population, routine screening in specific risk groups, such as adolescents, MSM, or HIV-infected individuals is recommended.

Cohen MS, Hoffman IF, Royce RA, et al. Reduction of concentration of HIV-1 in semen after treatment of urethritis: Implications for prevention of sexual transmission of HIV-1. AIDSCAP Malawi Research Group. *Lancet* 1997;349: 1868–1873. [PMID: 9217758]. (Classic article demonstrating the impact of urethritis on seminal HIV viral load.)

Pathogenesis

The transmission of *N gonorrhoeae* following a single episode of vaginal intercourse has been estimated to be approximately 70–80% from male to female partners, and 20–30% from female to male partners. Transmission through either receptive or insertive rectal intercourse may be less efficient than vaginal intercourse but data are limited. Penile-oral and oral-penile transmission is probably the least efficient means of transmission but does occur; again, data on the true frequency of transmission are limited.

Following introduction into a mucosal site, gonococci attach to the surface of columnar epithelial cells and colonize mucosal cells through parasite-directed endocytosis. The exuberant host immune response to gonococcal infection, while leading to control of infection, can account for many of the signs and symptoms of disease.

Edwards JL, Apicella MA. The molecular mechanisms used by Neisseria gonorrhoeae to initiate infection differ between men and women. *Clin Microbiol Rev* 2004;17:965–981. [PMID: 15489357]. (Thorough review of recent advances in understanding gonococcal infection, progression, and transmission from the molecular perspective.)

Prevention

Behavioral interventions remain crucial strategies for reducing the spread of gonorrhea. These include delaying sexual debut and reducing the number of new partners, in addition to consistent condom use.

Consistent male condom use significantly reduces transmission of gonorrhea. A female polyurethane condom is at least as effective as male condoms, but major drawbacks to either type of condom include noncompliance and unacceptability.

All patients with gonorrhea should be retested at 3 months. Sexual contacts must also be identified and given treatment. In most instances, partners are asked to notify their sexual contacts of the need for screening and treatment. Expedited partner treatment programs that allow patients to take medication to their sex partners are increasingly common in many areas.

Research is ongoing in the development of vaginal and rectal microbicides or antimicrobial gels that can be used during sexual intercourse to prevent the transmission of infection.

Howett MK, Kuhl JP. Microbicides for prevention of transmission of sexually transmitted diseases. *Curr Pharm Des* 2005;11:373–346. [PMID: 16305508]. (Good review of mechanisms of action of compounds at phase III or earlier development stages.)

Sanchez J, Campos PE, Courtois B, et al. Prevention of sexually transmitted diseases in female sex workers: Prospective evaluation of condom promotion and strengthened STD services. *Sex Transm Dis* 2003;30:273–279. [PMID: 12671544]. (Provision of periodic STD screening, treatment, condoms, and condom promotion demonstrated efficacy in reducing the burden of STDs in a group of female sex workers.)

Shain RN, Piper JM, Holden AF, et al. Prevention of gonorrhea and chlamydia through behavioral intervention: Results of a two-year controlled randomized trial in minority women. *Sex Transm Dis* 2004;31:401–408. [PMID: 15215694]. (Risk reduction efforts that included optional support groups reduced repeat infections over a 2-year period.)

Clinical Findings

A. Symptoms and Signs

The clinical manifestations of gonorrhea range from (most commonly) asymptomatic or mildly symptomatic disease to (more rarely) disseminated infection. The initial site of infection, infecting strain of *N gonorrhoeae*, host factors, and other coinfections all influence the spectrum of clinical disease experienced by the patient.

1. Men—Although almost half of all gonococcal infections in men are asymptomatic or minimally symptomatic, gonococcal urethritis is the most common manifestation of symptomatic infection. The incubation

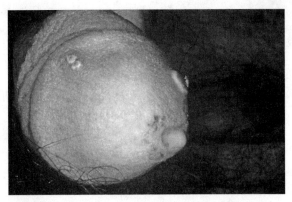

Figure 16–1. Copious mucopurulent urethral discharge is a hallmark of gonococcal urethritis.

period may range from 24 hours to 14 days, but most men develop symptoms (dysuria and discharge) within 4 days of infection (see Figure 16–1). Dysuria usually precedes the development of purulent discharge by approximately 24 hours. Untreated cases of gonococcal urethritis usually resolve over the course of several weeks, with the majority of cases becoming asymptomatic within 6 months.

Widespread availability of effective antimicrobial therapy since the 1940s has made rare most local genitourinary complications in men. Local complications include epididymitis, acute or chronic prostatitis, orchitis, seminal vesiculitis, posterior urethritis, and infection of the Tyson and Cowper glands.

Among MSM, the rectum is the only site of gonococcal infection in 40% of reported cases. Rectal infection may occur through direct inoculation by receptive anal intercourse and is usually asymptomatic. When symptoms occur, they are usually mild, producing only pruritus and painless rectal discharge. Rarely, more severe symptoms, including rectal pain and bloody mucopurulent discharge, may occur. External inspection may reveal few or no signs of infection, and anoscopy with collection of specimens for diagnosis is recommended (see Laboratory Findings, later). Without treatment the patient can carry the infection for months without symptoms.

Pharyngeal infection may occur in up to 10% of MSM who engage in oral-genital contact with an infected partner.

2. Women—The incubation period for gonorrhea in women is usually less than 10 days. Approximately 50% of women have asymptomatic endocervical infection. Clinical presentation includes nonspecific vaginal discharge, abnormal menstrual bleeding, and anorectal discomfort. However, many other sexually transmitted diseases (STDs) in women present with the same symptoms.

Endocervical infection may be accompanied by urethral infection, with dysuria as a symptom. Gonorrhea can be mistaken for acute bacterial cystitis and should be suspected in young, sexually active women with pyuria in the absence of bacteruria. Some experts recommend that all women who present with dysuria should have pelvic and urethral examination for inflammatory exudates, with visualization of the cervix for signs of endocervical involvement, and specimen collection.

Cervicitis is a clinical syndrome defined by the presence of cervical discharge, easy bleeding, or a yellow-greenish discoloration on a swab after insertion into the endocervix. Cervicitis can be caused by *N gonorrhoeae* and several other STDs (see Chapter 10).

Local infection of the endocervix ascends into the uterus, fallopian tubes, or adjacent structures in about 15% of women. Left untreated, this can result in upper reproductive tract infection or pelvic inflammatory disease (PID). Factors that may contribute to upper tract infections include menstruation, newly inserted intrauterine device, douching, adolescence, or previous PID. Clinical signs and symptoms of upper reproductive tract infection with gonorrhea are similar to those found with other intra-abdominal processes. None of the clinical signs and symptoms has both high sensitivity and specificity for PID, and the diagnosis is usually made on clinical grounds.

Pregnancy does not change the clinical presentation of gonorrhea in women. Pregnant women in the second and third trimester have demonstrated a lower incidence of PID. Whether this may represent a "barrier" effect of the products of conception or a change in sexual behaviors as the pregnancy progresses is unclear. Indeed, pregnant women have slightly higher rates of gonococcal pharyngitis that could be a marker for changing sexual behavior. Asymptomatic women may transmit infection throughout their pregnancy and postpartum periods to their sex partners.

Among women with endocervical infection, 10–20% also have pharyngeal infection likely associated with oral sexual exposure. Over 90% of pharyngeal infections are asymptomatic, but symptomatic disease includes an exudative pharyngitis or tonsillitis. Pharyngeal infection clears spontaneously in nearly all cases within 12 weeks of infection. All currently recommended treatment regimens are less efficacious against pharyngeal gonorrhea compared with uncomplicated genitourinary gonorrhea.

Peripartum transmission to the newborn may result in infection of the conjunctiva, rectum, or respiratory tract (see Figure 16–2). Genital or pharyngeal infection in young children is almost always an indication of sexual abuse.

The anorectal area may be the only site of infection in 5% of women. Symptoms are rare but when they occur are similar to those experienced by MSM (pruritus and painless discharge). Another less common presentation of gonorrhea in women is infection of the Bartholin gland duct, which produces local erythema and pus at the posterior third of the labia majora (see Figure 16–3).

3. Disseminated gonococcal infection (DGI)— DGI is a relatively rare manifestation of infection with *N gonorrhoeae*. Most cases occur in persons with asymptomatic mucosal infection and may be due to infection by a distinct strain that is prone to systemic dissemination. Host factors are important for development of DGI. In women, about 70% of disseminated gonococcal disease occurs during menses. Patients with terminal component complement deficiency are particularly susceptible to systemic infection with both *N gonorrhoeae* and *Neisseria meningitidis*.

The bacteremia of DGI typically causes skin lesions. The lesions begin as papules and pustules and sometimes

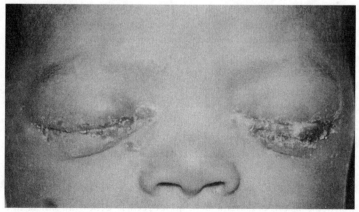

Figure 16–2. Gonococcal ophthalmia neonatorum with crusting and lid edema.

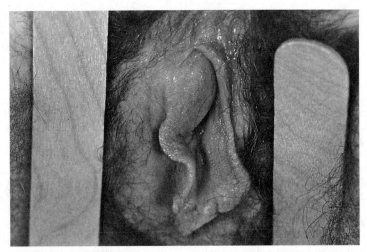

Figure 16–3. Bartholin gland infections may occur as manifestations of gonorrhea in women. Incision and drainage may be required along with antibiotic therapy.

include a hemorrhagic component with surrounding erythema (see Figure 16–4). Lesions are present in 50–75% of patients, but number fewer than 30 lesions in most cases. Other manifestations of DGI include arthritis, pericarditis, endocarditis, and meningitis (each of which is seen in fewer than 3% of patients with DGI). A later manifestation of the DGI-associated arthritis-dermatitis syndrome consists of migratory arthralgias followed by progressive arthritis in one or two joints.

B. LABORATORY FINDINGS

Definitive diagnosis for *N gonorrhoeae* can be made by Gram stain, culture, molecular probe assays, or nucleic acid amplification tests (NAATs). Test performance, available technology, cost, and prevalence of gonorrhea must be taken into account when selecting diagnostic tests to be used for identification of gonococcal infections. Ideally, the test should be highly sensitive, specific, rapid, and inexpensive.

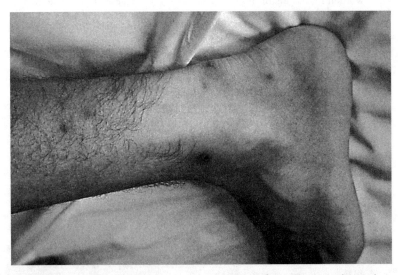

Figure 16–4. The hemorrhagic lesions of disseminated gonococcal infection are similar to those seen in other bacteremias. Culture of these lesions is usually not helpful in establishing the diagnosis.

1. Gram stain—Low cost and rapidity of diagnosis make Gram stain of urethral specimens an important test for the evaluation of gonorrhea, especially in men. A Gram stain is considered positive for *N gonorrhoeae* if neutrophils with intracellular gram-negative diplococci are observed under microscopy (see Figure 16–5). A Gram stain is considered negative in the absence of gram-negative intracellular diplococci, and is equivocal following the observation of extracellular gram-negative or morphologically atypical-appearing organisms.

The sensitivity and specificity of the Gram stain smear varies, depending on the site of infection and the presence or absence of symptoms. For symptomatic urethritis in men, the high sensitivity and specificity (95% and 98%, respectively), suffices for diagnosis. In asymptomatic men, sensitivity is significantly lower and requires culture or other diagnostic tests to rule out gonococcal infection.

Lower sensitivity (40–60%) also occurs in Gram stains of endocervical samples from symptomatic women, although it retains a high specificity in these cases. A presumptive diagnosis of gonorrhea can be made on the basis of a positive smear in women. However high intraobserver variability in preparing and reading endocervical Gram stains renders the finding of a negative Gram stain unreliable. Gram-stained smear of specimens from the rectum, pharynx, and other sites should be used only in conjunction with other diagnostic tests to confirm the diagnosis.

2. Culture—The "gold standard" for detection of *N gonorrhoeae* is culture, although widespread use of NAATs may signify a change in this long-standing standard.

The main benefits of culture are high specificity and the ability to perform antimicrobial susceptibility testing on culture isolates. The disadvantages of culture can be substantial in many areas because of stringent storage and transport requirements of culture media, fastidious growth requirements of *N gonorrhoeae*, and delays in obtaining results.

The yield of gonococcal culture is largely dependent on the anatomic site cultured and the culture media. Selective media contain several antibiotics to prevent the overgrowth of genitourinary, enteric, and oral flora. Modified Thayer-Martin (MTM) is probably the most widely used selective medium, with an overall sensitivity of 80–95% for isolation of *N gonorrhoeae*. Other selective media include NYC (New York City), Martin-Lewis, and GC-Lect. Nonselective media can be used for urethral specimens from men with symptomatic urethritis due to the high concentration of gonococci relative to that of other genital flora.

In women, a single culture of the endocervix is usually sufficient for isolation of gonococci because infection usually involves the cervix. For women who have undergone a hysterectomy, urethral cultures are indicated. Consideration of culturing the accessory gland ducts, pharynx, and rectum should be based on clinical presentation, site of sexual contact, and cost.

The overall yield of blood cultures is less than 30% for DGI, and decreases with duration of clinical illness. This may be due to intermittent, low levels of bacteremia, the extraordinary nutritional requirements of the disseminated gonorrhea strain, and the role of immune complex deposition as a cause of local inflammation. To confirm

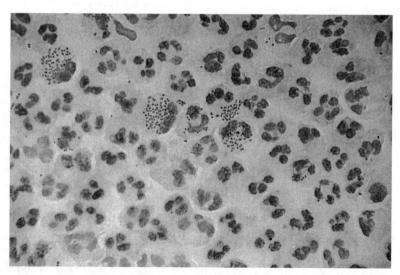

Figure 16–5. Gram-negative intracellular diplococci are visible within the polymorphonuclear cells on this urethral Gram stain.

the diagnosis of DGI, cultures should be obtained from all mucosal sites. In over 80% of patients, gonococci can be isolated from genital, rectal, or pharyngeal cultures. In cases where cultures are negative from all mucosal sites, isolation of *N gonorrhoeae* from sex partners may be the only means of confirming the diagnosis.

3. Molecular methods—Gonococcal infections can be diagnosed with other methods, including immunofluorescence assays and DNA probes. These diagnostic methods can offer quicker results and higher sensitivity than culture. DNA probe assays for *N gonorrhoeae* have reported sensitivity of 93–99% and specificity of 98–99.5%.

NAATs for *N gonorrhoeae* involve amplification of specific DNA or RNA sequences by polymerase chain reaction, strand displacement assay (SDA), or transcription-mediated assay (TMA). Commercially developed ligase chain reaction tests for *N gonorrhoeae* are no longer available.

The sensitivity and specificity of NAATs are comparable to urethral and endocervical culture. Advantages of NAATs are multiple and include decreased time to results; use with noninvasive urine specimens and self-collected vaginal swabs; identification of coinfecting *C trachomatis* (depending on manufacturer); and, for TMA and SDA, excellent performance diagnosing anorectal and pharyngeal infections. Urine-based testing permits screening of populations in nontraditional settings and may be more acceptable to patients. Self-collected vaginal swabs have also demonstrated good sensitivity and increased patient acceptability.

The primary disadvantage of NAATs is the inability to perform antimicrobial susceptibility testing for *N gonorrhoeae* from clinical specimens. In the future, commercially available NAATs may identify resistance genes.

With specificity less than 100%, NAATs can generate false-positive results when screening is performed in low prevalence populations. Caution must therefore be given to the interpretation of results when screening asymptomatic persons in low prevalence populations.

Garlan SM, Tabrizi SN. Diagnosis of sexually transmitted infections using self-collected noninvasive specimens. *Sex Health* 2004;1:121–126. [PMID: 16334994]. (Good review of the utility of self-collected specimens for various STDs.)

Katz AR, Effler PV, Ohye RG, et al. False positive gonorrhea test results with a nucleic acid amplification test: The impact of low prevalence on positive predictive value. *Clin Infect Dis* 2004;38:814–818. [PMID: 14999624]. (Demonstration of the importance of STD history and knowledge of local gonorrhea prevalence for interpretation of positive results in patients in whom the positive result was unexpected.)

Phipps W, Stanley H, Kohn R, et al. Syphilis, chlamydia and gonorrhea screening in HIV-infected patients in primary care, San Francisco, California, 2003. *AIDS Patient Care STDS* 2005:19:495–498. [PMID: 16124843]. (Excellent demonstration of the importance of screening for disease and obtaining specimens from multiple anatomic sites.)

Stary A, Ching SF, Teodorwicz L, et al. Comparison of ligase chain reaction and culture for detection of Neisseria gonorrhoeae in genital and extragenital specimens. *J Clin Microbiol* 1997; 35:239–242. [PMID: 8968915]. (One of the earliest reports demonstrating the superior sensitivity of NAAT methods compared with culture for genitourinary and extragenitourinary gonorrhea.)

Differential Diagnosis

The differential diagnosis for patients presenting with signs or symptoms of gonorrhea include other STDs and genitourinary syndromes (*C trachomatis, Trichomonas vaginalis, Mycoplasma genitalium, Ureaplasma urealyticum*). For women, the list also includes bacterial vaginosis, cervical herpes simplex infection, and candidiasis. Coinfection with other STDs further complicates the differential diagnosis.

For women presenting with vaginal or cervical symptoms, noninfectious causes to be considered in the differential diagnosis include retained foreign body, chemical irritation, allergic reaction, endocervical polyp, physical trauma, vesicovaginal or rectovaginal fistula, carcinoma, and leukorrhea of pregnancy. Additionally, hormones, age, and other factors can influence the presentation of vaginal discharge.

The differential diagnosis for men presenting with urethritis should include and urinary tract infection or prostatitis in men aged 35 years or older. The causes of prostatitis and prostadynia are beyond the scope of this chapter. Another genitourinary syndrome that can accompany urethritis in men in epididymitis, which may result from STDs, trauma or chemical irritation. Consultation with a urologist may be indicated.

For women presenting with PID, the differential diagnosis remains broad and includes ectopic pregnancy, urinary tract infection, pyelonephritis, appendicitis, proctocolitis, and endometriosis.

The differential diagnosis for patients presenting with DGI is extensive and must include meningococcemia, ecthyma gangrenosum, and other causes of bacteremia. Classic signs associated with bacteremia (high fever, leukocytosis, systemic toxicity) are usually absent in DGI.

The arthritis of DGI can be difficult to distinguish clinically from other causes of infectious arthritides (eg, staphylococcal, streptococcal). Synovial fluid cultures are usually sterile but demonstrate cell counts and chemistries consistent with septic arthritis. The chances of a positive culture increase when the synovial fluid is purulent.

Complications

PID requires prompt treatment to reduce the incidence of chronic infection and infertility (see When to Refer to a Specialist, later). The likelihood of infertility increases with the number of episodes of PID: 11% among women with one episode, 23% with two episodes, and

75% with three or more episodes of PID. Other sequelae include chronic pelvic pain and ectopic pregnancy.

Other urogenital complications from gonorrhea in women include perihepatitis (Fitz-Hugh-Curtis syndrome). This syndrome presents as acute right or bilateral upper quadrant tenderness, frequently with signs and symptoms of PID.

Ocular infection with gonorrhea in adults can threaten sight. Gonococcal conjunctivitis usually occurs with concomitant, or at least recent, genitourinary gonorrhea. Gonococcal ophthalmia resulting from accidental inoculation has shown excellent response to ceftriaxone, 1.0 g intramuscularly as a single dose.

Gonococcal arthritis, the most common complication of DGI, can present as monoarticular or pauciarticular arthritis. An important clinical finding that can distinguish gonococcal arthritis from other infectious causes is an accompanying tenosynovitis, which often occurs over the involved joint and may include erythema.

Bardin T. Gonococcal arthritis. *Best Pract Res Clin Rheumatol* 2003;17:201–208. [PMID: 12787521]. (Concise review of the clinical and diagnostic issues of gonococcal arthritis.)

Treatment

Treatment regimens for uncomplicated gonorrhea should cure at least 95% of genitourinary infections by a single dose of therapy (see Table 16–1).

Table 16–1. Recommended treatment regimens for gonorrhea based on US and European STD treatment guidelines.

	Drug	Special Considerations
Uncomplicated (cervical, urethral, rectal) infection	Ceftriaxone, 125 mg IM as a single dose[a] *or* Cefpodoxime, 400 mg PO as a single dose *or* Ciprofloxacin, 500 mg PO as a single dose[b] *or* Cefixime, 400 mg PO as a single dose[c]	Co-treat for *Chlamydia* unless excluded Any of these regimens may be used for gonococcal pharyngitis; few regimens reliably cure >90% pharyngeal gonorrhea

Pregnant women	Ceftriaxone, 125 mg IM as a single dose	Co-treat for *Chlamydia* using:
		 • Azithromycin, 1 g PO as a single dose
		    or
		 • Erythromycin base, 500 mg PO 4 times daily
		    or
		 • Amoxicillin 500 mg PO 3 times daily unless excluded
		 Use spectinomycin for women who cannot receive ceftriaxone
		 Obtain "test of cure" >7 d after treatment

Alternative regimens	Spectinomycin, 2.0 g IM as a single dose[c] *or* Kanamycin, 2.0 g IM as a single dose *or* Gentamicin, 240 mg IM as a single dose	Spectinomycin is not effective against pharyngeal gonorrhea

[a]Other single-dose second- and third-generation cephalosporins have no advantage over ceftriaxone.
[b]Other single-dose fluoroquinolones have no advantage over ciprofloxacin, although data regarding their use for gonorrhea is limited. Fluoroquinolones are not recommended for use in patients in California and Hawaii, or in men who have sex with men, due to increased incidences of fluoroquinolone-resistant *N gonorrhoeae* in these populations.
[c]Limited availability in the United States in 2006.

A. Antimicrobial Resistance

Reduced susceptibility to antimicrobials has been reported since the early 1950s and has continued to evolve and spread since that time. The reasons for the development of resistance are complex but can be attributed to four major factors: (1) poor compliance with prescribed therapy, (2) inadequate dosing of antibiotics, (3) circumstances causing low or inadequate antibiotic serum levels, and (4) conditions favoring the selection of resistance mutations (eg, widespread use of antimicrobial agents).

Treatment with penicillin and tetracycline is unreliable in much of the world due to the appearance of penicillinase-producing *N gonorrhoeae*, plasmid-mediated high-level tetracycline-resistant *N gonorrhoeae*, and chromosomally mediated penicillin and tetracycline-resistant *N gonorrhoeae*.

In reaction to widespread penicillin and tetracycline resistance, the Centers for Disease Control and Prevention in 1987 ceased to recommend these agents for treatment of gonorrhea and began advocating the use of third-generation cephalosporins and selected fluoroquinolones. Ceftriaxone continues to be effective, with no reported resistance. The only currently available oral third-generation cephalosporin in the US is cefpodoxime. Some oral second-generation cephalosporins may be used for therapy of uncomplicated gonorrhea (see Relevant World Wide Web Sites).

Fluoroquinolone resistance has been noted in the Far East, Australia, Africa, Europe, and, most recently, the United States. Ciprofloxacin-resistant strains are becoming more widespread throughout the United States. In 2006, fluoroquinolones are not recommended for gonorrhea treatment in Hawaii and California, nor are they recommended in MSM.

B. Treatment Recommendations

1. Uncomplicated infections—Specific treatment recommendations for uncomplicated gonococcal infections in patients are shown in Table 16–1. Because pharyngeal infections with *N gonorrhoeae* can be difficult to eradicate, few regimens reliably cure more than 90% of these infections.

All sex partners who have had contact with the infected patient (within 60 days of diagnosis) should be examined and treated. Additionally, patients and their sexual contacts should be offered HIV counseling and testing at the time of gonorrhea diagnosis. Routine "test of cure" is not indicated following treatment for uncomplicated gonorrhea with currently recommended cephalosporin regimens; however, patients who remain symptomatic after treatment should be reexamined and tested. Patients treated with a fluoroquinolone in areas with increased levels of fluoroquinolone resistance should also have a test of cure. All patients diagnosed with gonorrhea should be tested to rule out repeat infection

3–4 months after treatment. Unless coinfection with *C trachomatis* has been excluded, treatment for chlamydia is recommended as a part of all gonorrhea treatment regimens.

2. PID—Most PID is caused by *N gonorrhoeae, C trachomatis,* or gram-negative bacilli. Therapy should include drugs active against these organisms as well as anaerobes. Most women receive outpatient therapy that should be limited to nonpregnant, compliant women with mild to moderate disease. Women treated with outpatient regimens should be advised to return within 3 days to follow up response to therapy. Inpatient management of PID should begin with intravenous antibiotics that may be switched ultimately to an oral regimen.

3. Ophthalmia neonatorum—Gonococcal ophthalmia neonatorum can be prevented by routine screening for endocervical infection during pregnancy and by the prophylactic use of 1% silver nitrate, erythromycin, or tetracycline ophthalmic solution. These agents may not be available in developing countries. A single application of 2.5% povidone–iodine is an inexpensive alternative with a broad spectrum of activity against chlamydia, gonorrhea, HIV, and herpes simplex. Given the high rates of tetracycline-resistant *N gonorrhoeae*, tetracycline may no longer be adequate as prophylactic therapy.

4. DGI—Patients with DGI require hospitalization for observation of response to therapy and to assure adherence with the treatment regimen. The recommended initial regimen for DGI is ceftriaxone, 1 g intramuscularly or intravenously every 24 hours for 7 days. In patients with a prompt clinical response to therapy and whose adherence is likely, therapy can be completed on an outpatient basis. If a patient is allergic to cephalosporins, consultation with an infectious disease specialist is recommended (see When to Refer to a Specialist, later).

Isenberg SJ, Apt L, Wood M. A controlled trial of povidone-iodine as prophylaxis against ophthalmia neonatorum. *N Engl J Med* 1995;332:562–566. [PMID: 7838190]. (Classic article demonstrating the effectiveness of the less-expensive povidone-iodine solution for prevention of this serious gonococcal complication.)

Woods CR. Gonococcal infections in neonates and young children. *Semin Pediatr Infect Dis* 2005;16:258–270. [PMID: 16210106]. (Good review of gonorrheal infections in children, with a discussion of some of the medicolegal aspects involved in caring for infected children.)

When to Refer to a Specialist

Most uncomplicated genitourinary gonorrhea responds well to single-dose therapy. Consultation with an infectious disease specialist should be obtained for infections suspected of antimicrobial resistance, poor therapeutic response, or requiring repeated courses of oral or intravenous therapy, or when serious sequelae have developed.

Inpatient management of PID or of pregnant women with other complications of gonococcal infection should be carried out in conjunction with an infectious disease or obstetrician-gynecologist consultant to prevent further complications or adverse outcomes for the fetus. Most women with PID who have demonstrated clinical improvement (afebrile for 24 hours, able to tolerate oral regimens) may be switched to an oral regimen. Therapy should be continued to complete a 14-day course.

Ocular infections that do not respond to single-dose therapy should be referred immediately for ophthalmologic evaluation because of the risk of severe ulcerative keratitis and potential for visual impairment.

Patients with suppurative arthritis from gonorrhea should be hospitalized and managed in consultation with infectious disease and orthopedic specialists, especially in instances where the diagnosis is in doubt. Effusions may require frequent aspirations until they have ceased to accumulate.

Rare manifestations of DGI, meningitis, and endocarditis with *N gonorrhoeae* require high-dose intravenous therapy with a highly active agent that achieves adequate tissue levels in the site of infection. These systemic manifestations of gonorrhea infection should be managed in conjunction with an infectious disease specialist.

Prognosis

In general, cure rates for uncomplicated genitourinary gonorrhea exceed 95% with single-dose treatments. An important part of this high cure rate includes concomitant treatment of sex partners to prevent reinfections. However, it must be understood that high-risk sexual behaviors will continue to put the patient at risk of gonorrhea and other STDs, including HIV. Reinfection with

N gonorrhoeae is possible, because there is no conferred immunity from prior infections. Patients should be counseled on risk-reduction methods to prevent subsequent infections. Resolution of symptoms of PID or DGI usually occurs within 24–48 hours of initiation of therapy.

PRACTICE POINTS

- *All patients diagnosed with gonorrhea should be tested to rule out repeat infection 3–4 months after treatment. Unless coinfection with C trachomatis has been excluded, treatment for chlamydia is recommended as a part of all gonorrhea treatment regimens.*

Relevant Web Sites

[American Social Health Organization:]
http://www.ashastd.org
[Centers for Disease Control and Prevention, Division of STD Prevention:]
http://www.cdc.gov/std
[National Institute of Allergy and Infectious Disease, Division of Microbiology and Infectious Diseases:]
http://www.niaid.nih.gov/dmid/stds/
[World Health Organization, Sexually Transmitted Diseases Diagnostics Initiative:]
http://www.who.int/std_diagnostics/

Lymphogranuloma Venereum

17

Christopher S. Hall, MD, MS

ESSENTIALS OF DIAGNOSIS

- *In North America, lymphogranuloma venereum typically presents as a proctitis syndrome; elsewhere, genital ulcer disease followed by inguinal lymphadenopathy with or without bubo formation may predominate.*
- *Diagnostic tests include culture and typing for* Chlamydia trachomatis *and molecular assays.*
- *Patients should be asked about gender of sex partners and travel to areas of endemic disease or outbreaks, and behavioral risk assessment should be performed to elicit risks for transmission.*
- *In patients with suspected infection, screening for other STDs, including HIV, is warranted.*

General Considerations

Lymphogranuloma venereum (LGV) is a systemic sexually transmitted disease (STD) caused by L1, L2, and L3 serovars (subtypes) of *Chlamydia trachomatis*. LGV occurs worldwide as several clinical syndromes, the most common of which are characterized by papules or ulcers with inguinal lymphadenopathy, followed by proctitis (see Table 17–1). Although LGV is classically an invasive, inflammatory infection, patients may present without significant lymphadenopathy or with mild symptoms. Asymptomatic infection also has been observed.

LGV is endemic in some regions (Africa, Southeast Asia, Central and South America, and Caribbean countries) while occurring sporadically in others. It remains infrequent in the United States. However, case clusters have been reported in the northern hemisphere since 2002. Notably, an outbreak of 92 cases of proctitis caused by LGV was described among men who have sex with men (MSM) in the Netherlands in 2003–2004. Since then, case clusters have been reported in Belgium, France,

Sweden, and Canada, with fewer than two dozen confirmed cases reported throughout the United States by 2005.

Recent outbreaks and case clusters demonstrate the need for heightened awareness of this STD in the United States. LGV should be considered in those at risk for STDs, especially MSM and others reporting unprotected receptive anal intercourse who present with rectal complaints or lymphadenopathy. Such patients, along with any patient with a compatible clinical presentation, should be asked about travel to areas of endemic disease or outbreaks. Given the ulcerative nature of this more invasive chlamydial infection, the risk of facilitating HIV acquisition and transmission is thought to be higher.

In the United States, poorly standardized serologic tests lacking specificity and limited availability of tissue culture and molecular tests for rectal evaluation complicate both diagnosis and measurement of the true incidence of LGV. Although the incidence of fulminant LGV has dramatically decreased in industrialized countries since the advent of antibiotics, at least one researcher has suggested a low but persistent endemicity of LGV among those at risk for rectal chlamydial infection, particularly MSM.

Schachter J, Moncada J. Lymphogranuloma venereum: How to turn an endemic disease into an outbreak of a new disease? Start looking. *Sex Transm Dis* 2005;32:331–332. [PMID: 15912077] (Report demonstrating prevalent LGV infection in men in San Francisco since the 1980s and suggesting that recent case-finding, rather than transmission, may be contributing to the increased prevalence.)

Pathogenesis

C trachomatis is an obligate intracellular microorganism that is dependent on the host cell for ATP production and replication. The organism is surrounded by an outer membrane mainly composed of a major outer membrane protein (MOMP). Eighteen serovars of *C trachomatis* are classified according to the *Omp 1* gene encoding MOMP. The trachoma biovar includes serovars A through K and

Table 17-1. Characteristic syndromes associated with lymphogranuloma venereum.

Syndrome	Pertinent History	Symptoms
Lymphadenopathy syndrome		
Primary stage	Incubation 3–30 d	• Typically small, painless genital papule with or without urethritis or cervicitis that may ulcerate • Usually unrecognized by patient and resolves without treatment
Secondary stage	Occurs 2–6 wk after primary stage	• One or more regional lymph nodes that may ulcerate (ie, bubo); inguinal or femoral nodes may cause "groove" sign • One third of buboes may rupture • Genital ulcers may be manifest concurrently with lymphadenitis
Proctitis and proctocolitis	Risk factors include anal intercourse or other anal penetration	• Rectal discharge, bleeding, pain on defecation (tenesmus), and later, frank colitis; inguinal lymph node involvement is unusual • Fever or other constitutional symptoms (ie, weight loss, fatigue) may be present

is responsible for infections involving mucosa of the genital tract and the eye. Serovars L1, L2 (L2a/L2b), and L3 comprise the LGV biovar, which is more invasive, involving proliferation in lymphoid tissues.

Prevention

Prevention of LGV requires a multipronged strategy of promoting risk reduction among those likeliest to contract the infection, treating those diagnosed as well as those at high risk with a compatible clinical syndrome, and identifying and presumptively treating exposed sex partners who may have been infected.

Providers should assess sexual risk behaviors of patients by asking about number and gender of partners, sexual behaviors engaged in, and use of condoms. The primary risk factor identified for transmission of LGV is unprotected receptive anal intercourse or other penetration (eg, "fisting"), highlighting the importance of providers asking about such practices in routine, periodic sexual risk assessments. Tools to assist providers with risk assessment are available from the California STD/HIV Prevention Training Center (*http://www.stidhivtraining.org/pdf/ask-screen-intervene*).

HIV-infected MSM have been most often affected in recent outbreaks of LGV proctitis in Europe. For instance, in the well-characterized Netherlands outbreak in 2003–2004, 92 confirmed cases were observed, following a prior average of 5 LGV cases per year. All patients were MSM, and among those whose HIV status was known, 77% were HIV-positive. Most patients presented with lower gastrointestinal symptoms, including mucopurulent—sometimes bloody—anal discharge and other symptoms of proctitis. Only one patient had a genital ulcer or bubo. Six of 13 patients with concurrent STDs had gonorrhea, herpes simplex virus (HSV), syphilis, or chronic hepatitis B. In all cases, LGV was associated with serum antibodies to *C trachomatis* and rectal *C trachomatis* isolates of the L1–L3 serovar subtype, but chlamydial DNA was not found in urethral specimens, such that this common diagnostic approach would not have led to recognition of chlamydial LGV in these patients. Among the 62 cases reported in 2004, LGV was temporally associated with HIV seroconversion in 2 patients, and with recent acquisition of hepatitis C infection in 5 others.

Other European case clusters in 2004–2005 were observed in Paris, Antwerp, Hamburg, and elsewhere, including the United Kingdom. Similarly, all patients were MSM, and more than half were HIV-positive.

These case clusters and reports have demonstrated the significance of local sexual networks in transmission of this STD while highlighting the barriers to accurate diagnosis of rectal infections, including LGV. The potential facilitation of HIV acquisition and transmission in the setting of an inflammatory rectal infection has heightened concerns about possible increases in LGV incidence, while surveillance challenges—including the lack of a standard case definition—make sentinel detection of incipient LGV clusters difficult.

Following the northern hemisphere cases of LGV, the US Centers for Disease Control and Prevention (CDC) established a targeted surveillance effort to identify incident cases in the United States and to advise clinicians on appropriate diagnosis and treatment of LGV (*http://www.cdc.gov/std/lgv*). By 2005, fewer than two dozen cases had been identified in the United States, and case clusters driven by sexual networks and international travel had not been identified.

A. Significance of Rectal Infections

Notwithstanding the limited recognition of LGV in the United States in recent years, it should be emphasized that diagnosis of any sexually transmitted rectal infection in an HIV-uninfected individual should be considered a sentinel event with respect to elevated risk of HIV acquisition. Such a diagnosis necessitates education, ongoing risk assessment and risk reduction counseling, and screening for other STDs and HIV, with follow-up screening 3 months after diagnosis.

B. Reporting

In the United States, *C trachomatis* infection is a reportable disease, and LGV cases should be reported according to standard local regulations. In general, given the still rare incidence of LGV in the United States, providers should contact their local health departments to advise them of suspected cases.

C. Treatment of Sex Partners

Once the diagnosis is confirmed in infected individuals, sex partners within the prior 30 days should be clinically evaluated and, if symptomatic, managed as if potentially infected with LGV. If asymptomatic, sex partners should be treated with either oral doxycycline, 100 mg twice daily for 7 days, or a single 1-g oral dose of azithromycin.

Centers for Disease Control and Prevention (CDC). Lymphogranuloma venereum among men who have sex with men—Netherlands, 2003–2004. *MMWR Morb Mortal Wkly Rep* 2004;53:985–988. [PMID: 15514580] (Report of cases of LGV infection in European men who have sex with men.)

Nieuwenhuis RF, Ossewaarde JM, Götz HM, et al. Resurgence of lymphogranuloma venereum in western Europe: An outbreak of *Chlamydia trachomatis* serovar L2 proctitis in the Netherlands among men who have sex with men. *Clin Infect Dis* 2004;39:996–1003. [PMID: 15472852] (Outstanding epidemiologic, clinical, microbiologic report describing clinical and radiographic findings of new cases of LGV in men in Europe.)

Clinical Findings

LGV is a systemic infection that varies in its clinical presentation. Classic presentations include the rarely observed genital papular form accompanied by lymphadenopathy, as well as a proctitis syndrome. The infection may present without lymphadenopathy, and asymptomatic disease may also occur.

A. Signs and Symptoms

1. Primary stage—Primary LGV infection may present as a small genital papule or ulcer, appearing 3–30 days after exposure, and healing in several days to a week. The lesion may involve the glans or shaft of the penis, urethra, vulva or vagina, anus or rectum, or perineum and adjacent skin. Like the chancre of syphilis, the primary LGV lesion is typically painless and often may clear prior to recognition by the patient, often without leaving a scar. Case series suggest that patients are rarely identified at this stage of infection.

2. Secondary stage—Occurring days to weeks after primary infection, the secondary stage is systemic and involves extension to lymph nodes. When primary lesions are penile, vulvar, or perianal, inguinal or femoral lymphadenopathy is seen (see Figure 17–1). Nodal involvement is unilateral in two thirds of cases. Simultaneous enlargement of inguinal and femoral nodes leads to the pathognomonic "groove sign," formed by the delineation of these nodes by the inguinal ligament (see Figure 17–2). Initially discrete lymph node enlargement occurs, with tenderness; inflammation may then spread to adjacent tissue, with development of an inflamed mass and matting of nodes.

Abscess formation within such an inflammatory mass constitutes a bubo, which may rupture spontaneously or develop subcutaneous loculations or sinus tracts. Ruptured buboes may drain thick exudates for weeks prior to resolution, despite treatment. Nodes that do

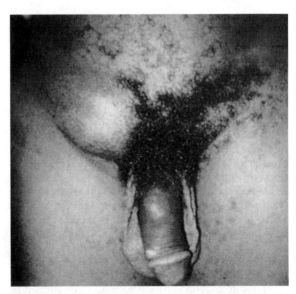

Figure 17–1. Early inguinal sign of lymphogranuloma venereum showing superficial, primary preputial erosion, dorsal penile lymphangitis, and right inguinal bubo. (Reproduced, with permission, from Holmes KK et al. *Sexually Transmitted Diseases*, 3rd ed. McGraw-Hill, 1999.)

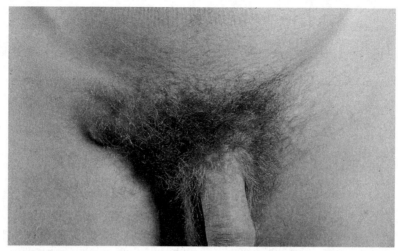

Figure 17–2. Striking tender lymphadenopathy occurring at the femoral and inguinal lymph nodes separated by a groove made by Poupart's ligament (groove sign) (Reproduced, with permission, from Wolff K, Johnson RA, Summond D. *Fitzpatrick's Color Atlas and Synopsis of Clinical Dermatology*, 5th ed. McGraw-Hill, 2005.)

not rupture may form indurated masses that resolve only in months.

At this stage, systemic manifestations may occur, including fever, chills, night sweats, headache, malaise, and myalgias. A mild leukocytosis may be observed. Although meningismus may be present and chlamydiae have been recovered from the cerebrospinal fluid of patients with secondary LGV, clinically significant neurologic site involvement is a rare feature.

3. LGV proctitis—The proctitis syndrome, more commonly seen in MSM, is characterized by rectal discharge, bleeding, and painful inflammation progressing to proctitis or proctocolitis. Symptoms may be mild, involving only perianal pruritus, scant rectal discharge, or constipation. Often patients describe frequent yet unsuccessful attempts at defecation that are painful (ie, tenesmus). Patients with such complaints in the primary care setting should undergo simple anoscopy, which may reveal exudates as well as diffuse friability and discrete ulcerations of the visualized rectal mucosa.

Symptoms may mimic those of inflammatory bowel disease and may be mistaken for Crohn disease, in particular; in such cases, the presentation often prompts referral and workup involving endoscopy, revealing findings similar to those seen on anoscopy. Of concern in such cases, gross pathologic changes on endoscopy are not specific for LGV, and rectal specimens for microbiologic evaluation may not be obtained uniformly, impeding the diagnosis of LGV. Histopathologic findings from rectal biopsies are not specific for LGV and include extensive inflammation, granulomata, and crypt abscesses, as observed in Crohn disease.

Nodal involvement accompanying proctitis also occurs, but affected nodes following rectal infection are iliac and thus unrecognized on physical examination. However, involvement of deep pelvic or lumbar nodes can give rise to lower abdominal and back pain.

B. Laboratory Findings

Given the limitations of current laboratory assays, the diagnosis of LGV in the United States is presumptive, relying on clinical recognition of suspected cases in patients with epidemiologic risk factors, supported by laboratory test evidence, along with exclusion of other causes of lymphadenopathy or proctitis syndromes.

1. Issues in laboratory diagnosis of LGV—In the United States, laboratory diagnosis of LGV is challenged by lack of availability of tests specific for LGV. Quantitative serologic tests have been the mainstay of LGV diagnosis in the past; however, the titer level specific to predict LGV infection is uncertain, and use of serology is being eclipsed by the rapid development of more specific and practical nucleic acid amplification tests (NAATs). Furthermore, there is no definitive serologic test specific for the L1–L3 serovars of *C trachomatis* responsible for LGV.

At present, commercially available NAATs for *C trachomatis* do not distinguish LGV serovars from the more common non-LGV chlamydial serovars (B and D–K); these tests are not yet cleared by the Food and Drug Administration (FDA) for use on rectal specimens, and their availability is limited albeit increasing. *C trachomatis* tissue culture cannot reliably distinguish LGV strains from other non-LGV strains; in addition, culture is less sensitive than NAATs. DNA sequencing by LGV-specific polymerase chain reaction (PCR) testing can be performed on culture isolates or the DNA extracted from a NAAT specimen but such tests are performed, to date, only by CDC and select research laboratories.

Timing of laboratory tests for LGV is problematic, because typical turnaround for serologic and other test results may exceed 7 days. Thus, clinicians must decide when to extend therapy beyond the typical 1-week course for non-LGV *C trachomatis* infection, often prior to receipt of test results that may support or confirm the diagnosis of LGV. Presumptive treatment of suspected LGV cases may by discontinued if all serologic and other test results for *C trachomatis* are negative prior to the conclusion of the 3-week course of treatment for LGV.

Importantly, standard procedure should be followed to conduct additional testing or screening in patients evaluated for LGV, including testing for *C trachomatis* and gonorrhea at appropriate sites and serum testing for syphilis, HSV, and HIV.

2. Swab specimens—In patients with suspected LGV, providers should collect swab specimens of the rectum (in those with proctitis) or other draining ulcers and nodes for laboratory testing. A swab specimen of a rectal lesion visualized by anoscopy is of greater microbiologic yield than a "blind" rectal swab. In addition, especially if *C trachomatis*- or LGV-specific NAAT testing is not available, serologic testing may aid in diagnosis, although cross-reactivity with non-LGV chlamydial species on some assays and turnaround time remain limitations. In patients with severe proctitis, HSV should be considered, especially in HIV-infected patients, and a rectal swab for HSV culture or PCR testing should be collected.

3. Serologic tests—Serologic tests for *C trachomatis* infection provide antibody evidence of systemic infection (see Table 17–2). These tests are not specific for LGV,

Table 17–2. Serologic tests for diagnosis of chlamydia.

Test	Description
Microimmunofluorescence	Species-specific test Titer ≥1:256 is suggestive of *Chlamydia trachomatis* infection
Complement fixation	Genus-specific test Positive 2 wk after infection Titer ≥1:64 is suggestive of lymphogranuloma venereum High background rate of low-titer reactors

although high titer results are commonly seen in LGV. As such, they provide indirect support for a clinical diagnosis of LGV. According to the CDC, serologic test criteria for LGV in a patient with a clinical presentation consistent with LGV include a high-titer positive result on serologic test for *C trachomatis*, such as microimmunofluorescence (ie, typically ≥1:256, but can vary by laboratory) or complement fixation (ie, titer ≥1:64). Most experts recommend use of a microimmunofluorescence assay employing purified elementary bodies as antigens. However, serologic tests available in the United States often are based on enzyme immunoassays that do not provide quantitative, titer-based results and are generally not recommended.

Furthermore, some experts believe that serologic tests for *C trachomatis* are of insufficient specificity for LGV to recommend their widespread use in diagnosing this infection, given cross-reactivity with non-LGV chlamydial species on some assays and questions about background *C trachomatis* antibody levels in persons at high risk for LGV infection.

4. Culture—Several tests are available to evaluate for the presence of *Chlamydia* (non-LGV and LGV; Table 17–3). *Chlamydia* culture can provide direct evidence of *C trachomatis* infection. However, this test is costly and may not be available in many clinical settings. If available, DNA sequencing of culture isolates by LGV-specific PCR and serotyping of isolates using a monoclonal antibody can be performed in research laboratories to determine whether a *C trachomatis* isolate is an LGV subtype.

5. Molecular methods—Commercially available NAATs for *Chlamydia* (eg, BDProbeTec [strand displacement amplification; SDA], Gen-Probe APTIMA [transcription-mediated amplification; TMA], and Roche Amplicor [PCR]) also provide direct evidence of *C trachomatis* but do not distinguish between LGV and more common chlamydial strains (serovars B and D–K). At present, these tests are not FDA-cleared for rectal (or pharyngeal) site specimens, limiting their widespread availability, yet select laboratories have internally verified the assays for testing these specimen types. DNA sequencing of isolates by LGV-specific PCR can be performed in research laboratories to determine whether a strain is LGV-related.

If the result on laboratory-validated *C trachomatis* NAAT is positive, LGV-specific PCR testing should be performed on a reflex basis. LGV-specific PCR testing is available through the CDC via public health laboratories, and real-time assays are being developed for use in regional laboratories.

Barring access to LGV-specific PCR testing to confirm LGV in a *C trachomatis*–positive rectal specimen (culture or NAAT), such a positive result itself is generally suggestive of LGV in a patient with severe proctitis when other etiologies (eg, *Neisseria gonorrhoeae* and

Table 17–3. Diagnostic tests of ulcers, buboes, and rectal site for direct identification of *Chlamydia* and lymphogranuloma venereum.

Test	Description
Swab specimen	Swab of rectal mucosa (on anoscopy or "blind") or exudate from ulcer or bubo
Chlamydia culture	Provides evidence of *C trachomatis* Costly and not often available in many local laboratories DNA sequencing of culture isolates to identify LGV is performed at select labs.

Nucleic acid–based tests for *Chlamydia*:
  BCProbeTec (SDA)
  Gen-Probe APTIMA (TMA)
  Roche Amplicor (PCR)
	Provide direct evidence of *C trachomatis*
	Commercially available NAATs are not specific for LGV, not yet FDA-cleared for rectal site, and thus not widely available, but select laboratories have validated these tests for this anatomic site

Nucleic acid–based tests for LGV: PCR for LGV	Provide direct evidence of LGV Not FDA-cleared for clinical use, but select reference laboratories (eg, CDC and some regional public health laboratories) conduct this test

LGV, lymphogranuloma venereum; NAAT, nucleic acid amplification test; PCR, polymerase chain reaction; SDA, strand displacement amplification; TMA, transcription-mediated amplification.

HSV) have been excluded. The spectrum of symptoms associated with LGV versus non-LGV *C trachomatis* infection of the rectum has yet to be precisely elucidated. In these cases, many practitioners would complete a 21-day course of therapy for LGV, given the impracticality of ruling out infection with an LGV-specific serovar of *C trachomatis*.

C. IMAGING STUDIES

In general, radiographic and ultrasonographic imaging modalities are not routine in the evaluation of patients with STDs. Given the atypical presentation of LGV compared with non-LGV *C trachomatis* infection, especially those stages characterized by ulcerative lymphadenopathy and proctocolitis, severe clinical presentations may result in workups that include such procedures. Lymphoid masses in severe disease may mimic lymphoma, especially in HIV-infected patients, and computed tomography (CT) is useful to ensure regional limitation of lymphadenopathy. In late-stage LGV involving fistula formation and strictures, CT scanning along with dye studies may be necessary to characterize anatomic defects.

D. SPECIAL EXAMINATIONS

Patients with severe proctitis may be referred for gastroenterologic evaluation, including lower endoscopy. Findings associated with LGV on sigmoidoscopy and colonoscopy include mucopurulent exudate, diffuse erythema and friability of rectal mucosa, discrete ulcerations, and inflammatory masses, although there is no constellation of findings that is specific for LGV.

Differential Diagnosis

Differential diagnosis includes a variety of entities, depending on the clinical stage of LGV. The typical LGV primary lesion differs from the chancre of primary syphilis in that the latter often is larger, with indurated edges, and may occur as multiple ulcers; both lesions are typically painless and can be accompanied by unilateral or bilateral regional adenopathy. The typical ulcer of chancroid is excavated and painful; extensive adenopathy may be seen in both LGV and chancroid.

In secondary LGV infection characterized by lymphadenopathy, the differential diagnosis includes syphilis, HSV, chancroid, and, especially in the case of HIV-infected individuals, lymphoma. HSV is more likely to manifest with vesicular, painful, and often multiple lesions; the regional adenopathy of HSV is often tender.

For disease characterized by proctitis and proctocolitis, the differential diagnosis includes gonorrhea, chiefly, as well as non-LGV *C trachomatis* infection and HSV. Classically, proctitis due to gonorrhea is thought to be severe, with copious, purulent discharge and pain; however, recent epidemiologic studies demonstrate that gonorrheal proctitis ranges widely in severity, and asymptomatic infection may occur in areas of high prevalence. The spectrum of symptoms in non-LGV *C trachomatis* rectal infection also ranges from mild to severe.

Complications

Compared with disease caused by non-LGV serovars of *C trachomatis* (eg, serovars B and D–K, which cause typical urogenital infection), LGV is known to produce a range of serious sequelae stemming from severe inflammation and scarring. Complications of LGV include chronic inflammation with development of fistulae from ruptured buboes (either cutaneous or to bladder or gastrointestinal tract), genital elephantiasis, and urethral or rectal strictures, which sometimes require surgical intervention.

These sequelae may occur years after initial infection in the absence of therapy. Secondary bacterial infection may play a role in late pathogenesis. Antimicrobial therapy may have a limited effect in resolution of strictures and other late sequelae once they have occurred.

Treatment

Recommended antimicrobial therapy for LGV (see Table 17–4) is a 3-week (21-day) course of oral doxycycline, 100 mg twice daily, or, alternatively, erythromycin base, 500 mg orally four times daily. Although data are lacking, some experts suggest azithromycin (1 g orally in three weekly doses) is effective in treating LGV. Patients with suspected LGV, especially those at high risk with compatible clinical syndromes for whom other causes have not been ruled out, should be treated empirically, and tests should be ordered on initial evaluation.

Pregnant and lactating women should be treated with erythromycin. No published data are available regarding its safety and efficacy for treating LGV in pregnancy; however, azithromycin may prove useful in the future. Doxycycline is contraindicated in pregnancy. HIV-infected persons with LGV should receive the same regimens as those who are not HIV-infected.

All patients should be followed clinically until signs and symptoms have resolved. Fluctuant buboes should be aspirated and may not fully resolve by the completion of the antimicrobial course. Although there is no standard recommendation for conducting a "test of cure" following treatment for this infection, an emerging consensus supports rescreening at 3 months for patients with *Chlamydia* infection—LGV or otherwise—because risk of reexposure, in general, is elevated among those with prior recent infection.

Sex partners within the prior 30 days should be clinically evaluated and, if symptomatic, treated as outlined earlier (see Prevention).

Centers for Disease Control and Prevention; Workowski KA, Berman SM. Sexually transmitted diseases treatment guidelines, 2006. *MMWR Recomm Rep* 2006;55(RR-11):1–94. [PMID: 16888612]

When to Refer to a Specialist

Consultation with an infectious disease or STD specialist is recommended in assessing patients who present with complicated genital ulcer or severe proctitis syndromes, given the complexities of accurate diagnosis of LGV as well as the potential for inflammatory sequelae should the diagnosis be missed. Moreover, the differential diagnosis of LGV includes other reportable infections, each with its own significant sequelae and implications for public health disease control. Thus, practitioners should have ready access to STD clinics or specialists in their local areas for consultation. The CDC, along with many state and local health departments, offers guidance to practitioners in recognizing and managing LGV. Specific training and other resources also can be accessed from the National Network of STD/HIV Prevention Training Centers (*http://www.depts.washington.edu/nnptc*).

Patients with severe proctitis of uncertain etiology should be referred to a gastroenterologist for lower endoscopy. Referral to a general surgeon is warranted for management of LGV involving nodal aspiration or drainage. A urologist or proctologist should be consulted to manage significant scarring of the genitourinary or gastrointestinal tracts, respectively, when late sequelae of LGV are encountered.

Prognosis

The prognosis for patients with LGV is excellent if infection is properly recognized and treated prior to the development of severe inflammatory sequelae, such as buboes and fistulae formation. Despite appropriate therapy,

Table 17–4. Treatment regimens for lymphogranuloma venereum.

Patient Population	Antibiotic Regimen
Diagnosed cases	
Recommended	Doxycycline, 100 mg PO twice daily for 21 d
Alternative	Erythromycin base, 500 mg PO 4 times daily for 21 d *or*
	Azithromycin, 1 g PO in 3 weekly doses
Sex partners in prior 30 d	Doxycycline, 100 mg PO twice daily for 7 d *or* Azithromycin, 1 g PO as a single dose

patients with buboes may require continued follow-up for aspiration and drainage. In general, scarring that results from late sequelae may require extended periods for resolution.

PRACTICE POINTS

- Given the limitations of current laboratory assays, the diagnosis of LGV in the United States is presumptive, relying on clinical recognition of suspected cases in patients with epidemiologic risk factors, supported by laboratory test evidence, along with exclusion of other causes of lymphadenopathy or proctitis syndromes.

- Patients with suspected LGV, especially those at high risk with compatible clinical syndromes for whom other causes have not been ruled out, should be treated empirically, and tests should be ordered on initial evaluation.

Relevant Web Sites

[California STD/HIV Prevention Training Center, provider resources for STD/HIV behavioral risk assessment:]

http://www.stdhivtraining.org/pdf/ask-screen-intervene

[Centers for Disease Control and Prevention, Lymphogranuloma Venereum (LGV) Project:]

http://www.cdc.gov/std/lgv

[National Network of STD/HIV Prevention Training Centers, training and other resources on LGV and related STD topics:]

http://www.depts.washington.edu/nnptc

Trichomoniasis

18

Jane Schwebke, MD

ESSENTIALS OF DIAGNOSIS

- In women, findings include motile trichomonads visible on vaginal wet mount, positive culture for Trichomonas vaginalis, *and Pap smear result that is positive for trichomonads.*
- In men, diagnosis is often presumptive, after failure to respond to standard treatment for nongonococcal urethritis (NGU).

General Considerations

Trichomoniasis is one of the three major causes of symptomatic infectious vaginitis, along with candidiasis and bacterial vaginosis, and is the only one known to be sexually transmitted. Despite being a readily diagnosed and treated infection, trichomoniasis is not a reportable one, and control of the infection has received relatively little emphasis from public health control programs for sexually transmitted diseases (STDs). The annual incidence of *Trichomonas vaginalis* infections in the United States has been estimated at 5 million cases. The World Health Organization has estimated that this infection accounts for almost half of all curable STDs worldwide.

Trichomoniasis is the exception to the rule that applies to most STDs in that it is more difficult to diagnose in men than in women. Currently available diagnostic methods for trichomoniasis in men lack sensitivity and availability. Therefore, most men are treated either as a result of sexual exposure to an infected woman or as part of an algorithm for persistent NGU.

Nanda N, Michel RG, Kurdgelashvili G, Wendel KA. Trichomoniasis and its treatment. *Expert Rev Anti Infect Ther* 2006;4:125–135. [PMID: 16441214] (Recent comprehensive review of trichomoniasis management.)

Schwebke J, Hook EI. High rates of Trichomonas vaginalis among men attending a sexually transmitted diseases clinic: Implications for screening and urethritis management. *J Infect Dis* 2003;188:465–468. [PMID: 12870131] (Study of the prevalence and association of *Trichomonas* with NGU in men).

Pathogenesis

T vaginalis, a flagellated parasite, is the causative agent of this infection. Although two other species of *Trichomonas* infect humans (*Trichomonas tenax* and *Trichomonas hominis*), *T vaginalis* is the only one that infects the urogenital tract. *Trichomonas* infects the squamous epithelium of the vagina and ectocervix and often causes an inflammatory response in the host manifested clinically by purulent discharge. The pathogenesis in men is poorly understood.

Prevention

As with any STD, unprotected sex is a risk factor for acquisition of infection. Limiting the number of sex partners or using condoms helps to prevent infection.

Clinical Findings

A. SYMPTOMS AND SIGNS

Symptoms of trichomoniasis in women include vaginal discharge, irritation, and pruritus; however, about half of all women infected with *T vaginalis* are asymptomatic. Occasionally women report vague lower abdominal pain. Signs of infection in women include vaginal discharge, odor, and edema or erythema, but these may be absent. Occasionally, erythematous, punctuate lesions may be seen on the ectocervix, the so-called "strawberry cervix."

In men, the prevalence and spectrum of disease is far less well characterized; the infection usually appears to be asymptomatic; however, it has been suggested as an increasingly important cause of NGU.

B. LABORATORY FINDINGS

Diagnosis of trichomoniasis in women is usually accomplished via direct microscopic examination of the vaginal fluid (wet mount); however, even when performed by skilled diagnosticians the sensitivity of this test is only 60% overall and may be less in asymptomatic women. In addition to motile trichomonads, white blood cells may be present. The vaginal pH may be elevated or normal. (Normal pH is generally associated with a low number of trichomonads.) Bacterial vaginosis is a frequent coinfection with trichomoniasis. Culture media is commercially available and is currently the "gold standard" for diagnosis (InPouch TV, BioMed Diagnostics, White City, OR). Polymerase chain reaction (PCR) techniques are under development but have thus far shown variable results.

Diagnosis in general is much more difficult in men, and the best culture results are obtained by combining urethral swabs and urine sediment for culture. Nonetheless, it is highly likely, as suggested by PCR results, that this approach lacks sensitivity.

A recently approved point-of-care antigen detection test (Genzyme Corporation, Cambridge, MA) has a sensitivity and specificity of 78% and 98%, respectively, compared with culture, which is superior to wet mount. This test may be of value in settings where microscopy is not possible.

C. SPECIAL TESTS

Trichomonads may be visualized on Papanicolaou (Pap) smears. A recent meta-analysis found the sensitivity and specificity of this technique to be 60% and 95%, respectively. Confirmation of the finding of trichomonads using another method has been recommended by some authors; however, most clinicians only have access to wet mount evaluation, which as stated lacks sensitivity.

Wiese W, Patel SR, Patel SC, et al. A meta-analysis of the Papanicolaou smear and wet mount for the diagnosis of vaginal trichomoniasis. *Am J Med* 2000;108:301–308. [PMID: 11014723] (Meta-analysis of the sensitivity and specificity of Pap smear for the diagnosis of trichomoniasis).

Differential Diagnosis

Other causes of vaginal complaints include yeast vaginitis, bacterial vaginosis, and atrophic vaginitis. Vaginal complaints should never be diagnosed without analyzing objective laboratory data.

Complications

Trichomoniasis has been associated with preterm birth in cross-sectional studies. Prospective trials on the treatment of trichomoniasis in pregnancy to prevent preterm birth suggested that such treatment may actually increase the risk of preterm birth rather than decreasing it, as predicted; however, there were limitations to both studies. One study, which used much higher doses of metronidazole than are recommended, was halted after the trend toward preterm birth was noted and thus did not enroll the number of women needed for a definitive analysis. The second study was a subanalysis of a study designed to answer questions relating to STD and HIV risk and thus was not primarily designed to answer questions regarding risks of preterm birth associated with treatment of trichomoniasis in pregnancy. Since the publication of these papers, the CDC has not revised its recommendations for treatment of trichomoniasis during pregnancy.

Acquisition of the human immunodeficiency virus (HIV) has been associated with trichomoniasis in several African studies, possibly as a result of local inflammation that is often caused by the parasite. Transmission of HIV also appears to be enhanced by coinfection with *T vaginalis*. In a study conducted in Malawi among men with urethritis, the median HIV RNA concentration in seminal fluid was significantly higher in men with trichomoniasis than in men with symptomatic urethritis due to an unidentified cause. In addition, successful treatment of trichomonal urethritis reduced levels of HIV RNA to levels similar to those seen in uninfected controls.

Goldenberg RL, Mwatha A, Read JS, et al; Hptn024 Team. The HPTN 024 Study: The efficacy of antibiotics to prevent chorioamnionitis and preterm birth. *Am J Obstet Gynecol* 2006;194:650–661. [PMID: 16522393] (Despite reducing the rate of vaginal infections, the antibiotic regimen [oral metronidazole, 250 mg, and oral erythromycin, 250 mg, three times daily for 7 days at 24 weeks' gestation and metronidazole, 250 mg, and ampicillin, 500 mg, every 4 hours during labor] used in this study did not reduce the rate of preterm birth, increase the time to delivery, or increase birth weight. Failure of this regimen to reduce the rate of histologic chorioamnionitis may explain the reason the antibiotics failed to reduce preterm birth.)

Klebanoff MA, Carey JC, Hauth JC, et al; National Institute of Child Health and Human Development Network of Maternal-Fetal Medicine Units. Failure of metronidazole to prevent preterm delivery among pregnant women with asymptomatic Trichomonas vaginalis infection. *N Engl J Med* 2001;345:487–493. [PMID: 11519502] (Treatment of pregnant women with asymptomatic trichomoniasis does not prevent preterm delivery, and routine screening and treatment of asymptomatic pregnant women for this condition cannot be recommended.)

Laga M, Manoka A, Kivuvu M, et al. Non-ulcerative sexually transmitted diseases as risk factors for HIV-1 transmission in women: Results from a cohort study. *AIDS* 1993;7:95–102. [PMID: 8442924] (Early study of the association of trichomoniasis with HIV.)

Okun N, Gronau KA, Hannah ME. Antibiotics for bacterial vaginosis or Trichomonas vaginalis in pregnancy: A systematic review. *Obstet Gynecol* 2005;105:857–868. [PMID: 15802417] (Contrary to the conclusions of three recent systematic reviews, these authors found no evidence to support the use of antibiotic treatment for bacterial vaginosis or *T vaginalis* in pregnancy to reduce the risk of preterm birth or its associated morbidities in low- or high-risk women.)

Treatment

A. STANDARD REGIMEN

In most patients, trichomoniasis is easily treated with a 2-g single dose of metronidazole. Resistant strains occur and may be increasing in prevalence. The resistance is relative and can often but not always be overcome with increased doses; however, side effects from metronidazole (eg, nausea and metallic taste) are common and may limit the dose. It has been reported that patients may experience a reaction similar to a disulfiram reaction, with nausea and flushing after ingesting ethanol. Although a review of the literature shows no convincing evidence for this type of reaction, this potential side effect is included in the manufacturer's warnings. Therefore, patients should be cautioned to avoid alcohol while undergoing treatment. Metronidazole may prolong the prothrombin time in patients who take warfarin, presumably by competing for binding sites on serum proteins. Rarely, transient black discoloration of the tongue may appear.

Tinidazole, which is also a nitroimidazole, was recently licensed in the United States to treat trichomoniasis using a 2-g single oral dose. It has a more favorable pharmacokinetic profile and is associated with fewer gastrointestinal side effects than metronidazole. Cost, however, may limit its routine use in this setting.

The reported cure rate with the recommended 2-g dose of metronidazole or tinidazole is 97%. Sex partners should also be treated. Infected women and their sex partners should be instructed to avoid intercourse until the patient and partner(s) are cured. An alternative regimen consists of metronidazole, 500 mg twice daily for 7 days. Metronidazole intravaginal gel has limited efficacy and should not be used. Although controversy persists about the safety of metronidazole in pregnancy, there has never been a documented case of fetal malformation attributed to its use, even in the first trimester. Occasionally patients are allergic to metronidazole (and to tinidazole, because it is a related nitroimidazole). In these patients, desensitization is the only option, because there is no other effective pharmacologic treatment.

Trichomoniasis should be considered in men with persistent NGU. Because there currently is no reliable commercially available test for *T vaginalis* in men, these patients should be empirically treated with metronidazole if they fail to respond to an initial course of doxycycline or azithromycin therapy for NGU.

Patients with trichomoniasis should be screened for other STDs, and STD prevention messages should be delivered. "Test of cure" examinations are not routinely indicated, because cure rates are high.

B. Antimicrobially Resistant Infection

An estimated 2.5–5% of all cases of trichomoniasis display some level of resistance to treatment with metronidazole. This resistance is relative and can usually be overcome with higher doses of oral metronidazole. For patients who do not respond to the standard treatment regimen and have not been reinfected, higher doses of metronidazole (eg, a 2-g single oral dose once daily for 3–5 days) can be tried. Some authorities recommend higher doses of oral medication in combination with

pharmacy-prepared intravaginal preparations. Intravenous formulations offer no advantage over oral drug formulations. There are limited anecdotal reports of success with paromomycin cream; however, this therapy may also be associated with a high incidence of local side effects. Tinidazole may be an effective option for patients with metronidazole-resistant infection. In one study of 20 patients with clinically refractory trichomoniasis (failure to respond to therapy with oral metronidazole, at least 500 mg twice daily for 7 days), high doses of oral and vaginal tinidazole (2–3 g orally plus 1–1.5 g intravaginally for 14 days) resulted in cure rates of 92%, and none of the patients discontinued therapy due to side effects.

Centers for Disease Control and Prevention; Workowski KA, Berman SM. Sexually transmitted diseases treatment guidelines, 2006. *MMWR Recomm Rep* 2006;55(RR-11):1–94. [PMID: 16888612] (Recommended guidelines for management of STDs).

Sobel J, Nyirjesy P, Brown W. Tinidazole therapy for metronidazole-resistant vaginal trichomoniasis. *Clin Inf Dis* 2001;33:1341–1346. [PMID: 11565074] (Use of tinidazole for resistant trichomoniasis).

When to Refer to a Specialist

Clinicians should consider referral to an infectious disease or STD specialist for women with trichomoniasis that is resistant to standard therapy.

Prognosis

Overall cure rates in treatment of trichomoniasis are high, and the prognosis is excellent. Occasionally patients with a highly resistant strain of *T vaginalis* require multiple courses of therapy.

 PRACTICE POINTS

- *For patients who do not respond to the standard treatment regimen for trichomoniasis and have not been reinfected, higher doses of metronidazole (eg, a 2-g single oral dose once daily for 3–5 days) can be tried.*

Relevant Web Sites

[Centers for Disease Control and Prevention fact sheet on trichomoniasis:]
http://cdc.gov/std/trichomonas/STDFact-Trichomoniasis.htm
[National Women's Health Information Center, National Institutes of Health, information on trichomoniasis:]
http://womenshealth.gov/faq/stdtrich.htm

Syphilis

Michael Augenbraun, MD

ESSENTIALS OF DIAGNOSIS

- *Sexually transmitted disease causing a wide range of systemic manifestations.*
- *Clinical disease occurs in well-characterized stages: primary (chancre), secondary (rash, swollen glands, systemic symptoms) and tertiary (dementia, neuromotor, gummatous, cardiovascular symptoms).*
- *Latent periods of variable duration occur between clinical manifestations of disease.*
- *Clinical disease is confirmed and latent disease diagnosed by two-stage serologic tests.*

General Considerations

Syphilis is a complex disease caused by the spirochete *Treponema pallidum*. It occupies an interesting place in the history of disease, appearing explosively as a virulent epidemic in Europe during the age of exploration, a time of intense scientific inquiry. Although syphilis incidence has waxed and waned over the centuries since, it has never really abated. Penicillin has been and remains the therapy of choice.

Unique among the sexually transmitted diseases, syphilis is characterized by a potential to cause a wide range of systemic manifestations. It can involve nearly every organ system in a variety of ways acutely or more commonly in an insidious and chronic fashion. Latent periods between clinical manifestations may be of variable duration. It has the potential to cause serious congenital disease and appears to enhance the transmission of human immunodeficiency virus (HIV).

Epidemiology & Pathogenesis

Syphilis is typically acquired sexually or congenitally. Rare cases of acquisition through contaminated blood products have been reported. Syphilis can also be spread by skin or mucosal contact with an infectious lesion (eg, through nonsexual direct contact such as skin to skin or kissing). The risk of syphilis following sexual exposure to an individual with infectious syphilis is probably about 30% and is dependent on a variety of factors, including the extent and location of disease in the source patient. Long-standing immunity following infection after treatment does not occur, and repeated infections are possible.

Prevention

Most syphilis infections are sexually transmitted; therefore, measures that prevent sexual exposure, such as condom use or reduction in the number of sex partners, are effective in reducing the risk of acquiring syphilis. Syphilis is unique among the sexually transmitted diseases because of a well-characterized prolonged incubation period during which infection can be aborted by prophylactic treatment. After sexual exposure infection may be prevented with penicillin G benzathine therapy.

Preventive treatment is highly effective and a mainstay of syphilis control programs. Persons who may have been exposed to syphilis are contacted and offered preventive therapy. Those who receive timely preventive therapy will not undergo seroconversion (see later discussion of serologic testing). Waiting for serologic test results before treatment is not recommended in patients who report syphilis exposure, because the opportunity to prevent infection may be missed. All persons who report exposure should receive preventive treatment, regardless of serologic test results.

Clinical Findings

A. SYMPTOMS AND SIGNS

Typical of syphilis is its clinical progression through several well-characterized stages, outlined below.

1. Primary syphilis—Incubation after exposure typically lasts from 1 week to 3 months. The initial manifestation is the chancre (Figure 19–1), an indurated, nontender lesion at the site of exposure. Several lesions may occur at once, but they are more often solitary. Disease is

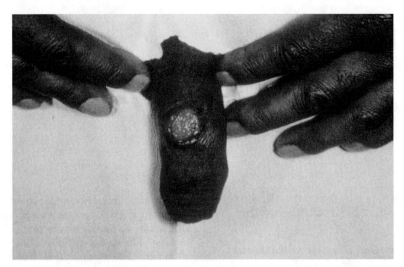

Figure 19–1. Syphilitic chancre on the shaft of the penis. (Courtesy of the Centers for Disease Control and Prevention.)

transmissible through contact with a chancre. In conjunction with the appearance of the chancre, patients usually develop nonsuppurative, nontender inguinal lymphadenopathy. Primary lesions can appear at any site of inoculation, including the perineum, vagina, cervix, anus, or rectum. Lesions can also appear on the lips or in the oropharynx.

2. Secondary syphilis—Without therapy the lesions of primary syphilis typically resolve over a period of about 3 weeks. By this time spirochetemia, first to regional lymph nodes and then systemically, has already occurred. Either coincident with the resolution of the primary lesion or more commonly several weeks later, the clinical manifestations of secondary syphilis develop. These have long been considered to be among the most diverse of all clinicopathologic phenomena. Most often they present as a diffuse maculopapular rash (Figure 19–2). Papulosquamous lesions with fine circumferential scaling may involve the palms and soles (Figure 19–3). Moist heaped-up lesions, termed *condylomata lata,* are seen in the intertriginous areas such as the buttocks and the upper thighs (Figure 19–4). Similar lesions, termed *mucous patches,* appear in the nasolabial folds and in the mouth. The moist lesions characteristic of condylomata lata and the mucous patch may transmit disease in a particularly efficient manner. Rashes covered in keratinized epithelium are less likely to transmit infection.

Patchy alopecia, diffuse lymphadenopathy, pharyngitis, or fever may also be present. Focal involvement of various organ systems, such as gastritis, uveitis, hepatitis, periostitis, meningitis, and cerebrovascular accidents, can occur as manifestations of secondary syphilis. The

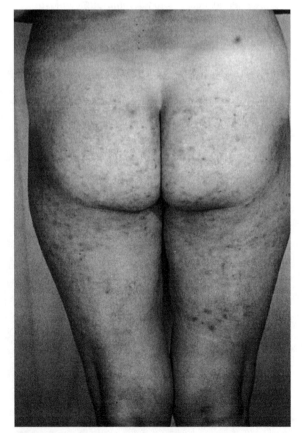

Figure 19–2. Generalized rash of secondary syphilis. (Courtesy of the Centers for Disease Control and Prevention.)

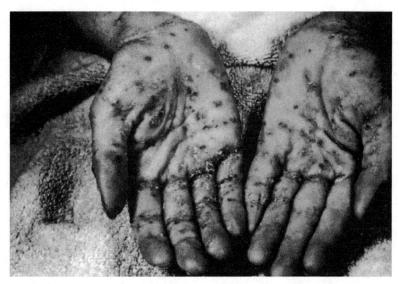

Figure 19–3. Palmar rash of secondary syphilis. (Courtesy of the Centers for Disease Control and Prevention.)

period of spirochetemia that is linked to the development of secondary syphilis is the most likely opportunity for transplacental transmission in the pregnant woman.

3. Latent syphilis—As in primary syphilis, the clinical manifestations of secondary stage disease abate with time (ie, weeks) even in the absence of specific therapy. At this point the disease is considered to have entered a latent period. Studies have demonstrated that about 25% of untreated persons with latent syphilis may have recrudescent secondary symptoms within a 4- to 5-year period

after their initial resolution. The majority of these events occur within 1 year. For the sake of convention this period within 1 year of exposure is regarded as the "early latent" period. Beyond this time frame a period of long-term or "late" latency develops in which there are no clinical manifestations of infection. For most of these patients, one of three outcomes can be anticipated: spontaneous resolution of infection, persistent latent infection with some level of immunologic control, or development of tertiary syphilis after a period of years or decades. As

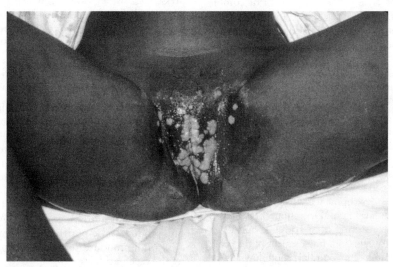

Figure 19–4. Condylomata lata of the vulvar and perineal areas. (Courtesy of the Centers for Disease Control and Prevention.)

many as one third of untreated patients with latent syphilis may go on to develop tertiary syphilis. Sexual transmission of syphilis in the latent stage is not likely.

4. Tertiary syphilis—This stage is characterized by an element of end-organ damage. There are three types of tertiary disease: neurosyphilis, cardiovascular syphilis, and gummatous (or late benign) syphilis.

a. Neurosyphilis—*T pallidum* appears to have a particular predilection for the nervous system. Even in early-stage disease, invasion of the central nervous system is well documented. Although usually asymptomatic, in some instances there may be ocular manifestations such as uveitis or even cerebrovascular accidents. Central nervous system disease that manifests after long periods of latency is characterized by either vascular compromise of some portion of the neuroaxis or chronic debilitating loss of function that correlates with parenchymal destruction.

General paresis is characterized by a combination of psychiatric and neurologic findings. The letters in the word PARESIS correspond to the prominent findings associated with this aspect of disease: Personality (emotional lability), Affect (flat), Reflexes (hyperreflexivity), Eye (Argyll-Robertson pupil), Sensorium (illusions, delusions, hallucinations), Intellect (memory, judgment impairment), and Speech (slurring). The classic Argyll-Robertson pupil of late neurosyphilis is characterized by a pupil that constricts upon accommodation but not to light.

Another classic late-stage neurosyphilis syndrome is **tabes dorsalis**. As a result of demyelination of the posterior columns of the spinal cord, patients develop abnormalities in gait, as well as various sensory abnormalities, including characteristic "lightening" pains, bladder and bowel dysfunction, and a positive Romberg sign. The clinical presentation is usually some portion or combination of these symptoms.

A host of inflammatory ocular and otic manifestations is also attributable to neurosyphilis, as are other cranial nerve abnormalities. It is more than reasonable to consider syphilis in the differential diagnosis of nearly any psychiatric or neurologic presentation. Neurosyphilis is discussed in more detail in Chapter 20.

b. Cardiovascular syphilis—Unlike neurosyphilis, and probably as a result of the widespread use of systemic antibiotics with activity against *T pallidum* for different clinical conditions, cardiovascular syphilis is not as common today as it once was. *T pallidum* damages the muscular intima of the aorta and with time the resultant weakening leads to the development of an aortic aneurysm, usually of the ascending arch. Dissection, however, is uncommon. Dilation resulting from syphilitic aortitis in turn leads to aortic regurgitation. Involvement of the coronary ostia may compromise myocardial blood flow.

c. Gummatous (or late benign) syphilis—Gummatous disease is also extremely uncommon and is characterized by indolent destructive lesions of skin, soft tissue, and bony structures. Significant scarring may result in disfigurement. Visceral organs and the central nervous system may also be involved. Gummas may vary widely in size from small defects to large tumor-like masses. Interestingly, treponemes cannot routinely be found in tissue specimens from these lesions. The process is suspected to be largely immune mediated.

B. Laboratory Findings

Under ordinary circumstances *T pallidum* cannot be cultivated in agar-based medium. Beyond clinical suspicion, diagnosis is made or confirmed through the use of darkfield microscopy, two-stage serologic tests, nucleic acid amplification tests (NAATs), direct antigen tests, or special tissue stains. The first two tests are the most commonly available. Clinicians should inform patients that reactive laboratory tests for syphilis are reportable to public health authorities.

1. Darkfield microscopy—*T pallidum* is too slender to be adequately observed by ordinary light microscopy and fails to take up usual stains. Instead it can be observed using darkfield techniques, which require a microscope equipped with a special condenser that angles light to allow only those rays reflected by the object of interest to enter the objective. The organism appears white against an otherwise black background, hence the term *darkfield*. Under such observation, the treponeme can be visualized as a corkscrew-shaped organism rotating along its long axis.

Darkfield microscopy is only useful when examining the moist lesions of primary syphilis or condylomata lata. For darkfield specimen collection, lesions must first be cleaned with saline-soaked gauze. Serous exudate is then pressed against a glass slide, which must be immediately examined before the specimen desiccates. Darkfield examination may also be used for aspirates from involved lymph nodes. The yield from resolving lesions is low.

2. Serologic tests—Traditionally, a diagnosis of syphilis of any stage should be confirmed through the use of two-stage serologic tests.

a. Nontreponemal tests—Initial testing is performed with a nontreponemal serologic test. These tests use a laboratory-prepared lecithin-cholesterol antigen to detect treponemal-directed antibody in the target serum specimen. The sensitivity of these tests (which include rapid plasma reagin [RPR], Venereal Disease Research Laboratory [VDRL], and toluidine red unheated serum test [TRUST]), is very good. Specificity is slightly less reliable. A variety of factors can produce false-positive reactions, including older age, autoimmune disease, intravenous drug use, and recent vaccination.

Nontreponemal tests can be performed both quantitatively and qualitatively. Repeated tests on serially diluted specimens allow for a determination of the strength of the reaction, which roughly correlate with the extent of infection. Conversely, treatment success can be measured by demonstration of declining nontreponemal test titers over time. Because up to 20% of nontreponemal tests may be nonreactive in primary syphilis, if that is a concern either repeat testing 1 week later or testing with a treponemal specific test is indicated.

b. **Treponemal-specific tests**—To rule out false-positive tests, when used for diagnosis, reactive nontreponemal serologic tests must be confirmed. This is done using treponemal-specific tests, which include the fluorescent treponemal antibody absorbed (FTA-ABS), *T pallidum* particle agglutination (TP-PA), and *T pallidum* hemagglutination assay (TPHA). The antigens for these tests vary, but all have in common the use of true treponemal antigen as a key reagent. The microhemagglutination–*T pallidum* (MHA-TP) test is no longer commercially available in the United States.

Treponemal tests tend to be labor intensive and expensive when compared with the nontreponemal tests. They are usually interpreted qualitatively and may remain reactive for the remainder of the life of the individual irrespective of the success of therapy. They are considered both sensitive and specific. The treponemal-specific tests may become reactive before the nontreponemal tests in the earliest stages of primary infection. That observation leads some experts to recommend the use of treponemal specific tests in the evaluation of a patient with suspected primary syphilis. Commonly, if the nontreponemal serologic test is nonreactive, the testing algorithm ceases.

Laboratories, particularly those processing large numbers of specimens, recently have been turning to enzyme-linked immunoassay technologies that make use of the treponemal-specific test as a screening test. Reactive tests by this method may be confirmed and quantitated by a traditional nontreponemal-specific test. Discordant tests may be further examined using a traditional treponemal test. The significance of an isolated reactive treponemal-specific test is unclear. It may reflect a false-positive test or a previously treated (knowingly or unknowingly) case of syphilis.

3. Nucleic acid amplification tests—The advantages of tests that rely on nucleic acid amplification techniques to diagnose infectious diseases are obvious. They are exquisitely sensitive as well as very specific. They do not rely on viable organisms yet directly assay those organisms. These techniques are available primarily as a research tool; however, in certain public health facilities or clinics connected to academic research centers, *T pallidum* nucleic acid amplification tests such as polymerase chain reaction are available to clinicians to help with syphilis diagnosis.

4. Biopsy and special stains—Treponemes can on rare occasions be visualized in tissue using special stains, including silver stain.

D. DETERMINATION OF SYPHILIS STAGE

The staging of syphilis is an important aspect of the clinical diagnosis. Identification of the disease stage determines the treatment, further management, and partner notification practices.

1. Incubating syphilis—Between the period of exposure until just before development of signs, serologic tests are not reactive. Diagnosis is purely presumptive and is based on a history of sexual exposure to someone with syphilis. Treatment at this stage will prevent seroconversion and development of clinical disease.

2. Primary syphilis—The chancre of primary syphilis is similar to yet unlike the ulcers of the other common causes of genital ulcer disease. Clinicians are highly likely to misdiagnose a genital ulcer purely on clinical grounds. Therefore, diagnostic tests for other etiologic agents of genital ulcer disease should be performed in addition to those performed for syphilis (eg, herpes simplex virus culture or PCR).

If darkfield microscopy is available, exudate from the lesion may be examined for spirochetes. The sensitivity of darkfield microscopy is somewhat operator dependent as well as dependent on the quality of the specimen. If characteristic corkscrew-shaped organisms are observed in a specimen from a patient who is likely to have syphilis, then the diagnosis is almost certain. Care must be taken, however, because nonpathogenic spirochetes are sometimes observed in the oral or rectal secretions of persons without syphilis. If a darkfield microscope is unavailable, then direct fluorescent antibody testing of the specimen may be appropriate.

Serologic testing supports the suspicion of syphilis. In the earliest phases of primary syphilis, the nontreponemal serologic test may be nonreactive while the treponemal-specific test is almost always reactive. However, within a short time (eg, days) both tests should be reactive.

3. Secondary syphilis—A rash of any type in a sexually active individual should be considered as potential syphilis until proven otherwise. The appearance of syphilis-associated rashes is so varied that reliance on some "characteristic" quality would be a mistake. Ordinarily, rashes of secondary syphilis do not present as ulcerative lesions and therefore do not yield moist surfaces for proper darkfield examination. The only exceptions are the perineal lesions of condylomata lata and mucous patches of the oropharyngeal area.

Reflecting the systemic nature of this stage of infection, nontreponemal test titers are high. Although truly nonreactive (or low-titer) nontreponemal test results in secondary syphilis have been reported, they are very uncommon. One situation that calls for caution in interpreting serologic tests is the so-called prozone phenomenon, which occurs when the concentration of antitreponemal antibodies is so high that the characteristic flocculation reaction that produces a reactive specimen cannot occur. This phenomenon is overcome by diluting the specimen and rerunning the test.

4. Latent syphilis—By definition latent syphilis is clinically inapparent. The only evidence of infection is a reactive serologic test. The nontreponemal serologic test titer is usually fairly low (ie, ≤1:8).

5. Tertiary syphilis—Diagnostic criteria for neurosyphilis are discussed in detail in Chapter 20. Reactive serologic tests in the setting of an aortic aneurysm may be construed as evidence of cardiovascular syphilis. A definitive diagnosis requires a pathologic specimen (ie, tissue biopsy). The range of tissues involved and the varying extent of inflammation that may be manifest in syphilitic gummas mean that almost any chronic destructive lesions of the body may be caused by syphilis. Serologic tests are usually reactive. Titers may range from reactive at only low dilution to reactive at very high dilutions. The prozone phenomenon was described earlier. Rare treponemes may be visualized on pathologic specimens.

Differential Diagnosis

Sir William Osler is often quoted on the topic of syphilis, which was a common diagnosis in his day. Nothing is more accurate than his reflection that, "Syphilis, which begins its pathological existence as a modest, inactive Hunterian chancre, soon enters upon a career that is unsurpassed for the inclusiveness and variety of its manifestation . . . it is almost impossible to describe its clinical symptoms without mentioning almost every symptom of every disease known."

In light of this it seems almost futile to devise a list of other diseases whose manifestations may suggest or be suggested by the symptoms of syphilis. Obviously the chancre of syphilis calls to mind the other common etiologies of genital ulcer disease, such as herpes simplex and chancroid. Lesions of herpes may be distinguished from syphilis by their superficial, nonindurated and painful nature. Viral culture of herpetic lesions is usually positive when lesions are open and moist. Chancroid is currently uncommonly seen in the United States. These lesions are painful like herpes but indurated like syphilis. Special culture media can be used for identification but is not readily available. Gram stain may demonstrate the characteristic gram-negative organisms. Polymerase chain reaction testing may also distinguish one etiology of genital ulcer disease from another but is also not commonly available. It should also be recognized that a genital ulcer may harbor more than one pathogen. The concomitant

lymphadenopathy may be confused with herpes, lymphogranuloma venereum, HIV, or lymphoma. Although classically characterized by hyperpigmented lesions on the palms and soles as well as fine scaling, the rash of secondary syphilis can be confused with almost any etiology of rash. Therefore, syphilis needs to be considered when evaluating a rash in any sexually active individual.

Neurosyphilis can appear early or as a late manifestation of syphilis. It can manifest with either motor or sensory deficits. Cranial nerves can be involved. There may be cognitive abnormalities or behavioral disturbances. Almost any disturbance of the central nervous system could be attributed to neurosyphilis. Cardiovascular disease should be considered in the development of aortic aneurysms, aortic valve regurgitation, and even the acute coronary syndrome. Gummatous disease may resemble a wide range of destructive or tumor-like lesions. Ulcers, inflammatory lesions, tumors, and fungal or mycobacterial processes may all bear some similarity to the gumma of syphilis.

Risk-taking behavior that predisposes individuals to acquire syphilis also predisposes them to other sexually transmitted diseases. All patients with syphilis need to be evaluated for other sexually transmitted diseases. For patients with early-stage syphilis, this should include screening for *Neisseria gonorrhoeae* and *Chlamydia trachomatis* infections. Evaluation for herpes simplex virus infection, human papillomavirus infection, and hepatitis B virus infection might also be warranted. In all instances of syphilis, whether early or late, patients should be tested for HIV infection.

Complications

Complications of syphilis develop in about one third of patients with untreated infection. As previously discussed, these can include progressive infection of the central nervous, cardiovascular, or musculoskeletal system, but any organ system can be involved.

Treatment

A. Pharmacotherapy

1. Penicillin G—Sixty years after it was demonstrated effective in the treatment of syphilis, penicillin G remains the treatment of choice for this infection. No other antibiotic has the proven track record of penicillin. The goal of therapy for syphilis is twofold: (1) render the individual noninfectious, and (2) halt disease progression and eliminate latency.

The use of benzathine G penicillin, or long-acting penicillin, is recommended in the treatment of early or latent syphilis. *T pallidum* has a slow metabolism, dividing more slowly than other bacteria but more quickly than mycobacteria, and the benzathine G penicillin formulation provides a long duration of antitreponemal therapy.

It is fairly obvious when penicillin or other antibiotics rapidly eliminate the risk of transmission of disease in the individual with communicable forms of syphilis such as the chancre of primary infection or condylomata lata and mucous patches of secondary disease. Within 24–48 hours of treatment, lesions begin to resolve and viable treponemes may no longer be recovered.

It is well documented that very early in the course of disease treponemes disseminate from even the most localized lesion, first to regional lymph nodes, and then elsewhere throughout the body, including distant lymph nodes and the central nervous system. Manifestations of infection in these areas may be subclinical. In this circumstance the only way to monitor the effectiveness of therapy is to serially repeat quantitative nontreponemal serologic tests with the goal of achieving at least a twofold dilutional decline or, in the best case, negative serologic tests. Unfortunately, the decline in test titers happens over a long period, up to 12–24 months. In some cases, serologic negativity may never occur; in these cases, patient titers are considered "serofast." Typical serofast titers are ≤1:8. Whether the persistence of a positive titer reflects continued treponemal infection after therapy remains to be demonstrated.

2. Other antibiotic agents—Although penicillin G remains the most commonly used agent in the treatment of syphilis, other antibiotics have demonstrated efficacy. Because of limited data and limited clinical experience, these agents remain alternatives to penicillin and when used are limited to early-stage disease. They include the tetracyclines, in particular doxycycline (because of its less-frequent dosing compared with tetracycline and its favorable side-effect profile). Another option is the third-generation cephalosporin ceftriaxone, which is easy to administer and provides excellent central nervous system penetration. Although there was interest in the use of erythromycin to treat syphilis, reports of failure, particularly in pregnancy, have led to its elimination as a treatment option.

Data from several randomized controlled trials suggest that the azalide antibiotic azithromycin is useful in the treatment of early-stage syphilis. Unfortunately there have been several concomitant reports of failure in patients who received this therapy along with in vitro data that demonstrates the presence of treponemal genetic elements encoding for azithromycin resistance. Azithromycin therapy for syphilis is not recommended by the Centers for Disease Control and Prevention (CDC), and, if used, should be administered cautiously with close follow-up. Caution should also be

exercised when using any of these alternative agents for the treatment of syphilis in immunocompromised individuals.

3. Stage-specific therapy—Treatment of syphilis depends on the stage of disease at diagnosis. Because of the long doubling time of the treponeme, antibiotics are usually administered either as a depot injection or orally over a prolonged period of time. Recommendations from the CDC are summarized in Table 19–1. There is no indication for adjunctive therapy.

a. Early-stage syphilis—Primary, secondary, and early latent syphilis can be treated with a single injection of 2.4 million units of intramuscular penicillin G. As an alternative in penicillin-allergic patients, doxycycline, 100 mg orally twice daily, may be used for 14 days. Ceftriaxone can also be used as an alternative to penicillin. It is active against *T pallidum* and is well tolerated. One to 2 g intramuscularly daily for 8–10 days has been recommended. Treatment of early latent syphilis follows the approach for primary and secondary syphilis because it is believed that the replicative capacity of treponemes at this stage is similar.

b. Latent and late latent syphilis—Treatment of late latent syphilis (including latent syphilis of unknown duration) requires a prolonged course of therapy. A dose of intramuscular benzathine penicillin, 2.4 million units, is given once and then repeated at weekly intervals two more times, for a total of three weekly injections. This assures up to 4 weeks of treponemicidal blood levels of penicillin. If a dose is missed, it has been suggested that the series of injection may be continued as long as no more than 14 days has passed between injections. If more time has elapsed, the series should be restarted. As an alternative, doxycycline (100 mg orally twice daily for 28 days) may be substituted, with the caveats as noted above.

c. Tertiary syphilis and neurosyphilis—Tertiary forms of syphilis are treated similarly to late latent disease except that evaluation of cerebrospinal fluid (CSF) should be performed before therapy is initiated. Neurosyphilis requires its own therapeutic approach. To achieve adequate penicillin levels in the central nervous system, it is recommended that patients receive intravenous penicillin G, 3–4 million units every 4 hours for 10–14 days. Many experts recommend that at the conclusion of this therapy patients receive two or three weekly doses of benzathine penicillin G, as previously noted, to eliminate the risk that latent forms of syphilis will persist. Procaine penicillin G, 2.4 million units intramuscularly once daily for 10–14 days, along with probenecid, 500 mg orally four times daily, is an acceptable substitute. As an alternative, ceftriaxone can also be used, but data as to efficacy are limited.

Table 19–1. Recommended treatment regimens for syphilis.

	Primary Therapy	Alternative Therapy[a]	Comment
Primary, secondary, and early latent syphilis	Benzathine penicillin G, 2.4 million units IM as a single dose	Doxycycline, 100 mg PO twice daily for 7 d *or* Ceftriaxone, 1 g IM daily for 8–10 d *or* Tetracycline, 100 mg PO 4 times daily for 7 d	
Latent of unknown duration and late latent syphilis	Benzathine penicillin G, 2.4 million units IM once weekly for 3 wk	Doxycycline, 100 mg PO twice daily for 28 d *or* Tetracycline, 100 mg PO 4 times daily for 28 d	
Neurosyphilis	Aqueous penicillin G, 18–24 million units IV daily administered as 3–4 million units every 4 hours or continuous infusion for 10–14 days	Procaine penicillin, 2.4 million units IM daily *plus* Probenecid, 500 mg PO 4 times daily, both for 10–14 d *or* Ceftriaxone,[b] 2 g IM once daily for 10–14 d	Follow-up treatment with 2 additional weekly injections of benzathine penicillin, 2.4 million units IM For further discussion, see Chapter 20
Tertiary syphilis (not neurosyphilis)	Benzathine penicillin, 2.4 million units IM once weekly for 3 wk		CSF evaluations should be performed before therapy

[a]In patients with penicillin allergy.
[b]Cross-reactivity in penicillin-allergic patients is possible but uncommon (<3%).
CSF, cerebrospinal fluid.
Based on Centers for Disease Control and Prevention; Workowski KA, Berman SM. Sexually transmitted diseases treatment guidelines, 2006. *MMWR Recomm Rep* 2006;55(RR-11):1–94.

B. Penicillin Allergy Testing and Desensitization

Although alternatives to penicillin are available, there are situations for which no good alternative exists. These situations include pregnancy, neurosyphilis, and to some extent HIV infection. Although patient reports of allergy to penicillin often turn out not to suggest risk of anaphylactic reaction, they remain a cause for concern. For such individuals, skin testing can be performed using the commercially available major determinants (Pre-Pen; Taylor Pharmacal Company, Decatur, IL) and penicillin G itself, which contains most but not all the minor determinants. Minor determinants are unfortunately not all commercially available (but can sometimes be obtained through the Allergy/Immunology section at some major medical centers). A small but real proportion of truly allergic patients (3%) may be misidentified when the panel containing Pre-Pen and penicillin G is used. There is cross-reaction with cephalosporins in individuals with penicillin allergy, but the frequency of that cross-reactivity appears to be low (<5%).

In cases of documented allergy where penicillin must be used, desensitization can be performed following any of several protocols (see Table 19–2). Desensitization lasts only as long as the penicillin is administered. Its effect does not persist beyond clearance of penicillin when therapy is complete. Both skin testing and desensitization should be performed in a controlled and monitored setting.

C. Response to Therapy

The efficacy of any syphilis therapy can be assessed by the resolution of clinical manifestations and the decline

Table 19–2. Oral desensitization protocol for patients with a documented allergy to penicillin.

Penicillin V Suspension Dose[a]	Amount (units/mL)	mL	Units	Cumulative Dose (units)
1	1000	0.1	100	100
2	1000	0.2	200	300
3	1000	0.4	400	700
4	1000	0.8	800	1500
5	1000	1.6	1600	3100
6	1000	3.2	3200	6300
7	1000	6.4	6400	12,700
8	10,000	1.2	12,000	24,700
9	10,000	2.4	24,000	48,700
10	10,000	4.8	48,000	96,700
11	80,000	1.0	80,000	176,700
12	80,000	2.0	160,000	336,700
13	80,000	4.0	320,000	656,700
14	80,000	8.0	640,000	1,296,700

[a]Doses diluted in 30 mL of water; 15-min interval between doses.
Reproduced, with permission, from Wendel G, Stark B, Jamison R, et al. Penicillin allergy and desensitization in serious infections during pregnancy. *N Engl J Med* 1985;312:1229–1232.

in serologic titers. Resolution of clinical manifestations by itself may be misleading, because even in the absence of therapy the clinical manifestations of syphilis (eg, chancre of primary disease or rash of secondary disease) will resolve. If clinical manifestations of early-stage disease respond to therapy, they do so quickly. Within 24–48 hours the chancre and rash should show clear evidence of resolution. Treponemes should no longer be observed in lesion exudates under darkfield microscopy.

Frequently following the treatment of secondary syphilis, and occasionally after treatment for primary syphilis, patients experience the rapid development of fever, headache, and myalgias. Signs may include hypotension and, if measured, an elevated white cell count. These findings are presumably secondary to an immunologically mediated process known as the *Jarisch-Herxheimer reaction*. This reaction is ordinarily self-limited and can be treated with antipyretics and analgesics. Because confusion with a reaction to penicillin therapy may occur, all patients treated for early syphilis should be made aware of the possibility of this immunologic reaction.

Current guidelines supported by decades of clinical experience recommend that successful therapy be followed by a fourfold decline (eg, 1:32 to 1:8) in the nontreponemal serologic test titer. The time course over which this can be expected to occur remains an area open to some conjecture. Clearly this cannot be reliably expected by 1 month after therapy. In early-stage syphilis, this decline should be seen within 6 months after therapy and certainly by 12 months. In latent forms of disease, such a decline can be seen by 12 months but may take even longer. The lower the titer when the patient begins therapy, the longer it may take to see a decline—if one is ever achieved. In either early or latent syphilis, the reactive nontreponemal test may never completely resolve, (ie, the "serofast" reaction). The clinical significance of this is unclear.

Sometimes titers may fail to decline or in fact even rise. Distinguishing failure of therapy from reinfection has long been one of the most vexing challenges in syphilis management. Obviously, the individual likely to have been reinfected simply needs retreatment. In the absence of evidence that this may have occurred, titers that do not decline sufficiently or those that rise after therapy should be considered evidence of treatment failure. In this situation, a lumbar puncture should ordinarily be performed to rule out neurosyphilis, and retreatment should be initiated, usually with the longer duration of treatment (three weekly injections).

The damage that occurs in tertiary disease is not likely to be reversed by any therapy. Halting progression of disease is a more realistic expectation. Declining serologic titers, as previously described, should occur. In patients with neurosyphilis, repeated examinations of CSF are necessary to assess proper response to therapy. By 6 months, improvement in lymphocytic pleocytosis should be seen as the earliest indicator of successful therapy. A decline in the CSF VDRL may take longer.

D. SPECIAL POPULATIONS

1. HIV-infected patients—It has been of concern for more than 20 years that patients who contract syphilis and have underlying HIV infection may manifest disease in unusual ways and may respond less well to therapy than those who do not have HIV infection. Despite several case reports describing rapid progression to tertiary disease, false-negative serologic tests for secondary syphilis, and failure of therapy, no well-collected data support the contention that these observations are anything other than random events. Although there seems to be no reason to require anything other than standard therapies for HIV patients found to have syphilis, it would be prudent to monitor serologic results in such patients more frequently than in non–HIV-infected individuals. Current recommendations suggest that this can be done every 3 months after treatment for early syphilis and every 6 months after treatment for latent forms of syphilis.

There continues to be some debate about the risk of progression to neurosyphilis in HIV-infected individuals, and hence the indication for lumbar puncture. Many experts continue to recommend CSF analysis in any HIV-infected patient with latent syphilis. Others extend this recommendation to those with early-stage syphilis despite the recognized fact that CSF abnormalities are common in early-stage syphilis for all patients. Yet others limit the recommendation for these invasive procedures to only those HIV-infected individuals with significant immunosuppression (ie, CD4 count <350/mL). Although most experts agree there is need for concern, there appears to be no consensus on what course to pursue.

2. Pregnant women—Syphilis can be readily transmitted to the unborn child of a pregnant woman at any stage of infection. The consequences of such infection for the infant can be severe and range from asymptomatic infection to neurologic disease, hepatitis, periostitis, and stillbirth. Screening for syphilis in all pregnant women is a routine part of obstetric care. Testing should be performed at the outset of prenatal care and in high-risk patients or high-incidence areas repeated at 28 weeks' gestation and again at delivery. Stillborn delivery after 20 weeks' gestation warrants syphilis testing in the mother.

Biologic false-positive tests (ie, reactive nontreponemal tests and a nonreactive treponemal-specific test) can occur in pregnancy. Care must be taken to confirm any reactive serologic test in this patient population. In the event of infection, treatment for the pregnant woman is exactly as it would be for the nonpregnant patient. As previously mentioned, penicillin G is the only recommended treatment for syphilis in pregnancy; there are no acceptable alternatives. Pregnant women with a history of penicillin allergy should undergo skin testing to confirm the allergy and then desensitization, if necessary, according to protocol. In pregnant women, the Jarisch-Herxheimer reaction (discussed earlier) may precipitate a miscarriage. To reduce that risk, pregnant patients are best treated in a monitored and controlled setting for 24–48 hours. Serologic testing after therapy in a pregnant woman should be performed frequently to determine both response to therapy and the possibility of reinfection.

3. Sex partners—A few simple rules should be followed for the management of sex partners of those with syphilis. Transmission of syphilis is most likely during the mucocutaneous manifestations of early disease (primary and secondary stages). All sex partners within 90 days of the diagnosis of early-stage syphilis (ie, primary, secondary, or early latent) in the index case should be treated presumptively with a single intramuscular dose of benzathine penicillin G. In this circumstance treatment of the partner is administered irrespective of the serologic test result in that individual. For partners with exposure occurring more than 90 days before diagnosis of syphilis in an index case, presumptive treatment is considered if follow-up cannot be assured. Otherwise, treatment can be guided by either clinical findings or serologic testing. For partners of patients with latent disease of unknown duration, late latent disease, or tertiary disease, treatment may be withheld pending serologic test results. Some experts recommend treating this last group presumptively if the serologic titers in the index case are 1:32 or higher.

Centers for Disease Control and Prevention; Workowski KA, Berman SM. Sexually transmitted diseases treatment guidelines, 2006. *MMWR Recomm Rep* 2006;55(RR-11):1–94. [PMID: 16888612]

Lukehart S, Godornes C, Molini B, et al. Macrolide resistance in T. pallidum in the United States and Ireland. *N Engl J Med* 2004;351:154–158. [PMID: 15247355] (Describes treatment failures associated with azithromycin-resistant syphilis, along with epidemiology and molecular characteristics.)

Mitchell SJ, Engelman J, Kent CK, et al. Azithromycin-resistant syphilis infection: San Francisco, California 2000–2004.

Clin Infect Dis 2005;42:337–345. [PMID: 16392078] (Epidemiology of azithromycin-resistant syphilis in San Francisco.)

Rolfs R, Joesoef M, Hendershot E, et al. A randomized trial of enhanced therapy for early syphilis in patients with and without human immunodeficiency virus infection. *N Engl J Med* 1997;337:307–314. [PMID: 9235493] (Classic randomized-controlled trial demonstrating that penicillin G benzathine is equal to enhanced therapy [penicillin G benzathine plus amoxicillin/probenecid] in the treatment of syphilis in HIV-infected patients. The study also demonstrated the low sensitivity of CSF VDRL in neurosyphilis and the lack of need to treat asymptomatic neurosyphilis, although follow-up was limited to 1 year.)

When to Refer to a Specialist

The management of both early and latent stages of syphilis should be within the purview of most clinicians. When serologic results fail to follow the expected course after therapy, patients are best referred to an infectious disease specialist. Referral is likewise probably best for the management of HIV-infected patients with syphilis and for the workup and treatment of other manifestations of syphilis, such as neurosyphilis, cardiovascular syphilis, and gummatous syphilis. Management of sex partners can often be handled most properly and expeditiously with the help of local public health authorities.

Early-stage, communicable syphilis is a reportable disease in all 50 states of the United States. It is the responsibility of all clinicians who diagnose syphilis to report such cases promptly to the public health authorities. Laboratories are routinely required to report cases to local public health authorities, and clinicians may be contacted by local public health authorities after the receipt of a laboratory-reported case.

Prognosis

When treated according to the guidelines outlined earlier and followed carefully with serial serologic tests, almost all patients should be assured of disease elimination with no serious long-term sequelae. Patients who have suffered end-organ damage as a result of tertiary syphilis may, after therapy, see a halt in the progression of signs and symptoms. Unfortunately, resolution of pathologic damage done to that point may not occur.

PRACTICE POINTS

- *Treponemal-specific tests may become reactive before nontreponemal tests in the earliest stages of primary syphilis infection. That observation leads some experts to recommend the use of treponemal specific tests in the evaluation of a patient with suspected primary syphilis.*

- *When interpreting serologic tests, clinicians should be aware of the prozone phenomenon, which occurs when the concentration of antitreponemal antibodies is so high that the characteristic flocculation reaction that produces a reactive specimen cannot occur. This phenomenon is overcome by diluting the specimen and rerunning the test.*

- *The lower the serologic titer when the patient begins therapy, the longer it may take to see a decline—if one is ever achieved.*

Relevant Web Sites

[Centers for Disease Control and Prevention:]
http://www.cdc.gov
[National Institutes on Health information about syphilis:]
http://www.niaid.nih.gov/factsheets/stdsyph.htm

Neurosyphilis

Roger P. Simon, MD

ESSENTIALS OF DIAGNOSIS

- *Central nervous system (CNS) or ophthalmic signs or symptoms of CNS syphilis (neurosyphilitic syndromes).*
- *Serologic evidence of syphilis infection (positive results on nontreponemal and treponemal tests).*
- *One of the following findings: positive cerebrospinal fluid (CSF) Venereal Disease Research Laboratories (VDRL) test result, CSF protein concentration greater than 40 mg/dL, or CSF white blood cell (WBC) count greater than 5 mononuclear cells per microliter.*

General Considerations

Approximately 7% of patients with primary and secondary syphilis, if untreated, develop some form of symptomatic neurosyphilis. In 1990, the number of cases of primary and secondary syphilis reported to the US Centers for Disease Control and Prevention (CDC) peaked at over 50,000. By 1996, the incidence had fallen dramatically, and in 1997, fewer than 10,000 cases were reported. Many counties, however, report an incidence of more than 4 cases per 100,000 population. As of 2006, cases of primary and secondary syphilis are again increasing in the United States, particularly in populations of men having sex with men, thus increasing the risk pool for neurosyphilis.

The nervous system is affected early in syphilis, and 10–25% of patients have CSF abnormalities at the time of the development of the secondary stage. CSF inflammation eventually occurs in approximately one-third of patients with syphilis, with the peak of CSF abnormalities seen 12–18 months after the primary infection. Of patients with CSF inflammation, 30% will develop some form of neurosyphilis. In those with normal CSF examination findings 5 years after the primary infection, the risk

of neurosyphilis is approximately 1%. Each of the clinical forms of neurosyphilis is a manifestation of this inflammatory response that continues, in reaction to *Treponema pallidum* invasion, over decades (see Figure 20–1).

Pathogenesis

There has been some experimental evidence regarding treponemal strain specificity and neuroinvasion. The sheath proteins of *T pallidum* have conserved and variable regions that differ between strains. Strain-specific differences in neuroinvasion in rabbits have been demonstrated, and the possibility that these proteins may explain *T pallidum* tropism is being studied.

Prevention

Neurosyphilis can occur in both early and later stages of syphilis. Prevention of neurosyphilis can be primary—through the prevention of sexual exposure and syphilis infection—or secondary—through treatment in early stages to prevent the progression of syphilis.

Clinical Findings

A. SYMPTOMS AND SIGNS

The inflammatory process in the subarachnoid space produces the classic spectrum of presentation, which comprises acute syphilitic meningitis, arteritis (meningovascular syphilis), meningoencephalitis (syphilitic dementia, general paresis), and dorsal root ganglionopathy (tabes dorsalis). These entities may overlap; however, relatively pure forms predominate, demonstrating a characteristic time course and presentation following the initial primary infection (see Figure 20–1).

Acute syphilitic meningitis is the earliest symptomatic subtype and often accompanies the rash of the secondary stage of syphilis. When the meningeal inflammation involves blood vessels in the subarachnoid space, vascular syphilis occurs, usually within the first 5 years. The parenchymal forms follow over a more protracted interval

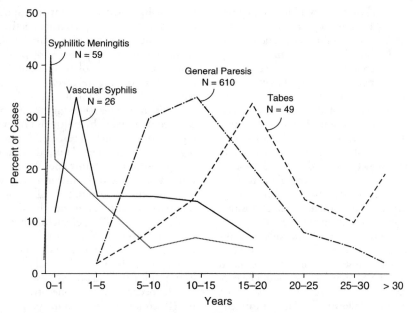

Figure 20-1. The interval between primary syphilis infection and symptomatic neurosyphilis. (Reproduced, with permission, from Simon RP. Neurosyphilis. *Arch Neurol* 1985;42:602.)

of several decades. The syndromes of neurosyphilis most commonly seen in recent years are syphilitic meningitis and cerebrovascular syphilis (see Table 20–1), because these are the earliest forms seen following a new infection.

B. LABORATORY FINDINGS

1. CSF analysis—CSF abnormalities are the hallmark of each stage of neurosyphilis. Lymphocytic pleocytosis with cell counts ranging from 10–500 WBCs/μL is

Table 20-1. Clinical findings in patients with early syndromes of neurosyphilis.[a]

	Acute Syphilitic Meningitis (n = 19)	Meningovascular Syphilis (n = 8)
HIV stage	Unknown 2, HIV-positive 7, AIDS 7, ARC 3	Unknown 2, HIV-positive 5, ARC 1
Serum VDRL	100% reactive; titer 1:8–1:1024	All positive at 1:32–1:1024
Neurologic findings	Headache 18, fever 4, meningeal signs 4, photophobia 4, altered mental state 1, CN defect (III, IV, VII, VIII, X)	Hemiparesis 5, dysarthria 3, CN VII defect 2, ataxia 2, tinnitus 1, headache 1, anisocoria 1
CSF cells (10^6/L)	9–892 (mean, 132)	33–653 (mean, 181)
CSF protein concentration (g/L)	0.29–2.29 (mean, 0.96)	1.02–3.84 (mean, 1.81)
CSF VDRL	100% reactive; titer 1:1–1:32 (mean, 1:4)	All positive at 1:1–1:32 (mean, 1.8)

[a]Data compiled from patients in San Francisco, 1984–1992.
ARC, AIDS-related complex; CN, cranial nerve; CSF, cerebrospinal fluid; VDRL, Venereal Disease Research Laboratories test.
Adapted from Flood JM, Weinstock HS, Guroy ME, et al. Neurosyphilis during the AIDS epidemic, San Francisco, 1985–1992. *J Infect Dis* 1998;177:931–940.

found in the most acute form, syphilitic meningitis. Decreasing numbers of cells are reported in syphilitic vascular disease, paresis, and tabes dorsalis. The glucose concentration may be mildly reduced in syphilitic meningitis. The protein concentration, the least specific of CNS parameters in neurosyphilis, is rarely greater than 200 mg/dL in syphilitic meningitis, syphilitic vascular disease, and paresis. Isolated protein elevations should be interpreted with caution. Protein concentrations of less than 100 mg/dL are the rule in tabes. The gamma globulin portion of the CSF protein is commonly elevated, and oligoclonal bands may be present, as is characteristic of any chronic meningitis. In late, "burned out" tabes dorsalis, after the period of inflammation, CSF findings may be normal, although positive CSF VDRL serologic test results may be retained.

Abnormal cellularity of the CSF defines disease activity, the potential amelioration of symptoms with therapy, and the adequacy of response to treatment (see Table 20–2). Therefore, repeat CSF examination should be performed after treatment (see later discussion). Persistence of CSF VDRL titer elevation following antibiotic treatment and cell count normalization is of uncertain significance.

2. Serologic tests—A negative treponemal serologic test result in blood (fluorescent treponemal antibody absorbed [FTA-ABS] or *T pallidum* particle agglutination [TP-PA]) excludes the diagnosis of neurosyphilis. A positive nontreponemal CSF serologic test result (CSF VDRL) establishes the diagnosis of neurosyphilis

(and an increased cell count in response to the spirochete documents the presence of active disease).

Whether true negative CSF VDRL serologic test results occur in the presence of presumed active neurosyphilis is an unresolved question. The classic literature relied on the relatively insensitive Wassermann reaction, and the clinical case series in patients with early neurosyphilis (meningeal and meningovascular) were contaminated by nonsyphilitic syndromes of viral meningitis and cerebral vascular disease that were unrecognized at that time. Thus, data from these clinical groups are of uncertain value. Where clinical diagnoses were clear in the older literature (eg, paresis and tabes dorsalis), the large numbers of reported cases suggest that seronegativity (even with the Wassermann reaction) was very rare. CSF serologic diagnosis in early syphilis remains a problem. For this reason, patients with a compatible clinical diagnosis and a mild elevation of cell count but nonreactive CSF VDRL are referred to as having "probable" neurosyphilis.

The occurrence of seronegative, active neurosyphilis in HIV co-infected patients has been suggested. However, spirochete penetration into the nervous system is not different in HIV-infected or-uninfected patients. Late serologic conversions in patients with secondary syphilis are well known, and the fact that the cellular response of the CSF may precede serologic positivity in early syphilis may explain many of these cases.

The role of the more sensitive treponemal test (FTA) in the CSF analysis remains uncertain, because the

Table 20–2. Cerebrospinal fluid findings observed in response to penicillin treatment in a patient with syphilitic meningitis.[a]

CSF Parameter	Day 0	Day 10 of Penicillin Treatment	6 Months Post-treatment
Opening pressure (mL CSF)	180	112	<20 (normal)
Cells/mL	140	19	2
Protein level (mg/d)	165	112	40
Glucose concentration (mg/dL)	45	42	52
CSF VDRL	Trace+	Positive	1:2
Blood VDRL	1:8	NR	NR

[a]Patient was a 38-year-old man with a history of bioccipital headache, fever, neck stiffness, photophobia, nausea and vomiting, left tinnitus, hearing loss, and brief blindness in the right eye on standing twice (1 d). On examination, patient had unilateral disk edema, mild hearing loss, and absent ankle reflexes. CT scan was negative. Treatment consisted of penicillin, 20 million units IV daily for 10 d. At day 2, resolution of headache and neck stiffness were noted. At 5 months, fundi were normal and hearing loss had improved.
CSF, cerebrospinal fluid; CT, computed tomography scan; NR, nonreactive; VDRL, Venereal Disease Research Laboratories test.

unabsorbed FTA test produces an unacceptably high false-positive response (4.5% of normal) and the addition of sorbent (FTA-ABS) decreases sensitivity to 75%. However, some laboratories now perform FTA-ABS and FTA tests of CSF to exclude neurosyphilis in at-risk patients in whom the CSF is abnormal but the CSF VDRL test is nonreactive.

C. CLINICAL DIAGNOSIS OF NEUROSYPHILITIC SUBTYPES

1. Acute syphilitic meningitis—Symptomatic syphilitic meningitis occurs during the first months to 2 years following the primary infection, and 10% of cases occur coincident with the secondary rash. The typical patient is afebrile, with headache, and may have some degree of confusion. Unilateral or bilateral swelling of the optic disk is common. Meningeal signs may be positive. The course is subacute. CSF examination demonstrates a lymphocytic pleocytosis (see Table 20–1). Currently, the most useful serologic test for the diagnosis of syphilitic CNS involvement is the CSF VDRL; rapid plasma reagin (RPR) or other nontreponemal testing of CSF has no role in CNS evaluation.

The meningeal inflammatory process may be concentrated at the vertex or base of the brain. Vertex involvement produces a communicating hydrocephalus, whereas basilar inflammation produces cranial nerve (CN) abnormalities, particularly CNs II and III and those of the cerebellopontine angle (VI, VII, and VIII); asymmetry is the rule. Meningeal enhancement may be seen on magnetic resonance imaging of the brain.

The diagnosis is made in patients with meningeal symptoms, cranial nerve abnormalities, and lymphocytic pleocytosis with a positive serologic test result. A negative CSF VDRL serologic result may occur in a patient with very early CSF sampling, because CSF inflammation precedes seropositivity. The meningeal symptoms may resolve without treatment but leave the patient at risk for later forms of neurosyphilis.

2. Meningovascular syphilis—When the CSF inflammatory process compromises arteries within the subarachnoid space, a syndrome of vasculitis involving mid-sized vessels is produced. The middle cerebral artery is most often affected, but any cerebral or spinal cord blood vessel may be involved, producing cortical syndromes or myelopathy in isolation or in combination. The clinical syndrome produced is distinct from that of thromboembolic stroke both in presentation and time course. Patients often have prodromal symptoms of headache, personality change, or emotional lability. The vascular occlusive syndrome is superimposed and, as is typical for a vasculitis, progresses over hours or days rather than occurring suddenly (see Table 20–1).

Increased white blood cell count in the CSF is uniformly seen. A positive CSF VDRL serologic result establishes the diagnosis. Neuroradiologic imaging most often shows involvement of the deep penetrating branches of the middle cerebral artery supplying the central white matter, particularly the white matter in the lenticulostriate distribution (see Figure 20–2A). Angiography shows concentric constriction of medium-caliber vessels (see Figure 20–2B). The angiographic features can be seen in a vascular bed prior to clinical symptoms (eg, cerebral arteritis in a patient being evaluated for a spinal presentation).

3. Syphilitic dementia—Parenchymal involvement of the brain by the spirochete produces a dementing syndrome (general paresis or dementia paralytica). This evolution occurs within 3–30 years after the primary infection, with a peak incidence between 10 and 20 years (see Figure 20–1). There is a male predominance. The clinical symptoms are notoriously nonspecific, being those of any organic brain syndrome (see Table 20–3). The classic features of psychosis with grandiose delusional states were uncommon even in the prepenicillin era.

Features useful in differentiating syphilitic dementia from other causes of progressive dementia (in a patient with a reactive treponemal serologic test) are the relatively early age of onset in syphilitic dementia (most commonly between 30 and 50 years) and the fact that untreated cases of syphilitic dementia are fatal within a few months to a few years. Furthermore, the CSF is always abnormal in syphilitic dementia, showing lymphocytic pleocytosis. The blood and CSF VDRL serologic results are positive. Several instances of unilateral or bilateral medial temporal lobe high-intensity magnetic resonance imaging T2 or fluid-attenuated inversion recovery imaging abnormalities, with or without associated atrophy, have been reported in patients with the mistaken diagnosis of herpes simplex encephalitis (see Figure 20–3). The high-intensity signals resolve with treatment, but the presence of atrophy may predict a fixed cognitive deficit. Seizures, including status epilepticus, may be the presenting manifestation of parenchymal syphilis, again offering a presentation similar to that of encephalitis.

4. Tabes dorsalis—Tabes dorsalis occurs within 5–50 years after a primary syphilitic infection, with a peak incidence 10–20 years after infection. This form of neurosyphilis in now uncommon. In the prepenicillin era, a marked male predominance occurred. The classic triad of symptoms—tabetic "lightning" pains, sensory ataxia, and bladder disturbances—are combined with a triad of signs—pupillary abnormalities, areflexia, and the Romberg sign. Lightning pains (localized, transient, agonizing, shooting pain, most often in the legs but affecting any body region) eventually occur in 75–90% of patients.

Either vibration or position sense may be affected out of proportion to the other. This proprioceptive sensory loss produces a wide-based gait with impaired balance that is exacerbated by eye closure (the Romberg sign). Whether the primary pathologic site is in the proximal

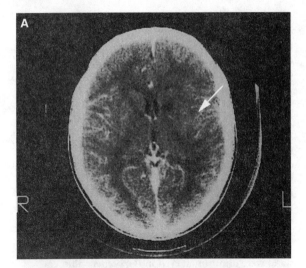

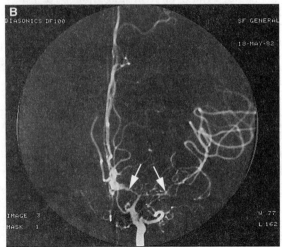

Figure 20–2. A: Contrast-enhanced computed tomography scan of the brain showing a small, low-density area in the left internal capsule (arrow). The patient was a 21-year-old man, 4 years after treatment for secondary syphilis, who presented with a 4-month history of personality change and progressive attenuation of language function over the preceding week. Neurologic examination showed mild right hemiparesis, denial, and mixed aphasia. CSF analysis showed lymphocytic pleocytosis, high protein concentration, and positive VDRL result. (Reproduced, with permission, from Holmes MD, Brant-Zawadski MM, Simon RP. Clinical features of meningovascular syphilis. *Neurology* 1984;34,553–556.) **B:** Anterior-posterior view of the left carotid digital angiogram in the same patient showing multifocal vascular narrowing of the proximal middle cerebral and anterior cerebral arteries (arrows).

Table 20–3. Symptoms and signs of syphilitic dementia (general paresis).

Symptoms
  Irritability
  Fatigability
  Personality changes
  Impaired judgment and insight
  Depression or elation
  Confusion and delusions
Signs
  Expressionless face
  Facial, lingual, and labial movement tremors
  Dysarthria
  Disordered handwriting (due to intention tremor)
  Hyperactive reflexes
  Rare focal signs

Based on Merritt HH. *A Textbook of Neurology*, 2nd ed. Lea & Febiger,1959:129–153.

dorsal root segments within the root entry zone or in the dorsal root ganglion remains an unresolved question.

Argyll-Robertson pupils are a characteristic finding but occur in only half of patients with tabes dorsalis. These pupils constrict to accommodation but not to light (the so-called light-near disassociation phenomenon). The typical pupils are small and irregular, bilaterally, but a host of other abnormalities can be seen. A lesion location involving the midbrain tectum has been proposed to explain this phenomenon. The differential diagnosis of these pupils includes diabetic autonomic neuropathy (pseudo tabes) and pineal region tumors or other lesions of the midbrain tectum.

The sensory impairment also results in the phenomenon of Charcot joints and distal ulcers. These phenomena and lightning pains may persist despite treatment.

5. Altered or atypical neurosyphilis—Modified or atypical presentations of the classic clinical syndromes of neurosyphilis have been suggested to be common in the antibiotic era, particularly in HIV-coinfected patients. Several series of patients confirm the classic spectrum of clinical presentations of neurosyphilis, in the setting of HIV although tabes dorsalis is now rare. In one series, no marked differences in clinical patterns were noted in 518 syphilis patients seen at the same hospital in 1930–1940 compared with 121 syphilis patients seen during 1970–1984. An increase in the number of cases of asymptomatic syphilis in the latter time period was attributed to the availability of more refined treponemal-specific tests. Another series, which compared neurosyphilis patients with and without HIV coinfection, found no clinical or serologic differences among patients, and a postmortem study concurred.

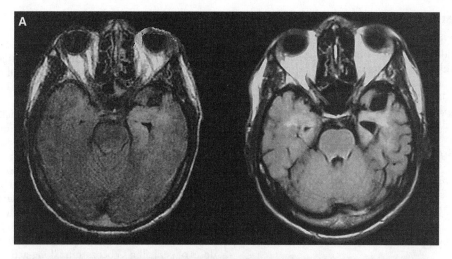

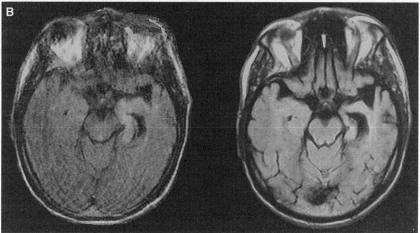

Figure 20–3. T2 high-intensity images of the medial temporal lobe in a patient with general paresis at the time of diagnosis (**A**) and 4.5 months later (**B**). (Courtesy of Drs Beau Ances and Toby Ferguson.)

The serologic response to treatment does not markedly differ in early syphilis patients with or without HIV coinfection. In CSF, normalization of pleocytosis (the marker of disease activity) does not differ in patients with or without HIV coinfection, although normalization of CSF VDRL results and protein concentration may be impeded in HIV patients. The significance of such serofast states in immunocompromised HIV-coinfected patients is uncertain.

Flood JM, Weinstock HS, Guroy ME, et al. Neurosyphilis during the AIDS epidemic, San Francisco, 1985–1992. *J Infect Dis* 1998;177:931–940. [PMID: 9534965] (Large and most recent retrospective report of 117 neurosyphilis patients from San Francisco hospitals during 1985–1992; meningitis was the most common presentation, followed by vascular syphilis.)

Marra CM. Neurosyphilis. *Curr Neurol Neurosci* Rep 2004; 4:435–440. [PMID: 15509443] (A recent review focusing on the problems of diagnosis and treatment in patients with HIV coinfection.)

O'Donnell JA, Emery CL. Neurosyphilis: A current review. *Curr Infect Dis Rep* 2005;7:277–284. [PMID: 15963329] (A recent, comprehensive review of diagnosis and treatment of patients with and without HIV coinfection.)

Timmermans M, Carr J. Neurosyphilis in the modern era. *J Neuro Neurosurg Psychiatry* 2004;75:1727–1730. [PMID: 15548491] (Discusses the spectrum of neurosyphilis in the postantibiotic era, including use of positive CSF FTA-ABS results in the setting of nonreactive VDRL to make the diagnosis.)

Wolters EC. Neurosyphilis: A changing diagnostic problem? Eur Neurol 1987;26:23–28. [PMID: 3545845] (Classic article comparing neurosyphilis presentation in the preantibiotic era [518 patients] with presentation during the antibiotic era [121 patients] at the same hospital.)

Differential Diagnosis

For acute syphilitic meningitis mimics include lymphocytic menigitides due to other infections agents, particularly tuberculosis and fungus as well as meningeal cancer. The angiographic differential diagnosis of meningovascular syphilis includes subarachnoid hemorrhage with spasm, tuberculous meningitis, and drug-induced vasculitis. Alzheimer's disease and degenerative dementing diseases can mimic paresis (see Table 20–3). MRI changes may be useful (see Fig. 20–3) As previously noted, the differential diagnosis of Argyll-Robertson pupils includes diabetic autonomic neuropathy (pseudo tabes) and pineal region tumors or other lesions of the midbrain tectum.

Complications

Although neurosyphilis is itself a complication of syphilis, untreated neurosyphilis can have its own complications, including permanent paralysis, dementia, and death. How reversible some complications may be depends on the duration and extent of untreated disease. Treatment of neurosyphilis can be lifesaving, so if neurosyphilis is suspected and cannot be excluded, most experts would recommend treatment.

Treatment

A. PHARMACOTHERAPY

Table 20–4 outlines recommended and alternative treatment regimens for neurosyphilis. Penicillin G remains the treatment of choice, administered as 12–24 million units daily via intravenous infusion or in six divided doses for 10–14 days; or as procaine penicillin, 2.4 million units by intramuscular administration once daily for 10–14 days with concomitant probenecid, 500 mg orally four times daily. A trial of ceftriaxone and penicillin (intravenous and intramuscular forms) produced similar results among the three treatment regimens. Treponemicidal drug concentrations have also been reported with tetracycline and doxycycline, and with chloramphenicol. After completion of the neurosyphilis treatment regimen, an additional one to three weekly doses of penicillin G benzathine (long-acting, 2.4 million units) is recommended.

A comparative trial of penicillin G and ceftriaxone (2.0 g intravenously or intramuscularly once daily for 10–14 days) for neurosyphilis in HIV-coinfected patients showed no difference in the improvement of CSF analytes between drugs. HIV coinfection did not alter the responsiveness of early syphilis to penicillin G benzathine, nor was the clinical responsiveness of

Table 20–4. Treatment regimens for neurosyphlilis.

Regimen	Description
Established regimen	Aqueous crystalline penicillin G, 12–24 million units IV daily (divided doses every 4 h) for 10–14 d; followed by penicillin G benzathine, 2.4 million units weekly for 1–3 wk
Alternative regimens[a]	Aqueous procaine penicillin G, 2.4 million units IM daily, plus probenecid, 500 mg PO 4 times daily, for 10–14 d; followed by penicillin G benzathine, 2.4 million units weekly for 1–3 wk *or* Ceftriaxone, 2.0 g IV or IM once daily for 10–14 d
Alternative regimens for penicillin-allergic patients[b]	Desensitize to penicillin (preferred) Tetracycline hydrochloride, 500 mg PO 4 times daily for 30 d *or* Doxycycline, 200 mg PO twice daily for 21 d
Recommended regimens for HIV-coinfected patients	Aqueous crystalline penicillin G, 12–24 million units IV daily (divided doses every 4 h) for 10–14 d; followed by penicillin G benzathine, 2.4 million units weekly for 1–3 wk *or* Aqueous procaine penicillin G, 2.4 million units IM daily, plus probenecid, 500 mg PO 4 times daily, for 10–14 d; followed by penicillin G benzathine, 2.4 million units weekly for 1–3 wk

[a]Probably equally effective but not CDC recommended.
[b]Based on published reports but not CDC recommended.
CDC, Centers for Disease Control and Prevention; CSF, cerebrospinal fluid.

primary and secondary syphilis patients to penicillin G benzathine, with or without amoxicillin and probenecid, affected by HIV coinfection.

Response to treatment is documented by the CSF results. The CSF cell count will normalize over weeks (see Table 20–2), with the CSF protein concentration and CSF VDRL titers normalizing more slowly. Serologic results may remain abnormal ("serofast"), a finding that may be more common in HIV-coinfected patients, particularly those with low CD4 T-cell counts. However, there is no known clinical significance to this finding. The CSF examination should be repeated at 6 and 12 months to document continued normalization. Although data in HIV-infected patients are not available, in the pre-HIV era, relapses did not occur if normalization persisted at 2 years.

B. TREATMENT OF ELDERLY PATIENTS WITH ABNORMAL SYPHILIS SEROLOGY

To make the diagnosis of neurosyphilis, CNS or ophthalmic signs or symptoms of CNS syphilis (neurosyphilitic syndromes) must be present. If neurologic signs are not present (eg, patient appears to be a normal 80 year old despite abnormal serologic results), the patient should be followed. Referral to a neurologist should be made if there is uncertainty about the diagnosis.

Patients who demonstrate signs of dementia require further evaluation, including CSF analysis for the presence of abnormal cells. Syphilitic dementia is progressive and fatal, leading to death in an average of 2.5 years if untreated. The absence of inflammation (WBC count <5 cells/μL) indicates no active disease and no need for treatment. If a diagnosis of syphilitic dementia is made, treatment for neurosyphilis is indicated. If there is no clear diagnosis, or if CSF analysis is not possible, some experts have given penicillin G benzathine, 2.4 million units per week intramuscularly for 3 weeks, although there is no clinical evidence of benefit and that form of penicillin has poor CNS penetration.

Marra CM, Maxwell CL, Tantalo L, et al. Normalization of cerebrospinal fluid abnormalities after neurosyphilis therapy: Does HIV status matter? *Clin Infect Dis* 2004;38:1001–1006.

[PMID: 15034833] (A comparison of neurosyphilis treatment with high-dose intravenous penicillin, intramuscular penicillin with probenecid, and intravenous ceftriaxone producing similar results.)

When to Refer to a Specialist

Patients with an uncertain diagnosis or those who have failed to respond to therapy should be referred to an infectious disease specialist or neurologist with experience in the management of neurosyphilis. For elderly patients with dementia and reactive serologic tests, consultation with an infectious disease expert or neurologist is recommended.

Prognosis

The prognosis for patients with neurosyphilis is good, if diagnosed and teated in the early stages before parenchymal manifestations occur. Syphilitic meningitis and ocular and otic disease respond to penicillin therapy. Residual neurologic symptoms or signs may occur but are uncommon. The response to treatment in patients with cerebrovascular signs, dementia, or tabes dorsalis is quite variable.

PRACTICE POINTS

- *Abnormal cellularity of the CSF defines disease activity, the potential amelioration of symptoms with therapy, and the adequacy of response to treatment in patients with neurosyphilis.*
- *A negative treponemal serologic test result in blood (fluorescent treponemal antibody absorbed [FTA-ABS] or T pallidum particle agglutination [TP-PA]) excludes the diagnosis of neurosyphilis.*
- *The CSF is always abnormal in syphilitic dementia, showing lymphocytic pleocytosis.*

SECTION III
Special Topics

Sexually Transmitted Diseases in HIV-infected Persons

21

Lisa A. Mills, MD, & Thomas C. Quinn, MD

ESSENTIAL FEATURES

- *Because new sexually transmitted diseases (STDs) are common in HIV-infected patients, regular screening and timely treatment are essential.*
- *Counseling of HIV-positive patients should include discussion of HIV-STD interactions and risks.*
- *Both genital ulcer–causing diseases and non–ulcer-causing STDs increase HIV transmission.*
- *Clinical and laboratory findings of syphilis in HIV-infected patients can be challenging to interpret, and these patients require close follow up.*
- *Prevention of human papillomavirus (HPV)–associated malignancies requires active surveillance in HIV-infected persons.*
- *Genital herpes and syphilis may increase HIV viral load, lower CD4 count, and hasten HIV disease progression.*

STD-FOCUSED CLINICAL EVALUATION OF HIV-INFECTED PATIENTS

Symptomatic Assessment

At the initial evaluation of a patient with HIV infection, the clinician should actively screen for typical symptoms and signs of STDs. These include the presence of genital, oral, or anal lesions; pain or burning with urination; new or unusual skin rash; lymphadenopathy and rectal symptoms of discharge, burning, or itching. In addition, men should be screened for urethral discharge or groin pain and women for bloody or foul-smelling vaginal discharge, itching, lower abdominal pain, missed menses, and pregnancy status. Any patient reporting symptoms and signs of STDs should have appropriate diagnostic testing regardless of reported sexual behavior or other risk factors.

Routine Laboratory Assessment

All HIV-infected patients should undergo serologic testing for syphilis, herpes simplex virus type 2 (HSV-2), and hepatitis as well as gonorrhea and chlamydia testing at all exposed anatomic sites (urogenital, anal, oral) at the initial visit. HSV-2 serologic testing should utilize newer, glycoprotein G–specific tests (see Table 21–1). HIV-infected women should undergo speculum-guided pelvic examination with microscopic evaluation of vaginal fluid (wet mount) and Papanicolaou (Pap) smear. Pap smears should be repeated at 6 months and then annually thereafter. Although no national guidelines exist, some experts recommend that HIV-infected men should also undergo regular anal cancer screening (anal Pap smear). Newly diagnosed HIV-infected patients should also receive a broad medical evaluation, which is beyond the scope of discussion in this chapter.

Repeat testing should be based on reported sexual risk behavior and may need to occur as often as every 3 months (see Table 21–2). Given recent increases in syphilis in HIV-infected men who have sex with men (MSM), most experts recommend syphilis testing for sexually active HIV-infected persons at 3- to 6-month intervals along with routine laboratory studies.

Table 21–1. Initial STD screenings in HIV-infected patients.

Patient Population	Test	Site or Source
All	RPR or VDRL	Serum
	HSV-2-specific antibody[a]	Serum
	Chlamydia trachomatis NAAT[a,b]	First-catch urine or urethral or cervical secretions, or both
	Gonorrhea culture or NAAT[a]	First-catch urine or urethral or cervical secretions, or both
Women	Wet mount or culture for *Trichomonas vaginalis*	Vaginal or cervical secretions
Patients engaging in receptive anal sex	Gonorrhea culture or NAAT (preferred), if available	Anal swab
	C trachomatis culture, if available or NAAT (preferred), if available	Anal swab
Patients engaging in receptive oral sex	Gonorrhea culture or NAAT (preferred), if available	Pharyngeal swab

[a]Test should be considered, but not routinely performed.
[b]Should be routine for all sexually active women aged 25 years or younger, and for any women at increased risk, even if asymptomatic.
HSV-2, herpes simplex virus type 2; NAAT, nucleic acid amplification test; RPR, rapid plasma reagin; VDRL, Venereal Disease Research Laboratories (test for syphilis).

Strategies for Effective Assessment of STD Risks in HIV-infected Patients

Discussing sexual practices with patients can be challenging, but it is essential to providing comprehensive care to HIV-infected patients. When discussing these topics, the mnemonic "Know the CODES" (**C**onfidentiality; **O**pen-minded approach and open-ended questions; **D**irect

Table 21–2. Patients who require more frequent screening for sexually transmitted diseases.

HIV-positive men who have sex with men
Patients with multiple or anonymous sex partners
Patients with a past history of any sexually treated disease (STD)
Patients with other STD or HIV risk factors
Patients who exchange sex for drugs or money
Sex or needle-sharing partners of people with these risks or behaviors
Patients with recent life changes leading to possible increases in risk behavior
Patients in areas with high prevalence of STDs
Patients who report substance use or dependence
Patients who use sildenafil (Viagra) or other erectile-enhancement drugs

questions about specific behaviors; **E**xplanation of implications of the elicited information; **S**pecific informations and advice) is a helpful guide.

Specific terms such as "men who have sex with men" should be used, rather than "gay." Assumptions about sexual behaviors and risk-taking should be avoided, including monogamy or heterosexuality among married people. Explanation of unfamiliar practices should be requested: "I don't know what you mean, could you explain ...?" Clinicians should ask about sex partners, including questions about number, where the patient meets sex partners, how well the patient knows the sex partners, HIV status (infected, not infected, or unknown) of sex partners, and any possible STD-related symptoms among sex partners. Questions should also focus on sexual activities and protection methods, use of condoms (and with what type of activities), use of drugs or alcohol, and sexual assault or coercion.

For patients acknowledging the use of drugs or alcohol, discussion of their impact on decision making and risk for further STDs or HIV transmission is appropriate and the responsibility of every treating medical provider. Use of drugs for enhanced erectile function (eg, sildenafil [Viagra]) may likewise be markers for sexual risk-taking behavior.

For injection drug users, discussion should include options to help with cessation or harm reduction, and advice regarding use of only sterile equipment and how to obtain such materials via needle exchange, local pharmacies, or harm reduction centers. Clinicians should ask the patient if all sex and needle-sharing partners have been informed of their possible exposure to HIV. Patients can be referred to appropriate services for facilitation of partner notification.

In women of childbearing age, clinicians should ask about pregnancy-related issues; these include possible current pregnancy (if so, test), past history of pregnancies and terminations, interest in future pregnancy, sexual activity, and contraception use.

Risk Reduction Counseling

The diagnosis of a new STD in a patient with HIV-infection should initiate a discussion about sexual risk behavior and the spread of STDs and HIV. The prevention of HIV transmission can be promoted during the patient visit by discussing safer behaviors to protect both the patient's own health and the health of sex and needle-sharing partners. Patients should be advised that there can be an significant adverse impact on their own health (increased HIV viral load or decreased CD4 T cell count, or both) as well as on the health of others should they practice high-risk sexual or injection behaviors.

The risk of HIV transmission to partners should also be discussed (see Table 21–3). Risks can be reduced in the following ways: abstinence from sexual or injection drug use; alteration of specific sexual behaviors for harm reduction (oral sex versus anal or vaginal sex; no ejaculation versus ejaculation); safer sex or injection practices (consistent and correct condom or barrier method use, bleaching or not sharing injection equipment); and sexual or injection activity only with others who are also HIV-infected (although as discussed later, this practice is not without risk).

Although effective highly active antiretroviral therapy (HAART) decreases plasma viral load and is thought to decrease risk of HIV transmission from the HIV-infected person taking HAART to an HIV-uninfected sex partner (see Table 21–4), it should be emphasized that even patients who are highly adherent to HAART regimens should not be thought of as unable to transmit HIV to others. HIV viral particles can be detected in the genital and rectal secretions of patients with an undetectable plasma viral load, and factors controlling viral load and infectivity in those anatomic compartments are currently being investigated.

In addition, patients should be counseled that antiretroviral drug interruptions, whether intentional or unintentional, increase both the risk of developing resistance to antiretroviral therapy and the risk of HIV transmission to sex or injection partners. Ultimately, virologic failure of HAART regimens can lead to asymptomatic increases in viral load and further increased infectivity among patients.

Table 21–3. Relative risk of HIV acquisition by sex act and condom use for HIV-negative sex partners of an HIV-positive person.

Sex Act	Relative Risk of HIV Acquisition[a]
Insertive fellatio	1
Receptive fellatio	2
Insertive vaginal sex	10
Receptive vaginal sex	20
Insertive anal sex	13
Receptive anal sex	100
Condom used	1
Condom not used	20

[a]Risks are multiplicative. If a condom is not used, the relative risk of the sex act is 20 times higher. Other factors, including presence of sexually transmitted diseases and HIV viral load of the infected partner, may also affect transmission risk. Adapted from Incorporating HIV prevention into the medical care of persons living with HIV. *MMWR Morb Mortal Wkly Rep* 2003;52(RR-12):9.

Table 21–4. Estimated risk of HIV transmission by HIV viral load of infected sex partner to uninfected partner.[a]

Serum Viral Load of HIV-infected Partner (copies/mL)	Risk of HIV Transmission to HIV-negative Partner (95% CI)
<3500	Reference risk
3500–9999	5.8 (2.26–17.80)
10,000–49,999	6.91 (2.96–20.15)
>50,000	11.87 (5.02–34.88)
Per 10-fold increase in viral load	2.45 (1.85–3.26)

[a]Patients in this study were not receiving antiretroviral therapy, and unknown factors may have caused untreated patients to have low viral loads. Risks may differ in treated patients with low viral loads. Serum viral load may not predict viral load in the genital tract, which may be more relevant in sexual transmission. Also see Quinn TC, Wawer MJ, Sewankambo N, et al. Viral load and heterosexual transmission of human immunodeficiency virus type 1. Rakai Project Study Group. *N Engl J Med* 2000;342:921–929.

Finally, there is evidence of transmission of drug-resistant HIV strains from infected patients with histories of antiretroviral therapy to HIV-uninfected persons who "inherit" the drug-resistance patterns of the person from whom they acquired their HIV infection. Numerous studies now demonstrate that a rising proportion of newly diagnosed cases of HIV infection are caused by viruses resistant to one or more antiretroviral drugs. Studies of the dynamics of transmission and clinical implications of drug-resistant HIV strains are ongoing.

Centers for Disease Control and Prevention; Workowski KA, Berman SM. Sexually transmitted diseases treatment guidelines, 2006. *MMWR Recomm Rep* 2006;55(RR-11):1–94. [PMID: 16888612] (The most recent national STD treatment guidelines, which include a special section on HIV.)

Incorporating HIV prevention into the medical care of persons living with HIV. *MMWR Morb Mortal Wkly Rep* 2003;52(RR-12). Available at: http://www.cdc.gov/ mmwr. (Rates the quality of evidence supporting recommendations for various preventive care strategies in HIV.)

Reynolds SJ, Quinn TC. Developments in STD/HIV interactions: The intertwining epidemics of HIV and HSV-2. *Infect Dis Clin North Am* 2005;19:415–425. [PMID: 15963880] (A recent review of the research demonstrating the intricate relationship between HSV-2 and HIV globally.)

Sangani P, Rutherford G, Wilkinson D. Population-based interventions for reducing sexually-transmitted infections, including HIV infection. Cochrane Database Syst Rev 2001;(2): CD001220. [PMID: 15106156] (A review of the seemingly conflicting results of multiple population-based trials in STD and HIV transmission.)

MANIFESTATIONS & TREATMENT OF STDS IN HIV-INFECTED PATIENTS

Syphilis

Syphilis and HIV affect similar at-risk populations, including MSM, injection drug users, and people who exchange sex for drugs or money. Many patients are dually infected. For example, among primary and secondary syphilis cases reported to the Centers for Disease Control

and Prevention (CDC) in 2002, 25% occurred in HIV-infected persons. Among MSM, rates of syphilis and HIV coinfection may be as high as 60%.

Clinical and laboratory findings of syphilis can differ in HIV-infected patients in several ways. Multiple chancres and atypical or florid skin manifestations are more common. HIV-infected patients are more likely to have chancres of primary syphilis at the same time as they manifest symptoms of secondary syphilis. In addition, more protracted and malignant constitutional symptoms and greater organ involvement have been reported. Studies also have demonstrated that HIV-infected persons appear to have a greater risk of central nervous system involvement at all stages of syphilis infection. Neurosyphilis presentations include meningitis and cranial nerve deficits, such as optic neuritis and deafness. Syphilitic uveitis, and particularly bilateral eye involvement, has been reported more frequently among HIV-infected patients than among those without HIV infection.

Because of the specific immune disturbances of B-cell function in HIV infection, antibody-based syphilis testing results in HIV-infected patients may be different in seemingly paradoxical ways (see Table 21–5). For example, HIV-infected patients in the early stages of HIV disease who have syphilis tend to have higher titers of antibodies than HIV-uninfected patients with syphilis. Also related to overexpression of B-cell activity in early HIV disease have been rare reports of falsely reactive nontreponemal test results. However, before defining a positive nontreponemal test as falsely positive (because a simultaneous treponemal test was negative), the clinician should repeat treponemal testing at least 1 week after the initial tests were performed. In cases where clinical suspicion is high in the face of negative serologic test results, alternative tests (eg, biopsy of skin lesions with silver staining) may be useful to confirm the diagnosis.

The rate of decline of nontreponemal titers following successful therapy may also be influenced by early HIV disease. In a large, randomized, prospective study of patients with early syphilis, HIV-coinfected patients had

Table 21–5. Results of serologic syphilis testing in early- and late-stage HIV infection.

	Early HIV versus non-HIV	Late HIV or AIDS versus non-HIV
Nontreponemal serologies (RPR, VDRL)	Higher titers in patients with syphilis Occasional false-positive results in patients without syphilis	Occasional false-negative results in patients with syphilis
Nontreponemal titers post-treatment	Higher rate of serologically defined treatment failures may be misleading due to slower decline of titers in patients who had meaningful clinical response	More frequent loss of prior reactivity

RPR, rapid plasma reagin; VDRL, Venereal Disease Research Laboratories test.

higher rates of serologically defined treatment failure, although patients had equal clinical responses to therapy, suggesting that the expected decline in titer in HIV-infected patients may be delayed.

Standard indications for lumbar puncture in HIV-infected patients with syphilis are as follows: neurologic, ocular, or auditory symptoms or signs; latent syphilis of unknown duration or late latent syphilis (>1 year); tertiary syphilis; or suspected treatment failure. However, some authorities recommend lumbar puncture in all HIV-infected patients with syphilis. Surveillance data from the CDC suggest neurosyphilis is two to three times more common in HIV-infected patients than in uninfected patients. In one study of 326 patients, many of whom had early syphilis, 20% who underwent cerebrospinal fluid (CSF) analysis had neurosyphilis. Those with serum rapid plasma reagin (RPR) titers of 1:32 or higher were 7.6 times as likely to have laboratory evidence of central nervous system involvement. A serum RPR titer of 1:32 or higher combined with a peripheral blood CD4 cell count of 350 cells/μL or lower conferred still higher odds of neurosyphilis in HIV-infected patients. Thus, a possible strategy to use in deciding whether to perform lumbar puncture in an HIV-infected syphilis patient without signs or symptoms of neurosyphilis might be to factor in serum RPR titer and a recent CD4 count.

The interpretation of CSF laboratory results in patients with syphilis and HIV infection requires careful consideration. Because mild pleocytosis (5–15 white blood cells [WBCs]/μL) can be attributed to HIV infection alone, especially when CD4 counts are higher than 500 cells/μL, most experts would consider more than 20 WBCs/μL to be indicative of a secondary process (ie, syphilis). Elevated CSF protein concentrations are highly nonspecific findings in HIV infection and should not be used alone to make a diagnosis of neurosyphilis. The CSF VDRL is not sensitive and may only be positive in 25–50% of patients with neurosyphilis. In the absence of inflammation (<5 WBCs/μL), the significance of a reactive CSF VDRL result is even less clear (see Chapter 20).

If available, the CSF fluorescent treponemal antibody absorbed (FTA-ABS) test may be helpful, because it is likely to be positive in HIV-positive patients with neurosyphilis who have falsely negative CSF VDRL results, as well as in many patients without other evidence of neurosyphilis. A negative CSF FTA-ABS test essentially excludes neurosyphilis, but a positive CSF FTA-ABS is nonspecific and the diagnosis should not be made if this is the only abnormal CSF result. If CSF evaluation is equivocal and neurosyphilis cannot be excluded, some experts would opt to treat patients for neurosyphilis while others would not. Such decisions are based in part on differing interpretations of the same data. Patient preferences, the likelihood of reliable follow-up, and other factors should also be incorporated in this decision-making process.

Similar treatment regimens are recommended for syphilis in both HIV-infected and uninfected patients; however, because of concerns about a modest increase in risk for treatment failure, closer follow-up is recommended for HIV-infected patients at 3, 6, 9, 12, and 24 months. All patients with neurosyphilis, regardless of HIV status, require repeat CSF analysis at 6 months to document improvement.

Among HIV-infected patients who contract syphilis, several studies have reported that CD4 concentration drops and HIV plasma viral load rises from previous levels. In studies where changes were observed, both markers tended to return toward baseline levels following syphilis treatment. The magnitude of CD4 and viral load changes was largest in patients not receiving HAART, and most of those data are drawn from patients with CD4 concentrations greater than 200 cells/μL. In the medical care of HIV-infected patients, an increase in HIV viral load or decrease in CD4 T cell count should prompt an evaluation for syphilis infection. The effect of advanced syphilis on HIV disease progression or of early syphilis on patients with advanced AIDS is less well characterized.

Human Papillomavirus–associated Genital Warts & Malignancies

HPV-associated genital warts may be more extensive and more difficult to treat in HIV-infected patients. Precancerous cervical lesions are much more common in HIV-infected women, and studies have reported up to ninefold increases in rates of cervical cancer in women with HIV. Among HIV-infected women with dysplasia, the severity of cervical disease correlates with the degree of immune compromise. Persistence of cervical cancer-causing HPV strains is also more common in women with HIV infection and correlates with the level of immunosuppression.

Anal cancer is similar to cervical cancer; it is associated with the same HPV strains, characterized by a predictable progression through stages of dysplasia to frank neoplasm, and can be detected by Pap smear techniques. The prevalence of HPV in MSM is 60–75%, and the frequency of anal carcinoma in men with HIV infection is 80 times that of the general population and increases with decreasing CD4 count. Some experts recommend regular anal cytology at three-year intervals for all HIV-infected men regardless of history of receptive anal intercourse. Patients with abnormal anal Pap smears should be referred for anoscopy and biopsy. The role of the new HPV vaccine in management of HIV-infected patients is being investigated and is currently unclear.

Herpes Simplex Virus Type 2

Much recent work has focused on the role of genital ulcer disease caused by HSV-2 in the sexual transmission of HIV infection. HSV-2 infection (with symptomatic genital ulcers or with positive HSV-2 serology) in an HIV-uninfected sex partner of an HIV-infected person increases the likelihood that the HIV-negative partner will acquire HIV. Similarly, HSV-2 infection (with or without a history of symptomatic genital ulcers) in an HIV-infected person also increases the risk that he or she will transmit HIV to uninfected partners. The mechanism of enhanced HIV transmission between an asymptomatic HSV-2–positive, HIV-coinfected person and his or her HSV-2–negative, HIV-uninfected sex partner may be related to the increased HIV viral loads observed in HSV-2– and HIV-coinfected individuals.

HIV-infected, HSV-2–positive patients experience both more frequent symptomatic herpetic outbreaks and more frequent and prolonged asymptomatic HSV-2 viral shedding than persons without HIV infection. At present, determinants of HSV-2 asymptomatic viral shedding are unknown. Clinical trials of chronic suppressive anti–HSV-2 therapy to decrease HIV transmission (from a coinfected partner to an HIV-uninfected partner) and HIV acquisition (by an HIV-uninfected person with HSV-2 from his or her HIV-infected partner) are ongoing.

Symptomatic HSV-2 lesions are more common in HIV-infected persons and may be more severe, numerous, painful, prolonged, or atypical. In fact, chronic HSV-2 ulcers of more than 1 month's duration are considered an AIDS-defining illness in HIV-infected individuals. HSV-2 ulcers appear frequently in the perianal area of HIV-infected people. In severely immunocompromised patients, HSV-2 may present as hyperkeratotic verrucous lesions that mimic condylomata.

Disseminated lesions, refractory disease, and acyclovir-resistant HSV disease are also more common in patients with advanced HIV infection. Neurologic complications of HSV-2 infection are rare, occur mostly in advanced AIDS, and develop rapidly. These complications can include aseptic meningitis, sacral radiculopathy, and transverse myelitis. If herpes is unresponsive to acyclovir or related agents, viral culture with testing of isolates for thymidine-kinase mutations should be undertaken and treatment using foscarnet or cidofovir should be considered. In HIV-infected patients, the treatment of HSV-2 infection can require higher doses and prolonged courses of therapy.

Among HIV- and HSV-2–coinfected patients treated with high-dose acyclovir therapy to suppress HSV reactivation, plasma HIV-1 RNA levels at a given CD4 cell count were decreased by about half, suggesting that HSV reactivation is associated with increased HIV replication in vivo. HIV-infected individuals who develop HSV-2 recurrences have a median HIV viral load increase of 3.4-fold, and increased viral load is sustained for 30–45 days following appearance of genital lesions.

HSV-2 has been shown to upregulate HIV replication at a cellular level. HSV-2 also likely plays a role in determining the steady-state HIV viral load of patients in the early stages of HIV disease following acute infection (the so-called viral set-point). HSV-2–seropositive patients with acute HIV infection have been found to have higher HIV viral loads more than 1 year following their estimated date of HIV acquisition than HSV-2–seronegative patients. Because of the role of HSV-2 in enabling HIV transmission, as well as its potential role in driving HIV disease progression, the overlapping global phenomena of HIV and HSV-2 can truly be considered a "syndemic."

We recommend routine, type-specific serologic testing for HSV-2 in all HIV-infected persons. Only tests that detect HSV glycoprotein G are truly type-specific and suitable for HSV-2 serologic screening. Patients with positive results should be informed of the increased risk of transmitting HIV during both symptomatic herpes episodes and phases of asymptomatic viral shedding. Such patients should be counseled regarding recognition of symptoms of early HSV-2 outbreaks, and may benefit from keeping anti–HSV-2 medications on hand to take when symptoms first develop. Consistent and correct condom use even when HSV symptoms are absent is advisable for maximal protection against transmission of HSV-2 or HIV to uninfected sex partners. Patients with negative HSV-2 serologic results should be counseled about measures to avoid HSV-2 exposure, and their sex partners should be offered serologic testing and counseling regarding chronic suppressive anti–HSV-2 therapy.

Consideration should be given to chronic suppressive anti-HSV therapy for HIV- and HSV-2-coinfected patients who experience recurrent symptomatic outbreaks. If a coinfected patient has an HIV-negative, HSV-2–negative, or dual-negative sex partner, the clinician could also consider chronic HSV-2 suppressive therapy for the patient to decrease the likelihood of HSV-2 and HIV transmission to the uninfected partner. Regimens recommended for chronic suppressive therapy of HSV-2 are acyclovir, 400 mg orally twice daily, or valacyclovir, 500 mg or 1000 mg orally daily (for further discussion, see Chapter 14). At this time, there is no direct clinical evidence to support recommending chronic HSV-2 suppressive therapy for HIV-infected patients to slow HIV disease progression; however, clinical trials addressing this question are now being performed.

Gonorrhea, Chlamydia, & Pelvic Inflammatory Disease

According to the CDC's 2006 STD treatment guidelines, whether the management of immunodeficient HIV-infected women with pelvic inflammatory disease requires more intensive treatment has not been determined. Such women were more likely to have tuboovarian abscesses but responded equally well to standard parenteral and oral antibiotic regimens when compared with HIV-uninfected women.

Similarly, gonococcal and chlamydial infections do not seem to cause differing illness or require different treatment in HIV-infected individuals. However, HIV-infected women more often have multiple concomitant reproductive tract infections, a fact that bears remembering when assessing and treating such patients.

Bacterial Vaginosis & Trichomoniasis

The clinical presentation and recommended treatment of these infections do not differ in HIV-infected patients. The reader is referred to detailed discussion of these diseases elsewhere in this text (see Chapters 11 and 18).

Vulvovaginal Candidiasis

Presentations of candidal vulvovaginitis are generally similar in HIV-infected and uninfected patients but are by definition considered "complicated" when occurring in immunosuppressed patients. Episodes may be more common and more severe among HIV-infected patients and may require longer duration of therapy (7–14 days or more) if standard courses are not effective for individual patients.

Lymphogranuloma Venereum

This infection is rare in developed countries but more common currently in HIV-infected people than in those without HIV infection. The manifestations and treatment of lymphogranuloma venereum are described elsewhere in this text (see Chapter 17), but the infection bears mentioning here because of its strong epidemiologic association with HIV-infected MSM, in whom outbreaks in urban areas have recently been reported.

Scabies & Norwegian Scabies

Norwegian (or crusted) scabies, a severe form of scabies that occurs in patients with advanced immunosuppression, is much more common in HIV-infected patients than in uninfected patients and, like all scabies, is highly contagious. It is best treated with oral ivermectin, 200 mcg/kg as a single dose, followed by a repeat dose 2 weeks later in conjunction with topical permethrin.

Molluscum Contagiosum

This skin and genital condition caused by a poxvirus is much more common in HIV-infected persons and has no apparent long-term adverse effects. It presents as scattered umbilicated papules, usually in the genital area, but can be disseminated in patients with advanced HIV infection. Treatment consists of ablative cryotherapy, as needed.

PRACTICE POINTS

- *The diagnosis of a new STD in a patient with HIV-infection should initiate a broad screening evaluation as well as a discussion about sexual risk behavior and the spread of STDs and HIV.*
- *In the medical care of HIV-infected patients, an increase in HIV viral load or decrease in CD4 T cell count should prompt an evaluation for syphilis infection.*

Relevant Web Sites

[Centers for Disease Control and Prevention information on HIV:]
http://www.cdc.gov/std/hiv/default.htm
[HIV Medicine Association:]
http://www.HIVMA.org
[National Institutes of Health up-to-date information on HIV:]
htpp://www.niaid.nih.gov/factsheets/hivinf.htm

Sexually Transmitted Diseases in Pregnancy

22

Natali Aziz, MD, MS, & Craig R. Cohen, MD, MPH

GENERAL CONSIDERATIONS

An estimated two million pregnant women are infected with sexually transmitted diseases (STDs) each year in the United States. These STDs are common complications in pregnancy. Physiologic—including immunologic and hormonal—changes during pregnancy may alter susceptibility to infection.

STDs can cause significant maternal and fetal complications. Adverse pregnancy outcomes directly and indirectly attributable to STDs include ectopic pregnancy, spontaneous abortion, fetal demise, perinatal infections, intrauterine growth restriction, congenital abnormalities, premature rupture of membranes, preterm birth, chorioamnionitis, puerperal infections, low-birth-weight infants, and neonatal infections. The immunologic mechanisms involved in STDs and adverse pregnancy outcomes are not well understood. Inflammatory cytokines, in response to infection, may be involved in the pathogenesis of preterm premature rupture of membranes and preterm labor, as well as adverse fetal conditions.

Diagnosis and management of STDs in pregnancy may decrease maternal and fetal morbidity and mortality. Most STDs are commonly asymptomatic or present with non-specific symptoms; without a high index of suspicion and low threshold for testing, a substantial number of STDs will be missed, potentially leading to adverse perinatal outcomes. Therefore, obtaining a complete STD history and performing appropriate screening studies of the pregnant patient at the first prenatal visit are essential.

STDs routinely screened for in pregnancy include syphilis, hepatitis B, HIV, and chlamydia. Leading authorities differ regarding STD screening recommendations in pregnancy (see Table 22–1). These variations arise from different risk stratification, cost-benefit, and prevention strategies. Of note, the Centers for Disease Control and Prevention (CDC) recommends chlamydia screening for all pregnant women at the first prenatal visit, whereas the American Academy of Pediatrics (AAP) and American College of Obstetricians and Gynecologists (ACOG), in their 2002 *Guidelines for*

Perinatal Care, recommend chlamydia testing only in high-risk pregnant women, given that evidence of prevention of adverse effects through screening in pregnancy is limited. High-risk individuals may be defined by numerous criteria, depending on the specific STD in consideration (see Table 22–1). Additionally, gonorrhea and hepatitis C testing are also recommended by the CDC for at-risk women during the first prenatal visit.

Testing for STDs, including HIV, syphilis, hepatitis B, chlamydia, and gonorrhea, should be repeated in the third trimester in any woman at high risk for acquiring these infections. Both the CDC and ACOG recommend that women younger than 25 years of age, regardless of risk profile, be retested for *Chlamydia trachomatis* in the third trimester.

Screening for bacterial vaginosis is not recommended as a routine component of prenatal care. Clinicians may consider such evaluation and treatment if indicated at the first prenatal visit for asymptomatic women with a history of preterm birth in order to potentially lower the risk of preterm premature rupture of membranes and low-birth-weight infants. Routine screening for *Trichomonas vaginalis* in asymptomatic pregnant women is not recommended.

In light of physiologic changes during pregnancy affecting the pharmacokinetics of medical therapy, drug exposure of the fetus, and breast-feeding safety considerations, treatment of STDs in pregnant and postpartum women may vary from guidelines for nonpregnant women (see Table 22–2). In addition, special concerns relating to the potential for transmission of some viral STDs need to be considered in determining the safety of breast-feeding (see Table 22–3).

ACOG committee opinion number 304. Prenatal and perinatal human immunodeficiency virus testing: Expanded recommendations. *Obstet Gynecol* 2004;104:1119–1124. [PMID: 15516421]

American College of Obstetricians and Gynecologists. *Antimicrobial Therapy for Obstetric Patients.* Educational Bulletin 245. ACOG, 1998. (Antimicrobial recommendations for safety in pregnancy by a leading organizational authority.)

Table 22–1. Screening guidelines for sexually transmitted diseases (STDs) in pregnancy.

	CDC	ACOG
First prenatal visit	HIV Syphilis Hepatitis B Chlamydia Pap smear[a] Trichomoniasis[b]	HIV Syphilis Hepatitis B Pap smear
First prenatal visit (high-risk)[c]	Gonorrhea Hepatitis C Bacterial vaginosis	Gonorrhea Hepatitis C Chlamydia
Third trimester	Chlamydia (<25 y)	Chlamydia (<25 y)
Third trimester (high-risk)[c]	HIV (before 36 wk) Syphilis (at 28 wk) Gonorrhea Chlamydia	HIV (before 36 wk) Syphilis Hepatitis B Gonorrhea
Delivery (high-risk)[c]	HIV Syphilis Hepatitis B	HIV

[a]If no Pap smear documented during preceding year.
[b]Women who are symptomatic with trichomoniasis should be evaluated to confirm diagnosis and treated to ameliorate symptoms.
[c]High-risk individuals may be defined by numerous criteria, depending on the specific STD in consideration; these criteria include maternal age (adolescent), use of illicit or intravenous drugs, history of STDs, diagnosis of STD in the current pregnancy, new sex partner, multiple sex partners during current pregnancy, current partner with an STD or high-risk behavior, blood product transfusion or exposure, undocumented HIV or syphilis infection status at time of delivery, history of adverse pregnancy outcome, and residence in areas with a high prevalence of specific STDs.
ACOG = American College of Obstetricians and Gynecologists; CDC = Centers for Disease Control and Prevention.

American College of Obstetricians and Gynecologists. *Breastfeeding: Maternal and Infant Aspects.* Educational Bulletin 258. ACOG, 2000.

American Academy of Pediatrics and the American College of Obstetricians and Gynecologists. *Guidelines for Perinatal Care,* 5th ed. AAP, ACOG, 2002. (STD screening guidelines for pregnant women.)

Centers for Disease Control and Prevention; Workowski KA, Berman SM. Sexually transmitted diseases treatment guidelines, 2006. *MMWR Recomm Rep* 2006;55(RR-11):1–94. [PMID: 16888612] (The most recent guidelines from the CDC, including recommendations for screening in pregnancy.)

CERVICAL INFECTIONS

Chlamydia

C trachomatis infection in pregnancy has been associated with various complications, including postpartum endometritis, spontaneous abortion, and possibly preterm

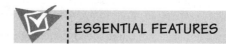

ESSENTIAL FEATURES

- *Genital chlamydia infection is most often asymptomatic.*
- *Adverse pregnancy outcomes include postpartum endometritis, ophthalmia neonatorum, and neonatal pneumonia.*

labor and delivery. Neonatal infections include conjunctivitis, otitis media, and pneumonia. The prevalence of chlamydia in pregnant women ranges between approximately 3% and 14%. Pregnant women infected with *C trachomatis* may present with vaginal discharge, spotting,

Table 22–2. Treatment recommendations for selected STDs in pregnancy.

Disease	Treatment Regimen
Bacterial vaginosis	Metronidazole, 500 mg PO twice daily for 7 d or Clindamycin, 300 mg PO twice daily for 7 d or Metronidazole, 250 mg PO 3 times daily for 7 d
Chancroid	Azithromycin, 1 g PO in a single dose or Ceftriaxone, 250 mg IM in a single dose or Erythromycin base, 500 mg PO 3 times daily for 7 d
Chlamydia[a]	Azithromycin, 1 g PO in a single dose or Amoxicillin, 500 mg PO 3 times daily for 7 d
Cytomegalovirus	Supportive care
Genital herpes	Acyclovir, 400 mg PO 3 times daily for 7–14 d (first episode) Acyclovir, 400 mg PO 3 times daily for 5 d (recurrent episode) Acyclovir, 400 mg PO 3 times daily (suppression after 36 wk) *Alternative regimen* (for women in whom adherence is an issue): valacyclovir, 500 mg daily
Genital warts	Cryotherapy and trichloroacetic acid
Gonorrhea[b]	Cefpodoxime, 400 mg PO in a single dose or Ceftriaxone, 125 mg IM in a single dose *Alternate regimen* (for women who cannot tolerate a cephalosporin: spectinomycin, 2 g IM as a single dose
Granuloma inguinale	Erythromycin base, 500 mg PO 4 times daily for at least 3 wk ± parenteral aminoglycoside
Hepatitis A	Immunoprophylaxis (immune serum globulin and hepatitis A vaccine) as needed
Hepatitis B	Immunoprophylaxis (HBIG and hepatitis B vaccine) as needed
Lymphogranuloma venereum	Erythromycin base, 500 mg PO 4 times daily for 21 d
Molluscum contagiosum	Curettage, cryotherapy, chemical cauterization, or laser therapies
Pediculosis pubis	Permethrin 1% cream rinse to affected areas, washed off after 10 min or Pyrethrins with piperonyl butoxide to affected area, washed off after 10 min
Scabies	Permethrin cream (5%) to all areas of body from neck down, washed off after 8–14 h
Syphilis[c]	Benzathine penicillin G, 2.4 million units IM in a single dose (primary, secondary, early latent) Benzathine penicillin G, 7.2 million units total, 2.4 million units IM once weekly for 3 weeks (late latent or latent of unknown duration)
Trichomoniasis	Metronidazole, 2 g PO in a single dose

[a]Repeat test 3 wk after completion of therapy.
[b]If chlamydia infection has not been excluded, then treat for presumptive co-infection.
[c]May consider second dose of benzathine penicillin 2.4 million units IM 1 week after initial dose for women who have primary, secondary, or early latent syphilis.
HBIG, hepatitis B immune globulin.

Table 22–3. Breast-feeding guidelines for women with STDs.

Breast-feeding contraindicated
  HIV infection
  Active herpes simplex virus lesion of the breast
Breast-feeding compatible
  Cytomegalovirus
  Hepatitis A[a]
  Hepatitis B[a]
  Hepatitis C

---

[a]After infant has received appropriate immunoprophylaxis.

dysuria, and pelvic pain. However, most women are asymptomatic. Pelvic examination may reveal findings consistent with cervicitis. Induced endocervical bleeding is also predictive of cervical infection in pregnancy.

Nucleic acid amplification tests (NAATs) are the standard diagnostic method for evaluation of chlamydial infection, because these techniques are more sensitive than culture and antigen-based assays. (For more detailed discussion, see Chapter 13.)

Doxycycline and ofloxacin, first-line treatments for chlamydial infection in nonpregnant women, are contraindicated in pregnancy. Instead, azithromycin and amoxicillin are recommended (see Table 22–2). Repeat testing for *C trachomatis* 3 weeks after completion of therapy is recommended for all pregnant women.

Gonorrhea

ESSENTIAL FEATURES

- *Almost half of all gonorrhea infections are asymptomatic.*
- *Adverse pregnancy outcomes include preterm labor, postpartum infection, ophthalmia neonatorum, and neonatal sepsis.*

The clinical course of *Neisseria gonorrhoeae* infection during pregnancy is similar to that in nonpregnant women. The prevalence of gonorrhea in pregnancy is approximately 1–10%. Almost half of infections are asymptomatic. Gonorrhea infection during pregnancy has been associated with pelvic inflammatory disease, predominantly in the first trimester before the chorion fuses with the decidua and obliterates the uterine cavity. Later in pregnancy, *N gonorrhoeae* is associated with

premature rupture of membranes, preterm labor, chorioamnionitis, and postpartum infection. Gonococcal conjunctivitis (ophthalmia neonatorum), the most common manifestation of perinatal infection, is usually transmitted during delivery. If untreated, this condition may lead to corneal perforation and panophthalmitis. Other more rare neonatal infections include meningitis, disseminated sepsis with arthritis, and genital and rectal infections.

Pregnant women infected with *N gonorrhoeae* may present with vaginal discharge, spotting, dysuria, or pelvic pain or be asymptomatic. Pelvic examination may reveal mucopurulent cervicitis, similar to that found in chlamydial infection, as well as urethral and rectal findings. A detailed examination of skin, pharynx, rectum, and joints should be performed when disseminated infection is suspected. Hospitalization and parenteral antibiotics are recommended for women with disseminated infection during pregnancy.

NAATs are the current standard diagnostic method for evaluation of gonorrhea infection, because these techniques are more sensitive than culture and direct microscopy. (For more detailed discussion, see Chapter 16.)

Pregnant women infected with gonorrhea should be treated with a recommended or alternate cephalosporin (see Table 22–2). They should not be treated with quinolones or tetracyclines, because these antibiotics are not recommended for use during pregnancy. Women who cannot tolerate a cephalosporin should be administered a single, intramuscular 2-g dose of spectinomycin. If recent chlamydia testing was not performed, it is recommended that pregnant women receive presumptive treatment for chlamydia. Although some authorities propose retesting women 3 months after treatment, given the adverse outcomes associated with gonorrhea in pregnancy it is reasonable to consider retesting 3–4 weeks after completion of treatment in pregnancy.

Differential Diagnosis of Cervical Infections

Mucopurulent cervicitis may be associated not only with chlamydia and gonorrhea but also with *Mycoplasma genitalium*, trichomoniasis, and genital herpes simplex virus (HSV) infection. Additionally, mucopurulent cervical discharge should be clearly distinguished from the normal increases in cervical mucous often seen during pregnancy. Inflammation of the cervix should be distinguished from the normal condition of the zone of ectopy (or ectropion) that results from the symmetric extension of the columnar cervical epithelium over the os and is frequently observed in high-estrogen states (eg, pregnancy, adolescence, and use of oral contraceptives). Patients with purulent cervical discharge may have either gonococcal or chlamydial infection, or both. The presence of mucopurulent discharge along with ulcerations and erythema of the ectocervix may indicate HSV infection. Other noninfectious causes of cervicitis include systemic illnesses such as autoimmune diseases, neoplasia, and mechanical or chemical trauma.

VAGINAL INFECTIONS

Bacterial Vaginosis

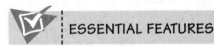

ESSENTIAL FEATURES

- *Bacterial vaginosis may be associated with preterm labor and preterm premature rupture of membranes.*
- *Testing may be conducted at the first prenatal visit in asymptomatic women who are at high risk for preterm delivery.*

Bacterial vaginosis has been associated with adverse pregnancy outcomes, including spontaneous abortion in the first and second trimesters, preterm labor, preterm premature rupture of membranes, preterm delivery, low-birth-weight infants, chorioamnionitis, postpartum endometritis, and postcesarean wound infections. Current evidence does not support routine screening for bacterial vaginosis during pregnancy in the general population. However, screening at the first prenatal visit is recommended for patients who are at high risk of preterm delivery (eg, those with a history of a previous preterm delivery or preterm premature rupture of membranes).

Most cases (50–75%) of bacterial vaginosis are asymptomatic or mild. Clinical presentation may include a fishy or ammonia-like odor of vaginal discharge, and thin, gray-white, nonclumping, homogenous vaginal discharge. Dysuria and dyspareunia are rare, and pruritus and inflammation are absent. The discharge associated with bacterial vaginosis originates from the vagina rather than the cervix.

The "gold standard" for diagnosis of bacterial vaginosis remains the Gram stain. This method distinguishes bacterial vaginosis from various categories of abnormal vaginal flora. Amsel criteria are used to make the diagnosis in clinical settings. Recently introduced point-of-care tests may be less reliable forms of diagnostic screening tests. (For further discussion, see Chapter 11.)

Both oral metronidazole and oral clindamycin are recommended for treatment of bacterial vaginosis in pregnant women (see Table 22–2). Clindamycin cream is not recommended during pregnancy because increased

adverse pregnancy outcomes were observed in trials using this therapy. Given that treatment of bacterial vaginosis in asymptomatic pregnant women who are at high risk for preterm delivery might prevent adverse pregnancy outcomes, a follow-up evaluation 1 month after completion of treatment should be considered to evaluate whether therapy was effective.

McDonald H, Brocklehurst P, Parsons J, Vigneswaran R. Antibiotics for treating bacterial vaginosis in pregnancy. *Cochrane Database Syst Rev* 2003;(1)CD000262. [PMID: 15674870] (Large meta-analysis evaluating the relationship of bacterial vaginosis with adverse perinatal outcomes.)

Trichomoniasis

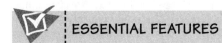

ESSENTIAL FEATURES

- *Trichomoniasis is associated with adverse pregnancy outcomes, and screening of asymptomatic high-risk pregnant women may be useful.*
- *Culture is more reliable than direct microscopic examination in the diagnosis of trichomonal infection.*

T vaginalis infection in the second trimester of pregnancy has been associated with preterm delivery, preterm premature rupture of membranes, and low-birth-weight infants. Transmission of *T vaginalis* to the neonate may also occur during passage through an infected vagina, resulting in vaginal infections in female infants. Clinical presentation and findings of acute and chronic trichomonal infection in pregnant women are similar to those in nonpregnant women. Many women are asymptomatic; however, half of these women may develop symptoms within 6 months.

Trichomoniasis may be diagnosed by microscopy on a wet mount of vaginal secretions in which the characteristic movements of *T vaginalis* can be identified (least sensitive); culture (more sensitive); point-of-care antigen detection testing, and NAATs (most sensitive). Of note, currently there are no commercially available NAATs for *Trichomonas*. Treatment can be with metronidazole, 2 g orally as a single dose, similar to the regimen for nonpregnant patients.

Differential Diagnosis of Vaginal Infections

Abnormal vaginal discharge in pregnancy may be a result of normal physiologic discharge of pregnancy, bacterial vaginosis, trichomoniasis, chlamydia, gonorrhea, mycoplasma, or HSV infection. Specifically, pregnant women with chronic trichomonal vaginitis may present with scanty vaginal discharge, mild pruritus, and dyspareunia. Additionally, in pregnant patients with an abnormal vaginal discharge but no obvious infectious cause, the differential diagnosis should include chemical or allergic vulvovaginitis, the presence of a foreign body in the vagina, and rupture of membranes. During microscopic evaluation, care should be employed to distinguish *T vaginalis* from sperm, as both findings are remarkable for movement.

GENITAL ULCER DISEASE

Genital Herpes

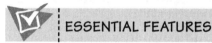

ESSENTIAL FEATURES

- *The vast majority of HSV-infected infants are born to asymptomatic mothers.*
- *Prophylactic acyclovir reduces the frequency of recurrent HSV infection and the need for cesarean delivery.*

HSV is common among women of childbearing ages and causes significant morbidity and mortality in the neonate. Both herpes simplex virus type 1 (HSV-1) and type 2 (HSV-2) may cause genital lesions, although HSV-2 is more likely to be associated with genital infection. Studies have shown that women with no prior HSV infection have a 3.7% chance of undergoing seroconversion to HSV-2 during their pregnancy compared with a 1.7% chance in those with prior exposure to HSV-1. Additionally, genital HSV infection recurs more often in HIV-infected pregnant women during labor compared with other pregnant women. Studies indicate that 10–20% of HSV-2–seropositive individuals report a history of genital herpes infection. As a result, the identification of pregnant women with genital herpes is important, but limited by patient history alone.

A. INITIAL CLINICAL EVALUATION

Evaluation includes a detailed history and careful examination of the genitalia for herpetic changes at the first prenatal visit and at time of delivery. Serologic testing is not currently recommended for universal prenatal screening because the benefit and cost-efficacy of such screening has not been proven. However, the CDC states that type-specific serologic testing may play an important role in the identification and counseling of women who,

because of partners with HSV infection, are at risk for HSV acquisition during pregnancy. Similarly, neither weekly genital cultures nor polymerase chain reaction (PCR) testing during late gestation is recommended, because these practices are not cost-effective and fail to predict poor neonatal outcomes.

Primary infection in pregnant women causes more severe symptoms and signs, is more prone to maternal dissemination, and has been associated with increased adverse pregnancy outcomes, including spontaneous abortion, preterm birth, and intrauterine growth restriction. Additionally, late acquisition of the infection is associated with low birth weight. Recurrent HSV has not been associated with spontaneous abortion or embryopathy.

The clinical manifestations of genital HSV infection are variable. Although HSV infections are common in pregnant women, they are rarely serious. However, disseminated HSV infection may cause fulminant hepatitis, with maternal and perinatal mortality approaching 40%. Primary infection or initial presentation of genital lesions in pregnant women is generally similar to that in nonpregnant women. Recurrent infection and prodromal clinical presentation are also similar in both pregnant and nonpregnant women.

The most common mode of vertical transmission is via direct contact of the fetus during delivery, either from viral secretions from active herpes lesions or by asymptomatic shedding. Congenital herpes, which occurs much more rarely, results from intrauterine transmission transplacentally or by ascending infection, especially in primary maternal HSV-2 infection. Congenital infection may cause neonatal skin vesicles, chorioretinitis, microcephaly, seizures, hepatosplenomegaly, bleeding diathesis, intrauterine growth restriction, and fetal demise. The risk of neonatal transmission is greater in women who acquire primary HSV infection during pregnancy compared with those having reactivation of previous infection: approximately 50% transmission in a primary infection, 20–30% transmission in a nonprimary first episode infection, and less than 1–5% transmission in a recurrent infection or infection acquired during the first half of pregnancy. Additionally, primary infection acquired near the time of labor is associated with the highest risk of transmission to the neonate during delivery. HSV infection in newborns usually develops in one of three patterns, which occur with roughly equal frequency: (1) localized infection of the skin, eyes, and mouth or mucosa; (2) central nervous system disease; and (3) disseminated disease involving multiple organs.

B. LABORATORY STUDIES

HSV infection can be diagnosed by viral culture, PCR, direct fluorescent antibody testing, and type-specific serologic assays. Detection of HSV by PCR is highly sensitive and superior to the other diagnostic tests. (For further discussion, see Chapter 14.)

C. TREATMENT

Treatment of primary infection, nonprimary episodes, and recurrent infection may be considered when clinically indicated, especially in the third trimester. Although first-episode genital HSV is self-limited, treatment with antiviral medication in pregnancy may be considered to reduce the duration of active lesions and viral shedding (see Table 22–2). Guidelines suggest that 400 mg of acyclovir be given twice daily for suppression of HSV in nonpregnant women. Valacyclovir, 500 mg daily, is a reasonable alternative for patients in whom adherence is a concern, although less data are available to support this regimen.

Suppressive therapy beginning at 36 weeks of pregnancy, an approach approved by ACOG, should be considered in patients with recurrent genital herpes during pregnancy. A recent meta-analysis found that in women with a history of recurrent genital herpes during pregnancy, acyclovir significantly reduced the risk of clinical HSV recurrence at the time of delivery by 75%, asymptomatic viral shedding at delivery by 91%, and cesarean delivery for clinically recurrent genital herpes by 70%. HSV suppressive therapy starting at 36 weeks should be considered for all women with a prior history of recurrent genital herpes regardless of whether the recurrences have occurred during pregnancy.

Experience with acyclovir therapy in both HSV infection and varicella pneumonia suggests that this drug is safe in pregnancy, including the first trimester, and even prolonged use of acyclovir has had no demonstrable risk to the fetus. Data are also accumulating on the use of valacyclovir and famciclovir in pregnancy. All three drugs are categorized as class B agents (no evidence of risk in humans) by the Food and Drug Administration.

Due to increased plasma volume in pregnant women leading to pharmacokinetic changes, studies evaluating HSV suppression in pregnant women have predominantly used acyclovir 400 mg 3 times daily compared to twice daily, the recommended suppressive dose in nonpregnant women.

Management of genital herpes in labor remains controversial. The CDC and ACOG recommend that cesarean delivery be offered to women in labor who have active lesions and to those with a history of herpes who report prodromal symptoms. Viral cultures or PCR testing during labor are not recommended because the results will not be available in a timely manner for clinical decision making. If the membranes have been ruptured for more than 6 hours, cesarean delivery should still be performed, although the benefit is not clearly proven. A prospective study of over 58,000 pregnant women indicates the effectiveness of cesarean delivery to reduce neonatal HSV transmission rates. In this study, cesarean delivery decreased the neonatal HSV transmission rate by 86% in comparison with vaginal delivery. However, the authors' analysis combined primary and recurrent cases of genital herpes, and patients did not receive prophylactic acyclovir during pregnancy.

Prophylactic cesarean delivery is not recommended for women with recurrent HSV who have no evidence of active lesions or prodrome at the time of delivery. Cesarean delivery is an expensive and morbid treatment that has no proven benefit for patients without active lesions. Cesarean delivery is also not recommended for women with active nongenital HSV lesions or lesions that have crusted fully at the time of labor. In summary, the risks of vaginal delivery for the fetus must be weighed against the risks of cesarean delivery to the mother.

Medically indicated, nongenital invasive procedures (eg, amniocentesis) need not be avoided but should be delayed if there is evidence of systemic disease. However, fetal scalp electrodes, which cause a break in the fetal skin, are potential risk factors for acquisition of neonatal HSV and thus should be avoided.

Mothers with active lesions, regardless of the lesion site, should use care when handling their infants (ie, ensuring that lesions are covered and hands have been washed before touching the infant). Breast-feeding is not contraindicated as long as there are no lesions on the breasts.

ACOG practice bulletin. Management of herpes in pregnancy. Number 8 October 1999. Clinical management guidelines for obstetrician-gynecologists. *Int J Gynaecol Obstet* 2000;68: 165–173. [PMID: 10717827]

Brown ZA, Wald A, Morrow RA, et al. Effect of serologic status and cesarean delivery on transmission rates of herpes simplex virus from mother to infant. *JAMA* 2003;289:203. [PMID: 12517231] (Highly quoted study of genital HSV management in pregnancy, demonstrating efficacy of cesarean delivery and prevention of maternal HSV acquisition in the reduction of neonatal herpes.)

Sheffield JS, Hollier LM, Hill JB, et al. Acyclovir prophylaxis to prevent herpes simplex virus recurrence at delivery: A systematic review. *Obstet Gynecol* 2003;102:1396–1403. [PMID: 14662233] (Significant systematic review demonstrating effects of acyclovir suppressive therapy for genital HSV in pregnancy.)

Syphilis

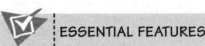

ESSENTIAL FEATURES

- *Pregnant patients with early syphilis are at greatest risk of delivering infants with congenital syphilis.*
- *Treatment of syphilis is not altered by pregnancy.*

Treponema pallidum has been associated with spontaneous abortion, fetal demise, intrauterine growth restriction, premature delivery, low birth weight, congenital anomalies, neonatal death, and early and late presenting congenital infection of the infant. The fetus is most likely to be infected transplacentally. More that 70% of infants born to mothers with untreated syphilis will be infected, compared with 1–2% of infants born to women who received adequate treatment during pregnancy. Vertical transmission can occur at any time during pregnancy and at any stage of the disease. However, approximately half of prenatal transmission occurs in patients with primary or secondary syphilis.

A. Initial Clinical Evaluation

Given the adverse outcomes associated with syphilis infection, screening is recommended for all pregnant women at the first prenatal visit, at 28 weeks' gestation, and at delivery in women who are at high risk for infection, live in areas of excess syphilis morbidity, are previously untested, or have positive serology in the first trimester. Women who deliver a stillborn infant after 20 weeks' gestation should also be tested for syphilis. Furthermore, it is important to verify a negative maternal syphilis serologic result, at least once during pregnancy and preferably at time of delivery, prior to discharge of the newborn from the hospital. Most women diagnosed with syphilis in pregnancy are asymptomatic. The natural course and clinical presentation of the different stages of syphilis are similar in pregnant and nonpregnant women. (For further discussion, see Chapter 19.)

B. Laboratory Studies

Screening for syphilis during pregnancy is performed with nontreponemal anticardiolipin antibodies. Two types of nontreponemal serologic tests for syphilis are available: the Venereal Disease Research Laboratories (VDRL) test and the rapid plasma reagin (RPR) test. (Refer to the detailed discussions in Chapters 19 and 26.) These tests remain positive for 6–12 months after treatment of primary syphilis, usually with progressively decreasing titers. In primary syphilis, serologic assays may be negative during very early infection, resulting in a lower sensitivity. These tests will become positive 1–2 weeks after the initial visit, and should therefore be repeated after appearance of the chancre in the adherent patient in whom the diagnosis cannot be made at first presentation. Of note, the RPR test is now available as a point-of-care assay, a screening tool that is particularly useful in populations in which prenatal follow-up is not optimal. A positive result must be confirmed with specific treponemal antibody studies, such as the fluorescent treponemal antibody absorbed (FTA-ABS) test and the *T pallidum* particle agglutination assay (TP-PA). The microhemagglutination test for antibodies to *T pallidum* (MHA-TP) is no longer available in the United States.

Alternatively, the most expedient and most direct method for diagnosing primary and secondary syphilis is visualization of the spirochete from moist lesions, such as skin lesions or mucous patches, by means of darkfield microscopy. However, in clinical practice, darkfield microscopy is generally limited to clinics that specialize in the diagnosis and treatment of STDs. Additionally, a multiplex polymerase chain reaction (M-PCR) assay can simultaneously detect *T pallidum*, *Haemophilus ducreyi,* and HSV. However, the M-PCR test has limited availability.

C. Treatment

1. Treatment of the mother—Treatment of syphilis is not altered by pregnancy. Seropositive pregnant women should be considered infected unless an adequate treatment history is documented. Treatment during pregnancy should consist of the penicillin regimen appropriate for the stage of syphilis (see Table 22–2 and Chapter 19). Some experts recommend additional therapy consisting of benzathine penicillin 2.4 million units IM administered 1 week following initial dose of antibiotic treatment for pregnant women who have primary, secondary, or early latent syphilis. Penicillin is effective for preventing maternal transmission to the fetus and for treating fetal infection. Evidence is insufficient to determine whether the specific, recommended penicillin regimens are optimal.

Pregnant patients who are allergic to penicillin should be desensitized and treated with penicillin. No alternatives to penicillin have been proved effective for treatment of syphilis during pregnancy. Skin testing may be helpful in documenting a true penicillin allergy. Tetracycline and doxycycline should not used during pregnancy. Erythromycin should not be used, because it does not reliably cure an infected fetus. Data are insufficient to recommend azithromycin or ceftriaxone.

In the second half of pregnancy, sonographic monitoring may be used for evaluation of congenital syphilis, but this should not delay therapy. Sonographic signs of fetal syphilis, including hepatomegaly, ascites, and hydrops, indicate a greater risk for fetal treatment failure. Evidence is insufficient to recommend specific regimens for these situations. Women treated for syphilis during the second half of pregnancy are at risk for premature labor or fetal distress if the treatment precipitates the Jarisch-Herxheimer reaction. Many experts treat these patients in a hospital or monitored setting, and women should be advised to seek obstetric attention after treatment if they notice any contractions or decrease in fetal movements. Although stillbirth is a rare complication of treatment, concern about this complication should not delay necessary treatment.

Coordinated prenatal care, treatment follow-up, and syphilis case management are important in the management of pregnant women with syphilis. Routinely, nontreponemal antibody serologic titers should be checked at 1, 3, 6, 12, and 24 months following treatment. During pregnancy, serologic titers should be repeated in the third trimester and at delivery, as well. Serologic titers may be checked monthly in women who are at high risk for reinfection or living in geographic areas in which the prevalence of syphilis is high. Titers should decrease fourfold by 6 months and become nonreactive by 12–24 months after completion of treatment. Most women will deliver before their serologic response to treatment can be assessed definitively.

In adequately treated women, a twofold increase in titers may be observed during pregnancy and is not necessarily an indication of recurrence, treatment failure, or reinfection. Management in such cases and decision to retreat a pregnant woman should be considered based on risk stratification, immune status, and serial monitoring of titers for a significant fourfold or greater rise. All patients who have syphilis should be tested for HIV infection. In geographic areas in which the prevalence of HIV is high, patients who have primary syphilis should be retested for HIV after 3 months if the first HIV test result was negative.

2. Treatment of the newborn—Routine screening of newborn sera or umbilical cord blood is not recommended for the diagnosis of congenital syphilis. Serologic testing of the mother's serum is preferred because the serologic tests performed on infant serum can be nonreactive if the mother's serologic test result is of low titer or if the mother was infected late in pregnancy. Additionally, the diagnosis of congenital syphilis is difficult due to the transplacental transfer of maternal nontreponemal and treponemal immunoglobulin G (IgG) antibodies to the fetus. This transfer of antibodies makes the interpretation of reactive serologic tests for syphilis in infants challenging.

All infants born to mothers who have reactive nontreponemal and treponemal test results should be evaluated with a quantitative nontreponemal serologic test (RPR or VDRL) performed on infant serum, because umbilical cord blood can become contaminated with maternal blood; examined thoroughly for evidence of congenital syphilis (eg, nonimmune hydrops, jaundice, hepatosplenomegaly, rhinitis, skin rash, or pseudoparalysis of an extremity); and undergo darkfield microscopic examination or direct fluorescent antibody staining of suspicious lesions or body fluids (eg, nasal discharge). Pathologic examination of the placenta or umbilical cord using specific fluorescent antitreponemal antibody staining is also suggested.

Treatment decisions often must be made on the basis of identification of syphilis in the mother; adequacy of maternal treatment; presence of clinical, laboratory, or radiographic evidence of syphilis in the infant; and comparison of maternal (at delivery) and infant nontreponemal serologic titers using the same test and, preferably, the same laboratory. Treatment of congenital syphilis in infants will depend on disease probability following a thorough clinical and diagnostic evaluation (see Table 22–4).

Chancroid, Lymphogranuloma Venereum, Granuloma Inguinale, & Other Causes of Genital Ulcers

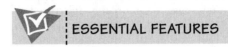

ESSENTIAL FEATURES

- *Genital ulcers have a wide variety of infectious and noninfectious etiologies.*
- *In general, empiric therapy should precede etiologic diagnosis.*

Genital ulcers may be caused by numerous infectious agents and other conditions. The most common causes of genital ulcers in sexually active young adults in the United States are HSV and syphilis. Other infectious causes of genital ulcers include chancroid (*H ducreyi*), lymphogranuloma venereum (*C trachomatis* serovars L1–L3), and granuloma inguinale or donovanosis (*Calymmatobacterium granulomatis*). Noninfectious etiologies include drug reactions, contact dermatitis, Behçet syndrome, neoplasms, and trauma. Presentation of specific genital ulcers is variable and may overlap. Pregnancy-related implications of syphilis and genital herpes infections are covered in detail earlier in this chapter, and treatment of pregnant women with other causes of genital ulcers does not differ from that described elsewhere in this text (see Table 22–2).

Differential Diagnosis of Genital Ulcer Disease

Infectious etiologies, including HSV, syphilis, chancroid (*H ducreyi*), granuloma inguinale (*C granulomatis*), HIV-specific ulcers (acute HIV infection or late HIV), and lymphogranuloma venereum (*C trachomatis* L1–L3 serovars) must be considered when evaluating patients with genital ulcers. Accurate clinical diagnosis may be challenging, because clinical presentations may vary and overlap. Additionally, multiple etiologic agents can cause ulcers at the same time and site. Therefore, obtaining a detailed history and performing a thorough examination are essential.

OTHER EXTERNAL GENITAL INFECTIONS
Genital Warts

Genital warts, also known as condylomata acuminata, are caused by the human papillomavirus (HPV). Lesions can proliferate during pregnancy but often spontaneously regress after delivery. There is no known association of HPV with pregnancy complications, such as spontaneous

Table 22–4. Treatment recommendations for infants of mothers with syphilis infection.

Physical Examination Findings	Serologic Findings and Maternal Treatment Status	Treatment
Infant with proven or highly probable disease or physical examination consistent with congenital syphilis	Serum quantitative nontreponemal serologic titer >4-fold the maternal or positive darkfield or fluorescent titer, antibody test of body fluid	Aqueous crystalline penicillin G, 100,000–150,000 units/kg/d, administered as 40,000 units/kg/dose IV q 12 h during the first 7 d of life and q 8 h thereafter, for a total of 10 d _or_ Procaine penicillin G, 40,000 units/kg/dose IM in a single daily dose for 10 d
Infant with normal physical examination	Serum quantitative nontreponemal serologic titer ≤4-fold the maternal titer, and: • Mother was not treated, was inadequately treated, or has no documentation of having received treatment • Mother was treated with erythromycin or other nonpenicillin regimen • Mother received treatment ≤4 wk before delivery • Mother has early syphilis and nontreponemal titer that has either not decreased 4-fold or has increased 4-fold	Same as above
Infant with normal physical examination	Serum quantitative nontreponemal serologic titer ≤ 4-fold the maternal titer, and: • Mother was treated during pregnancy, treatment was appropriate for the stage of infection, and treatment was administered >4 wk before delivery • Mother's nontreponemal titers decreased 4-fold after appropriate therapy for early syphilis or remained stable and low for late syphilis • Mother has no evidence of reinfection or relapse	Benzathine penicillin G, 40,000 units/kg/dose IM in a single dose
Infant with normal physical examination	Serum quantitative nontreponemal serologic titer ≤4-fold the maternal titer, and: • Mother's treatment was adequate before pregnancy • Mother's nontreponemal serologic titer remained low and stable before and during pregnancy and at delivery (VDRL ≤1:2; RPR ≤1:4)	No treatment required, but some recommend benzathine penicillin G, 50,000 units/kg as a single IM injection, particularly if follow-up is uncertain

RPR, rapid plasma reagin; VDRL, Venereal Disease Research Laboratories test.

ESSENTIAL FEATURES

- *Genital warts should be treated during pregnancy because the lesions may proliferate and become friable or may interfere with delivery.*
- *Cesarean delivery is not indicated for genital warts unless the pelvic outlet is obstructed or vaginal delivery would result in excessive bleeding.*

abortion or preterm delivery. Genital warts are rarely transmitted to the neonate, but there are reports of laryngeal and respiratory papillomatosis and perianal warts in infants. HPV types 6 and 11 can cause respiratory papillomatosis in infants and children. The route of transmission (ie, transplacental, perinatal, or postnatal) is not completely understood. It is thought that the HPV virus may be acquired during passage through the birth canal. The preventive value of cesarean delivery is unknown. Therefore, cesarean delivery is not recommended for prevention of HPV transmission to the infant and should only be considered in cases of obstruction of the pelvic outlet or if vaginal delivery would result in excessive bleeding.

Clinical diagnosis of genital warts is usually sufficient. Although serotyping for identification of HPV subtypes is available, it is unnecessary for the diagnosis and management of genital warts. (For further discussion, see Chapter 15.)

Therapy may be considered, especially in symptomatic patients, because lesions may become friable as they proliferate during pregnancy or may interfere with delivery. Cryotherapy and trichloroacetic acid are recommended treatments. Because the genital area is highly vascular during pregnancy and excessive bleeding may occur with electrocauterization, it is recommended that cautery therapy, if indicated, be performed in a hospital setting. Imiquimod, 5-fluorouracil, podophyllin, and podophyllotoxin are contraindicated in pregnancy.

Molluscum Contagiosum

ESSENTIAL FEATURES

- *Infection may be sexually transmitted.*
- *Molluscum contagiosum is not associated with adverse pregnancy outcomes.*

Molluscum contagiosum is spread by direct skin-to-skin contact and can therefore occur anywhere on the body. When it occurs in the genital region, it is classified as an STD. Pregnancy does not alter the clinical course of this infection, and molluscum contagiosum is not associated with adverse pregnancy outcomes.

Diagnosis of molluscum contagiosum can be made clinically by the characteristic appearance of the lesions. However, confirmatory diagnosis requires lesion biopsy for histologic or electron microscopic examination. (For further discussion, see Chapter 30.) Table 22–2 outlines treatment options in pregnant women.

Differential Diagnosis of Other External Genital Infections

Genital warts, molluscum contagiosum, malignant lesions, and condylomata lata should all be considered in evaluation of exophytic or atypical lesions located on the external genitalia. Condylomata lata (lesions of secondary syphilis), especially in an immunosuppressed individual, may resemble genital warts. Serologic testing for syphilis should be used to distinguish these lesions from condylomata acuminata. Skin lesions caused by cryptococcosis or histoplasmosis may clinically resemble molluscum lesions. Lesions may be further evaluated and distinguished through examination of biopsy specimens.

VIRAL INFECTIONS

Cytomegalovirus

ESSENTIAL FEATURES

- *Cytomegalovirus (CMV) is the most common perinatal viral infection, occurring in 1–2% of all live births.*
- *Congenital CMV infection may result in significant neurologic sequelae or even neonatal death.*

CMV may be sexually transmitted through the exchange of body fluids or intimate contact. By the age of 40 years, 50–85% of individuals in the United States are infected with CMV, and approximately 2% of pregnant women undergo seroconversion during pregnancy. In pregnant women, primary infection is either asymptomatic or presents as a self-limiting mononucleosis-like illness. Findings include fever, flulike symptoms, lymphocytosis, and elevated serum transaminase levels. CMV is the most common congenitally acquired infection, occurring in

0.2–2% of all neonates and causing approximately 40,000 neonatal infections in the United States each year.

Viral effects in the fetus depend on maternal immune status. Most studies suggest that gestational age has no apparent influence on the risk of transmission of CMV in utero. Transmission to the fetus during primary maternal infections occurs in 20–50% of cases, and up to one third of infected infants have clinical manifestation of CMV infection at birth or shortly thereafter. In a maternal viral reactivation or reinfection, fetal transmission is approximately 1% and fetal infection tends to be less severe.

Congenital CMV infection is symptomatic at birth in 5–20% of infected infants. Findings include intrauterine growth restriction, low birth weight, petechiae, hepatosplenomegaly, jaundice, chorioretinitis, motor disability, cerebral calcifications, lethargy, respiratory distress, seizures, and microcephaly. Infection is more severe in premature infants and when infection is acquired earlier in pregnancy. Of the asymptomatic infants, 5–15% will later develop sequelae. Most long-term defects in affected children are neurologic, including nerve deafness and mental retardation. CMV is the leading cause of congenital hearing loss in the United States.

Perinatal infection is usually acquired by exposure to maternal blood, cervical secretions, or breast milk. However, breast-feeding is not contraindicated. Although antiviral therapies for treatment of CMV infection in immunocompromised individuals are available, no therapies are currently recommended for maternal or fetal CMV infection.

Given that there is no effective treatment for CMV infection, screening is unnecessary in pregnancy. Serologic tests (IgM and IgG), as well as avidity testing, may be used to determine if an individual has had a recent or prior infection.

Hepatitis

 ESSENTIAL FEATURES

- *Pregnant women should be assessed for risk of acquiring hepatitis A or B infections and offered vaccination during pregnancy.*
- *Newborns born to mothers with chronic active hepatitis B infection (eg, hepatitis B surface antigen–positive) or to mothers with unknown hepatitis B status should receive hepatitis B immune globulin (HBIG) in accordance with local guidelines and the hepatitis B vaccination series.*

Viral hepatitis is the most common liver disease occurring in pregnancy. Approximately half of all cases of hepatitis are caused by hepatitis B virus (HBV) and one third by hepatitis A virus (HAV). HBV is most commonly transmitted sexually, whereas HAV and hepatitis C virus (HCV) are rarely acquired sexually.

A. HEPATITIS A

Approximately 1 in 1000 pregnant women has acute hepatitis A infection. Clinical manifestations include nausea, vomiting, fatigue, and low-grade fever. The infection is usually self-limited, and treatment is primarily supportive in the pregnant patient. Fulminant disease with encephalopathy and coagulopathy is extremely rare. Hepatitis A may be associated with preterm birth and perinatal death, especially in developing countries. Pregnancy does not affect the clinical course of this infection. Hepatitis A transmission to the fetus and newborn is extremely rare. Vaccination may be considered for pregnant patients at high risk of infection, including those traveling to endemic areas. Additionally, immune serum globulin administration may be considered for pregnant women in cases of close personal or sexual contact with an individual with hepatitis A infection. Newborns born to mothers with acute hepatitis A should receive immune globulin. Such infants may breast-feed after receiving appropriate immunoprophylaxis with immune globulin and vaccine.

B. HEPATITIS B

Approximately 1–2 in 1000 pregnant women have acute hepatitis B infection and 5–15 in 1000 develop chronic hepatitis B infection. Serologic tests for hepatitis B surface antigen (HBsAg) should be performed on all pregnant women at the first prenatal visit. HBsAg testing should be repeated late in pregnancy for women who are HBsAg-negative but who are at high risk for HBV infection (eg, injection drug users and women who have concomitant STDs). Fulminant infection resulting from acute HBV infection is rare, occurring in 1% of cases. Clinical manifestations include malaise, fever, fatigue, nausea and vomiting, hepatomegaly, and dark urine. Jaundice may also develop. Adverse obstetric outcomes include preterm delivery.

Perinatal transmission occurs primarily through exposure to blood and viral secretions during delivery. Transplacental transmission and transmission through breast-feeding are rare. Vertical transmission is approximately 20% in cases where the mother is HBsAg-positive and 90% in cases where the mother is positive for both HBsAg and HBeAg. Neonatal transmission risk is dependent on the gestational age of primary maternal infection, with 80–90% transmission risk in the third trimester compared with 10% in the first trimester.

HBV infection may cause significant morbidity and mortality in the neonate, with a majority of untreated neonates becoming chronic carriers. It is recommended that all newborns receive the hepatitis B vaccine at birth. Additionally, it is recommended that those born to seropositive mothers (HBsAg or HBeAg) or in some areas mothers with unknown HBV status receive HBIG. Neonatal infection can be prevented in up to 85–95% of cases with the use of the hepatitis B vaccine and HBIG. Vaccination may be considered for pregnant patients at high risk of infection. Additionally, hepatitis B vaccine and HBIG are recommended for pregnant women who are exposed to infection. Breast-feeding is not contraindicated, provided that the infant has undergone immunoprophylaxis.

C. HEPATITIS C

It is estimated that 1–3% of pregnant women are infected with hepatitis C. Testing for hepatitis C antibodies should be performed at the first prenatal visit for pregnant women at high risk of exposure (eg, a history of injection drug use, partner with hepatitis C, repeated exposure to blood products, prior blood transfusion before 1992, or organ transplantation). Symptoms may include jaundice, fever, malaise, and fatigue, similar to other forms of hepatitis. Screening for HCV during pregnancy is recommended in high-risk patients. During pregnancy, there may be lower rates of HCV-associated liver necrosis, perhaps due to immunosuppression.

Rates of vertical transmission range widely from zero to 40% and appear positively correlated with level of HCV viral load. Cesarean delivery may be considered in HCV- and HIV-coinfected pregnant women when HCV viral load is greater than one million copies per milliliter, regardless of HIV viral load. Fetal scalp monitoring, artificial rupture of membranes, and other invasive procedures should be avoided in labor, if possible.

HCV is usually mild and asymptomatic in infants and young children. There is no immunoprophylaxis for mother or neonate. Interferon alfa and ribavirin therapy are contraindicated in pregnancy. Similar to HBV, breast-feeding is not a significant risk factor for neonatal transmission and therefore is not contraindicated in mothers with HCV infection.

D. LABORATORY STUDIES

In HAV infection, liver function tests may be mildly elevated, and diagnosis is confirmed by anti-A IgM antibody. Elevated liver function tests are also present in HBV infection. Diagnosis is based on the presence of surface antigen (HBsAg), e antigen (HBeAg), and IgM antibody to core antigen (HBcAb). HCV is diagnosed by identification of the hepatitis C antibody.

Differential Diagnosis of Viral Infections

Clinical manifestations of CMV infection in adults resemble viral infection such as mononucleosis.

Additionally, CMV, HSV, and Epstein-Barr virus may all cause viral hepatitis. Flulike syndromes may also resemble mild cases of hepatitis. Preeclampsia, HELLP syndrome (hemolysis, elevated liver function tests, and low platelets), acute fatty liver of pregnancy, cholestasis of pregnancy, and autoimmune hepatitis must always be considered in the differential diagnosis of a pregnant patient with elevated serum transaminases.

American College of Obstetricians and Gynecologists. *Viral Hepatitis in Pregnancy.* Educational Bulletin 248. ACOG, 1998. (Hepatitis and pregnancy management guidelines.)

ECTOPARASITIC INFECTIONS
Pubic Lice & Scabies

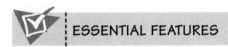

ESSENTIAL FEATURES

- *Patients with acute pruritus of the genitalia should be evaluated for public lice and scabies.*
- *Gamma-benzene hexachloride (Lindane) use is contraindicated in pregnancy.*

Pubic lice, caused by *Phthirus pubis*, generally affect the pubic and perineal areas. The infection is more common in women. Clinical manifestations include intense pruritus and dermatitis from the resultant scratching.

Scabies is caused by *Sarcoptes scabiei*. It is transmitted by close personal contact, often via sexual transmission. The "burrow" lesions are symmetric, initially occurring on the finger webs, the side of the hand digits, and the flexor surface of the wrist. Lesions may also occur on the elbows, axillae, breasts, buttocks, and genital region. Clinical manifestations include pruritus and an eczematous rash, resulting in secondary neurodermatitis.

Diagnosis of pubic lice is generally clinical, based on identification of nits attached to the hair shaft by use of a hand lens, or microscopic identification of an adult louse from a plucked hair. Scabies is clinically diagnosed by identification of characteristic skin burrow lesions. Confirmation is made by microscopic identification of mites or fecal pellets.

Treatment with gamma-benzene hexachloride (Lindane) for parasitic infections is not recommended for pregnant or lactating women. Although no studies have reported teratogenic effects in humans, 10% of the drug is absorbed systemically. However, it rarely causes central nervous system toxicity. Alternatively, pyrethrins, piperonyl butoxide combination, benzyl benzoate, and malathion may be used to treat pubic lice in pregnancy.

Additionally, crotamiton and sulfur in petrolatum may be used to treat scabies in a pregnant woman. Lindane should only be considered in extremely resistant or recalcitrant cases.

Differential Diagnosis of Ectoparasitic Infections

Scabies lesions may resemble secondary syphilis or other dermatologic disorders.

PRACTICE POINTS

- *Repeat testing for C trachomatis 3 weeks after completion of therapy is recommended for all pregnant women.*

- *Prophylactic cesarean delivery is not recommended for women with recurrent HSV who have no evidence of active lesions or prodrome at the time of delivery. Cesarean delivery is an expensive and morbid treatment that has no proven benefit for patients without active herpes lesions.*

Relevant Web Sites

[American College of Obstetricians and Gynecologists]
http://www.acog.org
[Centers for Disease Control and Prevention:]
http://www.cdc.gov/std
[Cochrane Database—excellent systematic reviews of the literature:]
http://www.cochrane.org
[National Institutes of Health web site for AIDS information with updated recommendations on HIV and pregnancy:]
http://www.aidsinfo.nih.gov

Sexually Transmitted Diseases in Adolescents

23

Renata Arrington-Sanders, MD, MPH, Jeri Dyson, MD, & Jonathan Ellen, MD

ESSENTIAL FEATURES

- *The biology of the developing cervix may increase the risk for STDs in young women.*
- *Adolescents have delayed health care–seeking behavior and may not be forthcoming in reporting sexual risk behavior.*
- *In most states, patients 12 years and older can give consent for confidential reproductive health care services.*

GENERAL CONSIDERATIONS

Nearly one quarter of all sexually transmitted diseases (STDs) occur in sexually active adolescents. A variety of biologic, cognitive, psychological, behavioral, and social factors contribute to the high rates of STDs observed in this population. To provide effective care for these patients, it is important that clinicians understand the issues that contribute to adolescents' increased STD risk.

Not all adolescents are sexually active. According to the 2003 Youth Risk Behavior Surveillance System (YRBS), 46.7% of high school students reported having had sexual intercourse during their lifetime. Only 28–63% of those who were sexually active reported having used a condom during their last intercourse. STDs commonly go undiagnosed in adolescents because (1) infections are often asymptomatic, (2) routine screening relies on appropriate health care–seeking behavior, and (3) adolescents must identify themselves as sexually active. STDs in adolescents result in complications such as infertility, ectopic pregnancy, HIV infection, and cervical cancer.

Centers for Disease Control and Prevention. Tracking the hidden epidemics: Trends in STDs in the United States, 2000. Available at: http://www.cdc.gov/std/ Trends2000. (Government report summarizing trends in STDs in 2000.)

Grunbaum JA, Kann L, Kinchen S, et al. Youth risk behavior surveillance—United States, 2003. *MMWR Morb Mortal Wkly Rep* 2004;53:1–96. [PMID: 15152182] (Survey of risk behaviors reported by high school students in the United States.)

EPIDEMIOLOGY

Adolescents have the highest age-specific rates for chlamydia and gonorrhea. In 2003, the highest age-specific chlamydial rates were among female adolescents aged 15–19 years (2687.3 per 100,000 females vs 9.8 per 100,000 males, Figure 23–1). As with chlamydia, gonorrhea rates are highest in female adolescents aged 15–19 years, and in men aged 20–24 years (see Figure 23–2).

Age-specific national prevalence estimates and case reporting data for genital herpesvirus infection, genital warts or other human papillomavirus (HPV) infections, and trichomoniasis are not available. The most common ulcerative disease among adolescents is herpes simplex virus type 2 (HSV-2). According to the National Health and Examination (NHANES) III data (1988–1994), seroprevalence rates among adolescents aged 12–19 years range from less than 10% to 17% in some reports. HPV is one of the most common STDs in adolescent and young adult women, with a prevalence of 30–50% in this population. Various studies report that trichomoniasis is found in 5–10% of the general population and in 18–50% of women with vaginal complaints.

Syphilis is typically not considered an adolescent disease. The incidence was highest among women aged 20–24 years (2.4 cases per 100,000 population) and among men aged 35–39 years (11.8 cases per 100,000 population) in 2003.

Nearly half of all new HIV infections in the United States occur in adolescents and young adults aged 13–24 years. It is estimated that as many as 100,000 adolescents are infected with HIV, of whom 25% are unaware of their status.

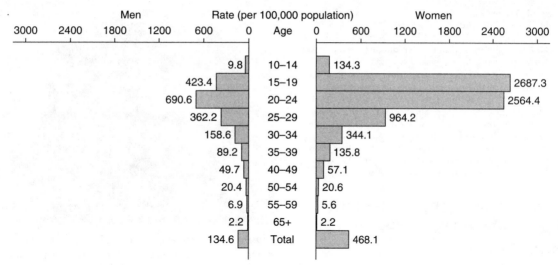

Figure 23–1. Chlamydia rates by age: United States, 1984–2003. Rate is per 100,000 population. (Source: STD surveillance, Centers for Disease Control and Prevention, 2003.)

STD rates have been disproportionately higher among African-American adolescents relative to same-age Caucasian counterparts. There does not appear to be a biologic basis for such differences, and the cause of this health disparity is unclear but may be attributable, in some degree, to higher rates of poverty, lack of access to quality health care, and living in high-prevalence communities. Reporting bias may also contribute to the high rates of STDs in minority communities, because minority populations are more likely to seek care at clinics that receive public funding, which may be in better compliance with reporting regulations than private providers. Additionally, sexual networks may explain why African-American adolescents who reside in a high-prevalence community are at increased risk of having sexual activity with a concurrent partner exposed to an STD.

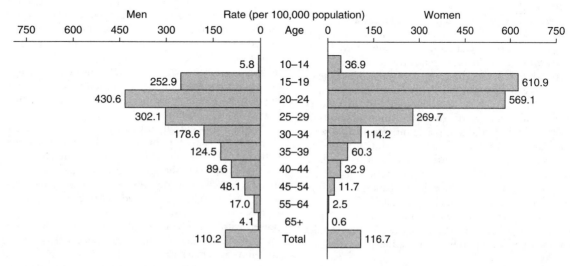

Figure 23–2. Gonorrhea rates by age: United States, 1984–2003. Rate is per 100,000 population. (Source: STD surveillance, Centers for Disease Control and Prevention, 2003.)

Centers for Disease Control and Prevention. Revised guidelines for HIV counseling, testing, and referral. *MMWR Morb Mortal Wkly Rep* 2001;50:1–57. [PMID:11718472] (Guidelines for HIV testing relevant to all sites but directed toward publicly funded programs and nonmedical settings.)

Ellen JM, Brown BA, Chung SE, et al. Impact of sexual networks on risk for gonorrhea and chlamydia among low-income urban African American adolescents. *J Pediatr* 2005;146: 518–522. [PMID: 15812456] (In addition to individual factors, network factors may explain why African-American adolescents are at increased risk for exposure to STDs. Multilevel community-based interventions may need to address network factors along with personal behaviors to prevent STDs among low-income urban African-American adolescents.)

FACTORS THAT INCREASE THE RISK OF STDS IN ADOLESCENTS

Biologic Factors

Overall, female adolescents appear to be more susceptible to STDs than male adolescents. Different pathogens preferentially infect different tissues: *Neisseria gonorrhoeae* and *Chlamydia trachomatis* preferentially attach to columnar cells, *Trichomonas vaginalis* and HPV attach to squamous epithelium, and *Treponema pallidum* infects squamous and columnar epithelial cells.

Many biologically plausible factors may contribute to increased adolescent susceptibility to infection. For instance, the cervix is physiologically immature in adolescent and young adult women, making it particularly vulnerable to STDs. During puberty, the epithelium lining the lower genital tract begins to thicken and undergo squamous metaplasia, the process during which readily infected, undifferentiated columnar (immature) epithelial cells transform into less susceptible squamous (adult) epithelium (see Figure 23–3). The junction of columnar and squamous epithelium is separated by squamous metaplastic epithelium referred to as the *transition zone*. In adolescents, this area on the exocervix is referred to as the *zone of ectropion*. The zone of ectropion is the preferential site of *C trachomatis* and *N gonorrhoeae* infections and thus biologically places female adolescents at risk for acquisition of multiple STDs, including HIV and pelvic inflammatory disease (PID), as well as abnormal Papanicolaou (Pap) smears.

In addition, during the first 2 years of menarche a relatively progesterone-deficient state of the vagina can occur, which may result in lower concentrations of hydrogen peroxide—producing lactobacilli. The resultant lack of hydrogen peroxide increases vaginal pH. Elevated vaginal pH has been associated in some studies with increased susceptibility to infection.

Behavioral Factors

All adolescents should be screened regarding sexual risk behavior, regardless of stated sexual orientation or

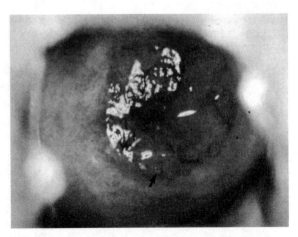

Figure 23–3. Presence of cervical ectopy. Endocervical columnar epithelium is present in an ectopic position on the exocervix, giving a bright-red circumoral appearance. Cervical mucus is clear, not purulent. (Reproduced, with permission, from Holmes KH et al. *Sexually Transmitted Diseases*, 3rd edition. McGraw-Hill, 1999.)

perceived risk. Specific discussion of behavioral risks and how to implement prevention strategies is an essential element of care for sexually active adolescents. Clinicians should clarify adolescents' definitions of sexual activity, using explicit examples (eg, vaginal, anal, and oral intercourse). Similarly, they should seek to obtain information about sexual debut, numbers of partners (both current and lifetime), partner concurrency, condom use, and douching. It is also important to discuss risk-taking behavior, gender of sex partners, and sexual orientation. These data can then be incorporated into discussions regarding sexual decision making related to STD risks; negotiation skills, including condom use or abstinence; partner risk; and substance use during or prior to sexual intercourse. Substance use may be associated with poor sexual decision making, including the choice of risky partners, which increases the likelihood of STD exposure.

Many adolescents are initiating sexual intercourse at an earlier age than in prior decades. The YRBS reported that over 7% of students surveyed had intercourse for the first time before the age of 13 years. Earlier coitus is, in turn, linked to greater numbers of lifetime partners, which are strongly associated with STD exposure. Female adolescents with older partners may have less power within the context of their relationships and more problems negotiating safer sexual behaviors. In addition, such behaviors as partner concurrency (having more than one partner at one time) and short-term "serial monogamy" (sequential partners over relatively short periods of time) can place adolescents at risk for STDs.

The benefits of condom use in adolescent patients are clear. Although condom use among sexually active young people has increased recently, it continues to be inconsistent. Condom use is dependent on both the adolescent's communication or negotiation skills and the partner in the relationship. Inconsistent condom use has been identified as resulting from inadequate communication, frequent sexual intercourse, and use of alcohol and other substances in conjunction with sexual activity. Adolescents tend to report more routine condom use with new or casual partners than with main partners. Consistent condom use has been associated with lower rates of chlamydial infection, gonorrhea, genital ulcer disease, HPV, bacterial vaginosis, and PID. Any "safe sex" benefits of condoms are maximized by consistent and correct use of condoms.

Douching behavior is very prevalent among adolescent women. The 1988 National Survey of Family Growth (1988 NSFG) showed that 31% of female adolescents aged 15–19 years reported douching. Cited reasons for douching included "feeling clean" after sexual intercourse or after menses, or for genital symptoms. Clinicians should recognize douching as a behavior to be discouraged in all women and adolescent girls, because douching may increase STD risk by altering vaginal flora or mechanically may lead to retrograde menses and facilitate the flushing of bacteria toward the endocervix.

Psychosocial Factors

A fundamental task of adolescence is identity formation. As adolescents' identities are being formed, they are forced to reconcile multiple psychological factors, including their sexual identity and the self-images that determine who they will become in adulthood. In addition, adolescents tend to be very concrete thinkers, limiting their ability to focus on long-term consequences of their actions. Even older adolescents, during periods of stress, may revert back to concrete thinking, compromising their capacity to make appropriate preventive decisions. This limitation, combined with the asymptomatic nature of most infections can impair an adolescent's understanding of the link between sexual behaviors and outcome. Thus, adolescents who are knowledgeable about condoms and STD prevention may still practice unsafe sex. Furthermore, misperceptions of a partner's or their own risk may also contribute to adolescents' decision to engage in sexually risky situations.

General psychological distress, including stigma, social pressure, and other mental health problems, has also been associated with increased sexual risk behavior and increased rates of STDs in adolescents. STD-related stigma may be a significant barrier to seeking health care for an STD. Adolescents who associate higher levels of stigma with STDs are more likely to anticipate negative reactions upon disclosing STD risk behaviors to a health care provider, less likely to have been tested for an STD in the previous year, and less likely to have sought STD-related care in the last year than their peers.

Adolescents frequently rely on social support from family and friends in seeking sexual health care. Real and perceived variation in social support has been associated with both positive and negative health practices, including sexual health care. Similarly, adolescents with perceived family support had more favorable attitudes toward condom use and were less likely to delay seeking care.

Differences in STD-related care of adolescents also derive from variations in access to care, care-seeking behavior among adolescents, availability of confidential services, and care providers' comfort in serving adolescents. Adolescents often lack knowledge of health insurance coverage or publicly funded facilities where free care is provided. Even very low copayments may discourage adolescents from seeking care. Others barriers include transportation problems, inconvenient clinic hours, inability to find clinical sites, and a clinic environment that is unwelcoming. Care-seeking behavior among adolescents appears to determine who seeks screening and obtains treatment for STDs. Adolescents have identified lack of confidential care as a barrier to seeking health care; they are more willing to seek and receive care from providers who assure confidentiality and are more willing to forgo care to prevent their parents from finding out.

Fortenberry JD, Tu W, Harezlak J, et al. Condom use as a function of time in new and established adolescent sexual relationships. *Am J Public Health* 2002;92:211–213. [PMID: 11818293] (Time to first unprotected coital event was significantly longer in new than in established relationships.)

Ness RB, Soper DE, Holley RL, et al. Hormonal and barrier contraception and risk of upper genital tract disease in the PID Evaluation and Clinical Health (PEACH) study. *Am J Obstet Gynecol* 2001;185:121–127. [PMID: 11483915] (No hormonal or barrier contraceptive method was related to a reduction in upper genital tract disease among women with clinical PID.)

Oh MK, Merchant JS, Brown P. Douching behavior in high-risk adolescents. What do they use, when and why do they douche? *J Pediatr Adolesc Gynecol* 2002;15:83–88. [PMID: 12057529] (In 104 rural southern young women, the following use of feminine hygiene products was reported: feminine suppository (9%), towelettes (33%), spray (40%), and feminine wash (67%). Only 18% reported no use of the feminine hygiene products listed. A history of ever having douched was reported by 79%; the mean first douching age was 14 years.)

PREVENTION

Primary prevention begins with reducing the behaviors that place adolescents at risk for infection. As adolescents age, dating patterns change from group dating to paired, unchaperoned dating for which adolescents may lack the required sophistication to handle intimate involvement. Most adolescents learn about sex from peer groups or school. The primary care setting provides an opportunity for physicians to discuss prevention.

Interactive counseling approaches should be directed at the adolescent's personal risk factors, identifying situations in which risk occurs and negotiating strategies to meet agreed upon goals to maintain sexual health. There is a range of sexual behavior that offers a means of expressing intimacy without having sexual intercourse, and this can be discussed as well.

Male and female condom use should be emphasized in sexually active adolescents for prevention of STDs. When used consistently and correctly, male latex condoms are highly effective in preventing the sexual transmission of HIV infection and reducing the risk of other diseases transmitted by fluids from mucosal surfaces (gonorrhea, chlamydia, trichomoniasis, and hepatitis B). Because condoms do not cover all exposed areas, they may be somewhat less effective in preventing diseases transmitted by skin-to-skin contact (HSV, HPV, syphilis, and chancroid). Recent data, however, demonstrate that condom use significantly reduces the transmission of HSV and HPV infection. Consistent and correct condom use is beneficial for STD and pregnancy prevention and should be emphasized with all sexually active patients.

INITIAL CLINICAL EVALUATION

Sexual History

The sexual history should be obtained in a nonthreatening, nonjudgmental manner. (For additional discussion, see Chapter 31.) Providers should be open to discussing sexual orientation, sexual activity, contraception, and fears or concerns the adolescent may have. We recommend that providers make it standard practice to routinely ask all adolescents if they have sex with boys, girls, or both. It should be emphasized that it is clinic policy to ask every adolescent to provide such information. This clarifies that sensitive questioning is reflective of clinical practice and not a value judgment about the adolescent by the provider.

Discussions should be appropriate for the developmental level of the patient and should identify risky behaviors (eg, sex and drug use behaviors). The clinician should inquire about condom use; number of partners; history of sexual activity with high-risk partners, including partners with a history of STDs; drug use, including intravenous drug use; and personal history of an STD. Sexual activity should be qualified as penile-vaginal, penile-anal, penile-oral, oral-vaginal, or with use of sex instruments. Additionally, it is important to elicit a thorough menstrual history. An irregular or painful menstrual history may be a clue to recent infection. Sexual activity during menses may increase the risk for acquiring an STD because of the reflux of menstrual blood

into the fallopian tubes, and the presence of relatively alkaline blood in the vagina.

The physical environment of the clinic should be appropriate for adolescents. Pamphlets that discuss sensitive topics should be available; these can be used to facilitate discussion as well as provide patient education. It is important to ask about care received outside of the traditional clinical practice, because adolescents are more likely to have received STD-related care in nontraditional venues such as school-based clinics, juvenile detention centers, national job training programs, drug treatment centers, and organizations that serve street youth.

When obtaining a sexual history, a contraceptive history should also be obtained. The use of barrier methods, including male and female condoms and diaphragms, have been found to be effective in reducing the risk of infection and acquisition of most, if not all STDs. Consistent condom use (using a condom every time one has sex) needs to be reinforced as the most effective means to reduce exposure and risk for acquiring an STD. When reviewing condom history, it is also important to ensure that adolescents know how to use condoms effectively. Having adolescents demonstrate placing a condom on a model, and reminding them to read the instructions and use the condom throughout intercourse, are all helpful measures. Hormonal contraceptive users may perceive less of a need to use condoms than nonusers and thereby expose themselves to STD acquisition. Clinical studies of spermicide use in women show various levels of protection against some STDs, and protection against HIV is unclear. Oral contraceptives and the use of depot medroxyprogesterone acetate (DMPA) have been associated with increased risk for acquiring chlamydial infection and protection from PID. Other studies have found no increased risk for cervical chlamydial infection among oral contraceptive users or among women using DMPA.

When obtaining historical information from adolescents, it is important to address confidentiality. Confidentiality is major concern for adolescents, because many are unaware that they are legally entitled to confidential services. However, the age for consent to STD-related care differs among states. Adolescents should also understand that both the clinician and laboratory are required to report some positive STD results to city and state health departments. If sexual abuse is considered to be the cause of an STD, clinicians should disclose this to the adolescent because reporting is required by law, regardless of the adolescent's age.

Clinical Findings

Although the symptoms of STDs in adolescents are similar to those in adults, when describing symptoms adolescents may use slang terms. Adolescent patients should be asked to be as specific as possible when describing symptoms and to clarify any unclear or colloquial descriptions.

Many adolescents with STDs are asymptomatic and do not seek medical care for an infection. Instead, the STD may be detected through a routine urine screening or the adolescent may seek care as the result of partner referral. Asymptomatic adolescents should be managed similarly to other adolescents who test positive for an STD.

Symptomatic adolescent girls who present for evaluation of an STD should have a thorough pelvic examination. In asymptomatic adolescent girls without a history of specific STD exposure who present for routine care, a pelvic examination is not necessary; these patients can be evaluated for chlamydial and gonococcal infection using a urine or self-collected vaginal swab specimen (if Nucleic Acid Amplification Test (NAAT) is available). In adolescent boys, urine-based testing should be performed.

In addition to genitourinary testing, patients engaging in oral or anal sex should have appropriate specimens collected from the throat and rectum. Patients should also be assessed for inguinal lymphadenopathy as evidence of genitourinary infection. This examination finding is helpful; however, negative findings do not exclude infection.

Pelvic Examination

Many adolescent girls are apprehensive before their first pelvic examination, and it may be difficult for the clinician to differentiate pain associated with infection from discomfort associated with anxiety. To minimize anxiety during specimen collection, the clinician should explain the procedure before and during the examination, and allow the patient to ask questions prior to the procedure. An experienced clinician who is examining an anxious adolescent patient will perform the examination when possible in a serene and calm atmosphere in the presence of a chaperone, because a negative experience during the initial examination may discourage the adolescent from seeking reproductive health care in the future. It is important to take the time to explain the anatomy of the genitalia to the patient, offer the adolescent patient a mirror to examine her own genitalia, and specifically communicate each step of the examination.

Cunningham SD, Tschann J, Gurvey JE, et al. Attitudes about sexual disclosure and perceptions of stigma and shame. *Sex Transm Infect* 2002;78:334–338. [PMID: 12407233] (Stigma about STDs may influence how female adolescents perceive reactions to disclosure of their sexual behavior to health care providers. It may also be an important factor in their decision to seek STD-related care.)

Ford CA, Millstein SG, Halpern-Felsher BL, Irwin CE. Influence of physician confidentiality assurances on adolescents' willingness to disclose information and seek future health care. *JAMA* 1997;278:1029–1034. [PMID: 9307357] (Large, randomized trial in high school students demonstrating that adolescents are more willing to communicate with and seek health care from physicians who assure confidentiality.)

TREATMENT

Measures to Increase Efficacy of Therapy

The outcome in treatment of STDs in adolescents is largely dependent on the patient's ability to adhere to the medication regimen that is selected. Allowing the adolescent an opportunity to be involved in the selection of medications may increase medication adherence. Thus, whenever possible, the patient should be involved in choosing the type of medication used for STD treatment.

In treating adolescents with cervicitis or trichomoniasis, single-dose directly observed therapy assures medication adherence. For management of PID, adolescents should be advised about the importance of appropriate 24- to 72-hour follow-up care for repeat examination. It is often helpful to provide adolescents with medications for PID therapy after starting the medications in clinic. This is particularly important for adolescent patients who are less compliant and less likely to return for follow-up visits.

When prescribing any medication, patient education is crucial to ensure adherence with the medication regimen and avoid treatment failure. Patients should be informed of the common side effects of prescribed medications and advised to contact the provider should any of these occur. Nausea and vomiting are relatively common side effects of some medications that are prescribed to treat STDs, and patients should be told to contact the provider if they are unable to tolerate therapy.

Abstinence during treatment is important in preventing recurrent infections. The patient should be encouraged to remain abstinent while taking medications for 7 total days after completion of therapy, including single-dose regimens. Partner notification and treatment reduces the risk of reinfection in the index patient and is an important public health intervention to reduce the continued transmission of infection (see Chapter 28). Depending on the jurisdiction, some health departments may contact the patient to help ensure recent partners (eg, prior 60 days) are notified and treated.

Risk reduction counseling should also be provided to all adolescents at the time of STD diagnosis and at follow-up. Results from randomized controlled trials have demonstrated that compared with traditional approaches, some brief risk reduction counseling approaches can reduce the occurrence of new STDs by 25–40% among STD clinic patients. As part of many risk reduction counseling programs, HIV counseling, testing, and referral services have been used to recommend HIV testing to adolescents with an STD. (Risk reduction counseling is discussed in detail in Chapter 27.)

Follow-up

The CDC guidelines for treatment of STDs do not recommend "test of cure" for nonpregnant patients who have received the appropriate treatment for gonorrhea or chlamydia unless symptoms persist or there is suspicion of reinfection or nonadherence. According to the CDC, a test of cure may be considered 3 weeks after completion of treatment for chlamydia infection with erythromycin. Testing sooner than 3 weeks after completion of therapy may lead to inappropriate false-negative or false-positive results.

In contrast to test of cure, providers are strongly encouraged to retest female adolescents with chlamydial infection at 3 months. Clinicians should have a system in place to recall treated patients at 3 months for repeat testing, because rates of reinfection in some studies were as high at 40%. Patients who have uncomplicated gonococcal infection do not need test of cure. If symptoms persist after treatment of gonorrhea, then patients should be evaluated by culture for *N gonorrhoeal*, and any gonococci isolated for antimicrobial susceptibility.

Symptomatic patients seeking medical attention should be tested as often as necessary to detect any STDs. Sexually active asymptomatic patients living in high-prevalence areas who have been diagnosed and treated for STDs should be routinely screened every 6 months. Because chlamydia is usually asymptomatic, annual screening is recommended for all sexually active girls and women 25 years of age and younger.

Counseling services should be provided to all adolescents who present with an STD. The style and content of counseling and health education should be appropriate for adolescents. It is important to have visual aids available, be direct about the information provided, and ensure that the adolescent understands the long-term and short-term complications associated with the STD.

In addition, history of an STD may have an important impact on the adolescents' ability to communicate, form future relationships, and seek STD-related care in the future.

Kamb ML, Fishbein M, Douglas JM Jr, et al. Efficacy of risk reduction counseling to prevent human immunodeficiency virus (HIV) and sexually transmitted diseases: Project RESPECT Study Group. *JAMA* 1998;280:1161–1167. [PMID: 9777816] (Large, randomized trial in heterosexual men and women attending STD clinics demonstrating that short counseling interventions using personalized risk reduction plans can increase condom use and prevent new STDs.)

 PRACTICE POINTS

- *In asymptomatic adolescent girls without a history of specific STD exposure who present for routine care, a pelvic examination is not necessary; these patients can be evaluated for chlamydial and gonococcal infection using a urine or self-collected vaginal swab specimen.*
- *In contrast to "test of cure," repeat testing is advised in all adolescent patients with chlamydial and gonococcal infection at 3 months. Clinicians should have a system in place to recall treated patients at 3 months for repeat testing, because rates of reinfection in some studies were as high as 40%.*

Sexually Transmitted Diseases in Men Who Have Sex with Men

24

William Wong, MD

ESSENTIAL FEATURES

- A thorough sexual history is requisite to identifying sexual risk behaviors and the subsequent risk for sexually transmitted diseases (STDs) in men who have sex with men (MSM).
- Epidemiology of STDs and individual risk behavior guide prevention, screening, and clinical management practices.

GENERAL CONSIDERATIONS

MSM are a diverse population defined by their sex and sexual behavior. They include men who identify as gay, bisexual, or heterosexual in their sexual orientation.

The epidemiology of STDs in MSM has changed considerably since the mid-1980s. Declines in the incidence of STDs that occurred in the late 1980s through mid-1990s have been followed by recent increases in the incidence of syphilis, gonorrhea, and HIV among MSM in the United States and Europe. These documented increases in STDs parallel the reversal in AIDS morbidity and mortality with the advent of highly active antiretroviral therapy (HAART).

Paradoxically, the success of HAART may have contributed to higher risk sexual behaviors as a result of reduced fears of HIV transmission among MSM who are infected with the virus and of HIV acquisition among MSM who are not infected. Decreases in condom use, increases in the number of sex partners, and changes in sex practices (from oral sex to anal intercourse) have been reported in MSM in major urban areas throughout the United States since the mid-1990s.

Changes in community norms resulting from HIV treatment optimism and the improved physical well-being of HIV-infected persons are some associated factors that may have contributed to these increases. Social factors that may have contributed to recent changes in sexual behaviors include the advent of the Internet as a means of meeting new sex partners, increased availability and use of methamphetamine and other drugs, and the use of the mass media for direct-to-consumer HIV medication advertising, mitigating the severity of HIV and AIDS.

INITIAL CLINICAL EVALUATION

Because some MSM are not gay-identified, it is essential that clinicians ask open-ended questions in a behavioral risk assessment and not make assumptions about the sex of a patient's sex partners. Building trust and rapport with patients will facilitate the disclosure of sexual behaviors. Every patient evaluation should include a risk assessment for STDs that includes a nonjudgmental and direct ascertainment of sexual behaviors. A thorough sexual history includes the delineation of anal, digital, oral, and vaginal sexual contact exposures (see Table 24–1; see also Chapter 31). The following sexual behaviors are associated with STD transmission in MSM: anal sex (insertive or receptive), oral sex (insertive or receptive), vaginal sex (insertive or receptive), oral-anal or anal-oral sex, and anal-digital or digital-anal sex. Sexually transmissible pathogens and associated syndromes that are most frequently identified in MSM are listed in Table 24–2.

Medical providers should understand the psychosocial contexts of increased sexual risk-taking among some MSM. Common factors associated with increased sexual risk-taking among some MSM include recreational drug use and the use of sexual venues. Alcohol and recreational drug use, such as methamphetamines, inhaled nitrates, ketamine, and MDMA (methylenedioxymethamphetamine) have been associated with high-risk sexual behavior

Table 24–1. Principles of sexual history taking in men who have sex with men.[a]

Principle	Example
Ensuring confidentiality	"Everything we discuss is strictly confidential."
Establishing trust and rapport	"In order to take the best possible care of you, I am going to ask a few questions about your sexual activity. I take a sexual history with all my patients as part of their health assessment."
Maintaining nonjudgmental attitude	"Are you sexually active?" "Do you have sex with men, women, or both?" "How many different sex partners do you have sex with"? "What types of sex do you have? Anal? Oral? Vaginal?" "I am trying to better understand the situations in which you engage in sex. Does alcohol or drugs play a role in your sexual activities?"
Using gender-neutral language when talking about sex or emotional partners	"Does your partner have other sex partners"? "How do you know the HIV status of your current partners?"
Asking open-ended questions	"What are ways you protect yourself from STDs, including HIV?" If HIV infected: "How do you prevent others from being exposed to HIV?"
Using the same language as patient when talking about sexual behavior and identity	"Are you a top (insertive anal), bottom (receptive anal), or both?" "Do you rim (anal-oral contact)?"

[a]Obtaining an adequate sexual history is a continual process between the clinician and patient. For further discussion of the sexual history, see Chapter 31.

and are prevalent among subpopulations of MSM. Additionally, some MSM use venues such as bathhouses, private sex parties, public sex areas, and the Internet to meet sex partners. Since sexual venues facilitate multiple sexual partnerships, anonymous sexual encounters, and are associated with higher risks sexual behaviors, clinicians should engage patients in discussions about venue use in the context of the individual's sexual health. Providers should talk about recreational drug use, both alone and in the context of sexual encounters, because these interactions may contribute to an increased risk for STD and HIV infection in some MSM.

Nevertheless, despite careful and nonjudgmental history taking by the clinician, some patients may not disclose their sexual behaviors, as it often takes time to build trust and rapport between a patient and the clinician. The key to conducting a successful sexual risk assessment includes creating a nonjudgmental and safe environment for the patient, making no assumptions about sexual behaviors, and making sexual risk assessments routine for all patients at the time of the initial visit and on a regular basis unreturned visits, as patients' circumstances and behaviors might change over time.

PREVENTION

Prevention of STDs in MSM includes primary and secondary prevention approaches. Primary prevention

focuses on reducing the potential exposures of MSM to sexually acquired infections through partner number reduction, increased condom usage, and encouraging behaviors that are less likely to transmit STDs such as oral sex and non-penetrative sex play. Primary prevention was successfully adopted by MSM in the mid- and late 1980s. As previously noted, these behavioral changes resulted in profound declines in the incidence of new STDs and HIV infections. With the reversal in safer sex practices observed in subpopulations of MSM, particularly HIV-infected MSM, following the advent of successful HIV therapy, intervention programs and affected communities have embraced secondary prevention strategies focused on increased health care-seeking behavior, increased screening, early detection of infection, and individual and partner treatment strategies.

As STDs declined during the AIDS epidemic, general awareness of STDs declined, along with their basic knowledge of signs and symptoms of STDs, STD transmission, and the value of routine screening for STDs. With noninvasive, accurate, and even self-collected screening tests now available for gonorrhea and chlamydia, MSM and their providers can screen for and treat these infections at an early stage, thereby reducing the duration of infection and the subsequent prevalence of these diseases. Reductions in prevalence should be followed by declines in incidence. However, for screening

Table 24–2. Selected sexually transmissible pathogens and syndromes in MSM.

Causative Pathogen	Syndrome or Disease
Bacterial	
Calymmatobacterium granulomatis	Donovanosis, granuloma inguinale
Campylobacter spp	Enteritis, proctocolitis
Chlamydia trachomatis	Pharyngitis, proctitis, urethritis, epididymitis, Reiter syndrome
C trachomatis serovars L1, L2, L3	Lymphogranuloma venereum-inguinale, proctocolitis, urethritis
Haemophilus ducreyi	Chancroid
Neisseria gonorrhoeae	Pharyngitis, proctitis, urethritis, epididymitis, conjunctivitis, disseminated gonococcal infection
Shigella spp	Enteritis
Treponema pallidum	Syphilis
Viral	
Cytomegalovirus	Mononucleosis; systemic disease, including blindness in immunosuppressed patients
Hepatitis A, B, and C	Acute and chronic liver disease
Herpes simplex virus types 1 and 2	Initial and recurrent genital herpes, orolabial herpes, proctitis
HIV types 1 and 2, and subtype 0	Chronic HIV infection, AIDS
Human papillomavirus	Condylomata acuminata, laryngeal papilloma, anal dysplasia, anal carcinoma
Molluscum contagiosum virus	Genital molluscum
Fungal	
Candida albicans	Balanitis
Ectoparasitic	
Phthirus pubis	Lice
Sarcoptes scabiei	Scabies
Protozoal	
Cryptosporidium parvum	Enteritis
Entamoeba histolytica	Enteritis
Giardia lamblia	Enteritis, proctocolitis
Trichomonas vaginalis	Urethritis

measures to be effective, medical providers and public health departments need to engage the gay community as partners in STD prevention efforts that include enhanced health promotion and awareness, the building community coalitions, increasing access to medical and laboratory services, and enhancing awareness of STDs among community organizations, and health providers.

Several groups, including the California STD Controllers' Association, the Seattle-King County STD Program, and the Centers for Disease Control and

Prevention (CDC), have developed screening recommendations for STDs in HIV-infected MSM and MSM in general. These guidelines recommend screening at least twice a year in sexually active MSM based on sexual behaviors that place MSM as risk for infections at specific anatomic sites. The guidelines recommend pharyngeal gonorrhea screening, urine-based gonorrhea and chlamydia screening, rectal gonorrhea and chlamydia screening, and serologic tests for herpes simplex virus type 2 (HSV-2), syphilis, and HIV. Guidelines from the Infectious Disease Society of America and the Department of Health and Human Services echo these recommendations in HIV-infected persons in care. A summary of current screening recommendations appears in Table 24–3.

Centers for Disease Control and Prevention; Workowski KA, Berman SM. Sexually transmitted diseases treatment guidelines, 2006. *MMWR Recomm Rep* 2006;55(RR-11):1–94. [PMID: 16888612]

STD Control Program and the HIV/AIDS Control Program, Public Health—Seattle & King County, Seattle, Washington, USA. Sexually transmitted disease and HIV screening guidelines for men who have sex with men. *Sex Transm Dis* 2001;28:457–459. [PMID: 11473217] (Set of recommendations for STD screening in MSM, including routine rectal screening and HSV-2 antibody testing.)

BACTERIAL INFECTIONS

Gonorrhea

Neisseria gonorrhoeae causes infections of the pharynx, urethra, and rectum (uncomplicated gonococcal infection), classically presenting as pharyngitis, urethritis, and proctitis, respectively. Asymptomatic infection with gonorrhea has been increasingly recognized as important, although the natural history of asymptomatic infections is largely unknown. Additional research into the pathogenesis of gonococcal infections may elucidate our understanding of the duration of asymptomatic carriage, the rate at which asymptomatic infections become symptomatic, the sequelae of untreated asymptomatic

Table 24–3. STD screening recommendations for MSM.

	Recommendation
Frequency	Screening tests should be performed at least annually or more often based on the number of new sexual partners for sexually active MSM: • HIV serology, including HIV RNA testing, if HIV negative or not previously tested • Syphilis serology by RPR or VDRL • Herpes simplex virus type 2 serology • Urine NAAT for gonorrhea • Urine NAAT for chlamydia • Pharyngeal NAAT or culture for gonorrhea in men with oral-genital exposure • Rectal gonorrhea and chlamydia NAAT or culture in men who have had receptive anal intercourse • Hepatitis A and B immune status, with immunization against hepatitis A and B if susceptible[a] More frequent STD screening (eg, at 3- to 6-month intervals) may be indicated for MSM at highest risk, including: • Patients who acknowledge having multiple anonymous partners or having sex in conjunction with illicit drug use • Patients whose sex partners participate in those activities
Indications	Screening tests usually are indicated regardless of a patient's history of consistent use of condoms for insertive or receptive anal intercourse
Additional considerations	Appropriate diagnostic tests should be performed for any MSM whose sex partner has an STD, and for the following manifestations of symptomatic STDs in MSM: • Urethral discharge or dysuria • Anorectal symptoms (eg, pain, pruritus, discharge, and bleeding) • Genital or anorectal ulcers • Other mucocutaneous lesions • Lymphadenopathy • Skin rash

[a]Prevaccination serologic testing may be cost-effective in MSM, among whom the prevalence of hepatitis A and B infection is likely to be high (>25%).
NAAT, nucleic acid amplification test; RPR, rapid plasma reagin; VDRL, Venereal Disease Research Laboratories test.

infections, and the differences in bacterial load that may alter transmission.

Increases in rectal and urethral gonorrhea among MSM have been reported in Boston, Denver, Los Angeles, San Francisco, and Seattle since the mid-1990s, mostly in older MSM (30–40 years of age) and in those who are HIV-infected. Risk factors identified for rectal gonorrhea included meeting partners on the Internet and methamphetamine use. Studies have documented the high prevalence of pharyngeal gonorrhea by nucleic acid amplification testing (NAAT): 6% among MSM seeking anonymous HIV testing and 11% among MSM seen in an STD clinic in San Francisco.

The diagnosis of gonorrhea continues to be made predominantly by culture, particularly for pharyngeal and rectal infections. A recent study in the San Francisco Department of Public Health demonstrated the superiority of NAAT over culture (sensitivity 93% vs 64%) in detecting pharyngeal infections. Current studies show similar improvement in the detection of rectal gonococcal infections by NAAT. In many practice settings, simplified gonorrhea screening by NAAT on urine specimens has replaced culture and the need for urethral specimen collection, resulting in increased detection of asymptomatic infection. In urethritis, diagnosis by culture is often preferred because the discharge is readily accessible and the isolation of the organism allows for antimicrobial susceptibility testing. Antimicrobial susceptibility monitoring is a critical component of public health surveillance, which allows for timely and evidenced-based therapeutic recommendations. Recent reports have documented the increased prevalence of the decreased susceptibility of gonococcal isolates to ciprofloxacin in Hawaii and California, resulting in changes in treatment recommendations (from fluoroquinolones to third-generation cephalosporins such as ceftriaxone injection or cefpodoxime by mouth). The emergence of fluoroquinolone-resistant gonococci among MSM in the United States has prompted changes in national treatment guidelines.

The recommended treatment for uncomplicated gonococcal infection in MSM is cefpodoxime, 400 mg orally as a single dose, or ceftriaxone, 125 mg intramuscularly as a single dose. With these regimens, treatment success is about 95%; therefore, a follow-up "test of cure" is not necessary. In patients in whom coinfection with *Chlamydia* has not been ruled out, chlamydial therapy is warranted. Recent data in MSM demonstrate a 15% chlamydial coinfection rate in gonococcal urethritis and proctitis. All sex partners within the past 60 days of patients diagnosed with gonorrhea should be evaluated and treated for gonorrhea. In circumstances where it may be unlikely that sex partners will return for evaluation and treatment, patient-delivered partner therapy is recommended. Treatment of recent sex partners prevents reinfection and may decrease continued transmission in the community. In patients treated for gonorrhea, repeat testing at 3 months is recommended to rule out reinfection.

Geisler WW, Whittington WL, Suchland RJ, Stamm WE. Epidemiology of anorectal chlamydial and gonococcal infections among men having sex with men in Seattle: Utilizing serovar and auxotype strain typing. *Sex Transm Dis* 2002;29:189–195. [PMID: 11812458] (Prevalences of anorectal chlamydial and gonococcal infections increased from 4.0% and 6.3%, respectively, during 1994–1996 to 7.6% and 8.7%, respectively, during 1997–1999. Serovar and auxotype analyses indicate these increases are not clonal but are due to the spread of unique distributions of strains that differ from those causing urogenital infections in the same community.)

Kent CK, Chaw JK, Wong W, et al. Prevalence of rectal, urethral, and pharyngeal chlamydia and gonorrhea detected in 2 clinical settings among *men who have sex with men: San Francisco, 2003. Clin Inf Dis* 2005;41:67–74. [PMID: 15937765] (The prevalence of infection varied by anatomic site as follows: for chlamydia, rectal, 7.9%; urethral, 5.2%; and pharyngeal, 1.4%; for gonorrhea, rectal, 6.9%; urethral, 6.0%; and pharyngeal, 9.2%. Approximately 85% of rectal infections were asymptomatic, supporting the need for routine screening. Because 53% of chlamydial infections and 64% of gonococcal infections were at nonurethral sites, these infections would be missed and not treated if only urethral screening was performed. In addition, more than 70% of chlamydial infections would be missed and not treated if MSM were tested only for gonorrhea.)

Chlamydia

Similar to *N gonorrhoeae, Chlamydia trachomatis* causes infections of the pharynx, urethra, and rectum in MSM. Chlamydia is better recognized as an asymptomatic or minimally symptomatic infection. Recent data on rectal chlamydial infections in MSM show increases over the past 5 years and a 10% prevalence of asymptomatic infection. Additionally, studies in MSM show that chlamydia may cause up to 20% of cases of nongonococcal urethritis (NGU), similar to the proportion of NGU attributable to chlamydia in heterosexual men. In asymptomatic populations of MSM undergoing urine screening for urethral chlamydial infection at anonymous HIV testing sites, 0.5% had chlamydial infection in Denver and 3% in San Francisco. Data on pharyngeal chlamydia suggest the prevalence is low, ranging from 0.5% to 2%.

Before the advent of NAAT for the diagnosis of rectal chlamydial infection, the role of chlamydia in proctitis was underappreciated. One study using NAAT showed that 12% of MSM with clinical proctitis who attended an STD clinic had chlamydial infection. Another recent study demonstrated that 20% of MSM with rectal symptoms were infected with *C trachomatis*. Comparison of NAAT versus culture identified six rectal specimens positive for chlamydia by NAAT and none by culture in that study. In a research cohort of

MSM, 4.2% had rectal chlamydia using the polymerase chain reaction (PCR) assay, while only 0.5% of this population had urethral chlamydia. Another study in Seattle compared different methods of processing rectal specimens for the PCR assay and found no differences by the means of specimen processing. Other verification studies in individual laboratories have confirmed the adequate performance of NAATs for the detection of rectal chlamydial infection.

To date antimicrobial resistance has not been a significant problem in the management of chlamydial infections. One reported case in 2000 documented *C trachomatis* resistant to azithromycin and doxycycline, but the extent of resistance at the population level appears limited. Routine surveillance for decreased antimicrobial susceptibility of *C trachomatis* is not performed, however, and monitoring relies on case reports. Because isolation of *C trachomatis* depends on tissue culture systems that are less sensitive than NAAT, defining antimicrobial susceptibility is largely dependent on independent research laboratories and has not been a public health priority.

The recommended treatment of uncomplicated chlamydial infection is doxycycline, 100 mg orally twice daily for 7 days, or azithromycin, 1 g orally as a single dose. Doxycycline is significantly less expensive than azithromycin, is equally efficacious, and offers the patient a continuous reminder to abstain from sexual activity until treatment is completed. In addition, doxycycline is effective against incubating syphilis. Azithromycin can be given under directly observed therapy to assure adherence, and because of its excellent safety profile is easily amenable to being provided to patients to give to their recent sex partners, either through prescription or by directly providing additional doses. Azithromycin, however, is not recommended for the prevention or treatment of syphilis, because the prevalence of azithromycin-resistant syphilis in some areas is 80%. In an effort to augment the control of chlamydia in California, as of January 2001 state law authorized medical providers to dispense additional chlamydial therapy for partners of patients with chlamydial infection.

Lymphogranuloma Venereum

Lymphogranuloma venereum (LGV) is a systemic STD caused by an invasive type of *Chlamydia trachomatis* (serovars L1, L2, and L3) that is prevalent in parts of Africa, Asia, South America, and the Caribbean, but rare in industrialized countries. Since 2003, outbreaks of LGV proctitis reported among MSM, most of whom were HIV-infected, were first identified in the Netherlands, followed by neighboring European countries and then the United States and Canada.

Common clinical manifestations of LGV include tender, unilateral or bilateral inguinal or femoral adenopathy, often becoming fluctuant; and hemorrhagic proctitis or proctocolitis associated with receptive anal intercourse, often mimicking manifestations of inflammatory bowel disease. Because anal infection with LGV may also present asymptomatically, scientists have debated whether LGV reemerged as a new epidemic in industrialized countries or whether it was present but undiagnosed prior to the first reported outbreak. Recent outbreaks of LGV infections in major US cities are most likely attributable to increased testing and enhanced surveillance for this disease.

The diagnosis is based primarily on clinical findings, because laboratory confirmation may not be readily available. Diagnosis of LGV is challenged by the lack of a commercially available assay that distinguishes between LGV serovars of *C trachomatis* and less-invasive serovars of this pathogen. Confirmatory tests using real-time PCR technology are in development.

Patients with LGV infection are treated with doxycycline, 100 mg orally twice daily for 21 days. Alternative treatment is erythromycin base, 500 mg orally four times daily for 21 days. Sex partners who had contact with patients infected with LGV should be clinically evaluated; if asymptomatic, they should be treated with azithromycin, 1 g orally, or doxycycline, 100 mg orally twice daily for 7 days.

Centers for Disease Control and Prevention (CDC). Lymphogranuloma venereum among men who have sex with men—Netherlands, 2003–2004. *MMWR Morb Mortal Wkly Rep* 2004;53: 985–988. [PMID: 15514580] (Report of cases of LGV proctitis in MSM in Europe.)

Syphilis

After becoming a common infection in MSM in the late 1970s, the incidence of syphilis dramatically declined during the early AIDS epidemic to levels consistent with disease elimination by the mid-1990s. The recent resurgence in sexual risk behaviors that led to increases in STDs in MSM has also precipitated outbreaks of syphilis in Boston, Chicago, Houston, Fort Lauderdale, Los Angeles, Miami, New York City, Philadelphia, San Francisco, southern California, and Seattle. In San Francisco, about two thirds of cases have occurred in HIV-positive men with a mean age of 38 years. Cases have been associated with public sex environments, including bathhouses, sex clubs, adult bookstores, and meeting places such as the Internet. Methamphetamine use has been associated with about 25–50% of cases. A recent survey in Chicago among MSM attending a community event showed only about 25% of respondents knew a rash was a symptom of syphilis, and more than 50% incorrectly identified urethral discharge as a symptom.

Several studies have shown that MSM are more likely to be diagnosed at later stages of syphilis illness and less likely to be diagnosed at the primary stage. Primary syphilis lesions may remain occult when they occur in the mouth or the anus, thereby causing delay in the recognition of infection and contributing to the further transmission of disease among sex partners. Therefore, in the physical examination of MSM, it is essential to perform a thorough oral and anal examination. Anoscopy is not routinely recommended unless symptoms are present.

The diagnosis of syphilis is reliably made by the use of darkfield microscopy of exudates from primary or secondary lesions or serologic tests in both HIV-uninfected and HIV-infected persons. Both the rapid plasma reagin (RPR) and the Venereal Disease Research Laboratories (VDRL) tests are commercially available. Although the RPR may be slightly more sensitive, the VDRL is the only assay approved for testing of cerebrospinal fluid specimens. Older case reports suggesting the unreliable nature of syphilis serology in HIV-infected patients have not been substantiated. HIV-infected patients with syphilis should undergo close follow-up at 3, 6, 9, 12, and 24 months. A fourfold decline in titer at 6 months in patients with early infection and at 12 months in patients with late infection is usually consistent with adequate response to treatment.

Chen JL, Kodagoda D, Lawrence AM, Kerndt PR. Rapid public health interventions in response to an outbreak of syphilis in Los Angeles. *Sex Transm Dis* 2002;29:277–284. [PMID: 11984444] (Of the 89 outbreak cases identified, 40% were detected by HIV/AIDS early intervention providers and 26% by private clinicians or health maintenance organizations. Other case identification sources included public STD clinics [10%], STD program case-management contacts [7%], mobile van screening [7%], and correctional facility screening [10%]. Screening at high-risk venues detected a syphilis prevalence of less than 1% and an HIV prevalence of 6%. Weekly calls to the STD hotline increased 600% during the outbreak, and 80% of surveyed individuals cited the media as the source of their awareness of syphilis.)

Nongonococcal Urethritis

Because chlamydia or gonorrhea is recovered in only about 40% of cases of urethritis in MSM, nongonococcal, non–*C trachomatis* urethritis (NGC/NCTU) is the most common diagnosis in urethritis. Overall, NGC/NCTU is MSM is poorly studied, and one can only extrapolate from data from heterosexual populations. Since sexual exposures in MSM are primarily oral or rectal, whereas in heterosexuals exposures are primarily oral or vaginal; extrapolations from these data are limited.

In heterosexual men, common etiologic agents recovered in NGC/NCTU include *Trichomonas vaginalis, Mycoplasma genitalium, Ureaplasma urealyticum*, herpes simplex viruses, adenoviruses, *Streptococcus* species, *Haemophilus* species, and anaerobes. Recent studies have implicated *Mycoplasma genitalium* in heterosexuals with NGC/NCTU, but the role that this agent plays in MSM is unknown. Noninfectious etiologies of NGU should also be considered; these include inflammatory reactions to urethrally inserted drugs (eg, cocaine), chemicals in lubricants (eg, nonoxynol-9), devices such as metal urethral dilators used in certain sex play, postcatheterization after medical procedures, and immunologically mediated conditions such as Reiter syndrome.

Despite the lack of data on causative agents in NGC/NCTU, after the clinician rules out noninfectious causes by history, most cases respond to traditional therapy for NGU: doxycycline, 100 mg orally twice daily for 7 days, or azithromycin, 1 g orally as a single dose. After 7 days, a small proportion of patients may present with persistent symptoms. These patients should be reevaluated for urethritis using microscopic examination of urethral discharge or urine sediment, questioned about treatment adherence and the possibility of reinfection, and then retreated with a different antimicrobial effective against NGU. Persistent urethritis after retreatment would indicate continued urethral inflammation for more than 14 days, which is rare, and consultation with an infectious disease specialist or urologist would be recommended.

VIRAL INFECTIONS

Genital Herpes

With the recent advent of type-specific serologic assays for the determination of herpes simplex virus type 1 (HSV-1) or HSV-2 antibody and the role that genital and rectal herpes infections play in HIV transmission, there has been a renewed interest in herpes epidemiology in MSM. Recent studies have documented higher prevalence levels of HSV-2 antibody in MSM as compared with heterosexual men (31% vs 18%) and a higher proportion of initial genital herpes infections attributable to HSV-1 infection among MSM as compared with women and heterosexual men (47% vs 21% and 15%, respectively). In a Canadian study, 54% of genital herpes infections were caused by HSV-1, and a San Francisco study showed that 22% of genital herpes infections among STD clinic attendees resulted from HSV-1.

Genital herpes infections cause a substantial amount of morbidity in MSM, with symptoms ranging from recurrent itching, redness, or burning sensations to blisters and sores and genital neuropathic pain. These manifestations can involve the penis, scrotum, perineal area, anus, or rectum. Definitive diagnosis is often difficult because it requires isolation by culture of HSV from the affected area. Most laboratories upon isolation of HSV will routinely confirm the subtype using direct fluorescent type-specific antibody. Serologic testing may be helpful to rule out infection, because the seropositivity of HSV-1 and HSV-2 in the general population is about

70% and 22%, respectively. A negative antibody test for both subtypes thus makes infection unlikely. Recent data show that asymptomatic viral shedding is common in HSV-2–infected MSM, similar to prior data in women, occurring in more than 50% of men an average of 1 day a month.

The most significant recent advance in the treatment of genital herpes has been the approval by the Food and Drug Administration of valacyclovir, 500 mg orally twice daily for 3 days, for recurrent infections. Clinicians can prescribe the 1-g dose and order it scored or split. The average wholesale cost of three 1-g tablets of valacyclovir ($23.25 in 2004) is less or similar to the cost of the recommended dosage of acyclovir for recurrent infections (400 mg orally twice daily for 5 days, [$30.90]; and 800 mg orally three times daily for 2 days [$24.00]).

Given the known role that HSV infection plays in the increased risk of acquisition and spread of HIV infection, several studies are underway to determine whether chronic herpes suppression (twice daily acyclovir therapy) will reduce HIV transmission. Although suppressive herpes therapy (valacyclovir, 500 mg by mouth daily) was recently approved by the FDA for chronic suppression and reduction of HSV transmission based on studies in heterosexual couples, chronic suppressive therapy is likely effective in reducing HSV transmission between MSM, as well.

Hepatitis

Hepatitis infections are a major concern for MSM, because both hepatitis A and hepatitis B are sexually transmitted via oral-anal sex and anal intercourse. Current CDC guidelines for preventive care in MSM recommend routine immunization against hepatitis A and B; however, immunization coverage of this population has been low. The recently FDA-approved combination hepatitis A and B vaccine provides a simpler delivery system for immunization, given over several months in three separate doses. Various immunization schedules of 0, 1, and 4 months or 0, 2, and 6 months have been shown to be equally immunogenic, and data demonstrate that even after a single dose more than 50% of patients have demonstrable seroprotection.

Hepatitis A is most often a self-limited infection with rare fatalities. The morbidity, however, can be substantial and, recently, hepatitis A immunization in MSM has been shown to be cost-saving.

Treatment for chronic active hepatitis B is evolving. Recent clinical data suggest that therapy with antiviral agents such as lamivudine, 100 mg daily, and interferon alfa, 10 million units three times per week, can suppress viral replication in 30–40% of patients. The recent FDA approval of the oral drugs adefovir and entecavir offers a promising new addition to treatment options for patients with chronic hepatitis B.

Hepatitis C is an important sexually acquired infection for MSM, particularly for HIV-infected MSM, because population-based prevalence data document a higher risk of infection than in the general population. Recent data controlling for past injection drug use suggest limited risk for MSM and that the sexual transmission of hepatitis C virus is rare among MSM. Hepatitis coinfections with type A or B virus may accelerate the course of hepatitis C; thus, it is imperative that persons with hepatitis C infection receive immunizations for hepatitis A and B.

Human Papillomavirus & Anogenital Warts

Over 70 oncogenic and nononcogenic subtypes of human papillomavirus (HPV) are associated with sexual transmission. In MSM these infections can cause asymptomatic infection, external genital warts, internal rectal warts, and anorectal (and rarely, penile) carcinoma. Exposure to HPV through sexual activity is common, and population-based prevalence studies document that more than 80% of sexually active persons have been exposed to HPV. There is a clear relationship between the number of sex partners and increased prevalence of HPV and infection with an increasing number of different HPV subtypes.

External genital warts are a major reason why MSM present for clinical care and evaluation. In men may present with warts on various areas of the penis and anus. Anal condylomata acuminata should be a clinical cue to receptive anal sex and should prompt further discussion of risk behaviors and appropriate screening (ie, rectal gonorrhea, rectal chlamydia, and syphilis testing). Most external genital warts can be adequately diagnosed by visual inspection, but if the diagnosis is uncertain biopsy may be indicated.

Patients may also complain of internal rectal warts, either self diagnosed or recognized by a sex partner. Symptomatic rectal warts, rectal obstruction, or significant bleeding are indications for referral to a colorectal specialist for wart removal.

Treatment for external genital warts includes provider- or patient-applied therapy such as liquid nitrogen, podophyllin 25%, trichloroacetic acid, imiquimod 5%, or podofilox gel. Patient-applied topical applications appear more efficacious on mucosal sites and other areas that are less keratinized. One advantage of imiquimod 5% is that it may be associated with a reduced recurrence rate, because it activates host immunologic mechanisms to clear infection rather than simple ablation of the wart.

Several observational studies have shown the relationship between oncogenic subtypes of HPV and anorectal carcinoma. These studies have led some experts to recommend routine anal Papanicolaou (Pap) smear testing as a means to reduce the rate of anorectal carcinoma in MSM. The current rate of anorectal carcinoma, at 50 cases per 100,000 MSM per year, is similar to the rate of cervical cancer before the implementation of cervical cancer screening programs. Although HIV-infected persons may have higher rates of abnormal anal Pap smears, the impact of HAART on the reversion of abnormal anal Pap smears is currently under study. Because HIV-infected patients are living longer, one might expect the incidence of anal carcinoma to increase in this population if HAART has no effect.

Anorectal carcinoma is a treatable, albeit not curable, condition with substantial treatment-associated morbidity. At present there are no national recommendations regarding male screening for anorectal carcinoma (anal Pap smear testing).

PARASITIC & ENTERIC INFECTIONS

Enteric Infections

Since the original seminal paper describing enteric infections in MSM by Quinn and colleagues, there have been a few reports contributing to the epidemiology of these infections. *Giardia lamblia*, *Entamoeba histolytica*, *Shigella* species, and *Cryptosporidium parvum* are important causes of gastroenteritis, particularly colitis (characterized by cramping, tenesmus, and diarrhea in the former three and voluminous, loose, watery diarrhea in the latter). Recent studies have documented continued population-based outbreaks of shigellosis in MSM related to oral-anal or digital-anal contact.

Bacterial stool culture for enteric pathogens, as well as ova and parasitic examination with *Giardia* antigen testing of stool, should be performed on MSM who present with abdominal pain and diarrhea. Although one stool specimen may be sufficient to rule in infection, three stool specimens collected on different days are usually required to obtain adequate sensitivity to rule out infection.

Both giardiasis and amebiasis are treated with metronidazole, 750 mg three times daily for 10 days. Amebiasis treatment is followed by treatment with a luminal agent (eg, paromomycin or iodoquinol) for 21 days to eradicate amoebic cysts. Successful therapy for cryptosporidiosis is limited, and most infections in immunocompetent hosts resolve without treatment. Treatment with supportive care includes fluid and electrolyte replacement along with an antimotility agent. Recent reports of treatment include the use of paromomycin and azithromycin, alone or in combination with other antibiotics. Nitazoxanide, twice daily for 3 days, a broad-spectrum antihelminthic drug, is effective in reducing clinical symptoms and oocyte shedding in cryptosporidiosis and in the treatment of giardiasis. Nitazoxanide has been FDA-approved for treating cryptosporidiosis and giardiasis in children (3-day course). The usual adult dose is 500 mg orally twice daily for 3 days.

Shigella and other bacterial causes of gastroenteritis are also important to rule out. Shigellosis often presents in MSM as abdominal pain and diarrhea with or without blood. Diagnosis is by stool culture and treatment is with a fluoroquinolone antibiotic (eg, ciprofloxacin, 500 mg orally twice daily for 5 days). Recent reports of *Shigella* species resistant to trimethoprim-sulfamethoxazole and ampicillin make those antimicrobials less useful in routine management.

Pubic Lice & Scabies

Pubic lice (*Phthirus pubis*) and scabies (*Sarcoptes scabiei*) are commonly encountered in clinical practice in MSM. Symptoms of pubic lice include itching in the pubic area and often patient identification of lice or nits on hair shafts. Diagnosis is made by visual inspection and identification of the lice or by finding small red macules in the skin around the hair follicles. Treatment is with several different topical shampoos including permethrin (1%) cream, pyrethrins, or piperonyl butoxide applied to the affected area.

Scabies can cause more morbidity than pubic lice. Often patients complain of itching around the waist, wrist, and in the webbed area between the fingers. Warmth often exacerbates the symptoms, and patients may complain of itching that is worse at night, when under the bedcovers, or after a hot shower. Raised papular lesions can also occur on the scrotum or penis, mimicking secondary syphilitic lesions or epidermoid cysts.

The diagnosis of scabies is made on the basis of history and physical findings. Rarely, lesions can be scraped and mite or mite feces identified by microscopy under oil immersion. Treatment is with permethrin 5% cream (Elimite or Acticin) applied overnight. Rare complications of Elimite use include seizures. Some experts recommend repeat treatment at 1 week.

HIV & STD INTERACTIONS IN MEN WHO HAVE SEX WITH MEN

Over the past two decades a large body of evidence has emerged to describe the relationship between STDs and HIV transmission, from early epidemiologic studies showing increased risk for HIV acquisition among those with ulcerative STDs to intervention studies demonstrating reduction in HIV transmission with control of STDs. The data in MSM, however, are limited. Because most HIV infections in MSM are acquired through receptive anal intercourse, the role of rectal gonococcal infections has been most studied. One study showed a threefold increased risk for HIV seroconversion in MSM with rectal gonorrhea. A more recent study showed compounding increases in risk of HIV acquisition with the number of rectal infections. Intervention studies to demonstrate the effect of rectal

STD treatment in reducing HIV acquisition, however, are lacking.

Biologic data in persons with HIV infection have shown increased local HIV viral replication in anatomic sites with concurrent bacterial STDs. Studies have further elucidated the role of immunologic mechanisms, including the role cytokine production may play in increasing HIV viral replication after bacterial infection. Recent studies have demonstrated that newly acquired syphilis infection in a patient with chronic HIV infection can lead to increased HIV viral replication and decreased CD4 counts. The impact on HIV disease progression remains to be determined.

FUTURE DIRECTIONS

STD management in MSM requires clinicians to be conversant with sexual risk assessments, clinical presentations and current diagnosis of prevalent infections, and new therapeutic agents. Successful STD care of MSM is rewarding, because many infections are easily diagnosed and curable with simple, single-dose therapy. The current challenges lie in achieving effective risk reduction and optimizing preventive care in a cost-effective manner. New molecular-based diagnostic studies will offer insights into the etiology of several clinical syndromes, but the basis of care will always rely on the same critical components of medicine—listening and talking with the patient.

 PRACTICE POINTS

- *The key to conducting a successful sexual risk assessment includes making no assumptions about the sexual behaviors of patients, and making sexual risk assessments routine for all patients at the time of the initial visit and on a regular basis on return visits, because the patient's circumstances and behaviors might change over time.*
- *Primary syphilis lesions may remain occult when they occur in the mouth or the anus, thereby causing delay in the recognition of infection and contributing to the further transmission of disease among sex partners. Therefore, in the physical examination of MSM, it is essential to perform a thorough oral and anal examination.*

Sexually Transmitted Diseases in Women Who Have Sex with Women

Jeanne M. Marrazzo, MD, MPH

 ESSENTIAL FEATURES

- Transmission of common sexually transmitted diseases (STDs), including trichomoniasis and human papillomavirus (HPV), has been reported in women who have sex with women (WSW).
- Transmission likely is mediated through exchange of infected cervicovaginal secretions or direct contact.
- Most WSW, including self-defined lesbians, have had sex with men.
- Barriers to care exist for many WSW, including lack of provider education about relevant issues.
- Papanicolaou (Pap) smear screening should be performed in WSW according to routine national guidelines.

GENERAL CONSIDERATIONS

Relatively few data are available to inform estimates of the risk of female-to-female sexual transmission of STDs. The available data come primarily from four sources.

First, review of records from clinics that provide STD services (STD clinics) has provided estimates of some outcomes, including diagnosis of STD syndromes, laboratory results, and risk reporters. Such studies have the advantages of capturing a reproducible population of women who can be characterized relative to heterosexual women attending the same venue and of relying on clinician-based or laboratory-defined reports of outcomes, but are limited primarily by the relatively small number of WSW who attend these clinics.

Second, several studies have recruited women who either self-identify as lesbian or who report recent same-sex behavior, regardless of stated identity. Although this type of study may capture a more representative sample of WSW and frequently includes laboratory diagnosis of STDs, the sample of women included is likely biased due to self-selection for enrollment.

Third, although population-based surveys attempt to enroll a more representative sample of women, including WSW, because these surveys are generally expensive and complex to undertake, most do not include laboratory-confirmed assessment of STDs but rely on self-reported STD history.

Finally, case reports of STD transmission between women provide the only documented evidence available for some STDs. Despite their obvious limitations, these reports are valuable in that they can demonstrate the potential for STD transmission between women and, as such, help to emphasize the need for more robust, population-based data to inform WSW patients and their providers about the true risks associated with same-sex behavior between women.

Numerous studies have demonstrated that important barriers to health care exist for WSW. These barriers include, but are not limited to, lack of patient educational materials aimed at their specific risks and circumstances, lack of knowledge among providers, low socioeconomic status, absence of spousal benefits, and impact of negative experiences within the health care system. Among the latter are included outright instances of homophobia and general invisibility. For example, many office registration materials still list options for marital status as "single" or "married"—terms that do not apply to WSW who may be in domestic partnerships, particularly those that are not recognized by regulatory authorities. Even providers who are comfortable assessing STD-related risks may not be knowledgeable about the sexual practices engaged in by many WSW, or about the limited disease-specific information in the literature. For these reasons, education of providers in this area is paramount.

Because recent national surveys indicate that same-sex behavior among women is relatively common, providers should familiarize themselves with information about this patient population, and be aware of referral options for more detailed information. Available information on transmission of specific STDs in WSW is discussed later, under Laboratory Studies.

O'Hanlan KA, Dibble SL, Hagan JJ, Davids R. Advocacy for women's health should include lesbian health. *J Women's Health* 2004;13:227–234. [PMID: 15072737] (This excellent editorial review summarizes much of the data detailing barriers to preventive care for WSW, and outlines key areas of which providers should be aware.)

INITIAL CLINICAL EVALUATION

Risk Assessment

Risk assessment in WSW should begin the way all STD-related risk assessment begins in every patient: with a thorough sexual history. Most importantly, providers should not make assumptions about sexual practices based on the patient's self-reported identity—in this case, specifically, as a lesbian. Assuming that a self-identified lesbian has not previously been or is not currently sexually active with men is usually incorrect. In one study, 74% of self-identified lesbians had male partners in the past, and of self-identified bisexual women, 98% had prior or current male partners. Among lesbians recruited for studies in Seattle, 80–86% reported prior sex with men, 23–28% had had sex with a man in the last year, and the median number of male and female lifetime partners was the same. In a sample of women evaluated at a London STD clinic, 69% of those identifying as lesbian had prior male partners, and at another London clinic specializing in the sexual health of lesbians, 91% had prior male partners. Heterosexual intercourse transmits the full range of STDs, some of which (notably, chronic viral infections, including HPV, genital herpes, hepatitis B virus, and HIV) may remain undetected for years.

Important components of the sexual history include number of recent (prior 2 months and 1 year) and lifetime sexual partners, both male and female. Other key components should include types of sexual practices that could pose a risk of transmission of STDs. Some sexual practices—including oral-genital sex; vaginal or anal sex using hands, fingers, or penetrative sex toys; and oral-anal sex—are practiced commonly between female sex partners. Practices involving digital-vaginal or digital-anal contact, particularly with shared penetrative sex toys, present a plausible means for transmission of infected cervicovaginal secretions.

In several studies, women who report sex with both men and women report more sex partners over their lifetimes than women who have sex exclusively with either men or women. One population-based survey in low-income neighborhoods found that women who had sex with men only reported a mean of 16 lifetime partners, whereas women reporting sex with men and women reported a mean of 307 lifetime partners. Similarly, among patients attending an STD clinic in Seattle, women with only female partners in the previous 2 months reported 3.4 partners in the past year; women with only male partners, 5.3 partners in the past year; and women with male and female partners, 16.5 partners in the past year. Women who report sex with both men and women are likely to be at higher risk for STDs than women who report sex with women or men only.

WSW may have male partners who are at higher risk for HIV and STDs than the partners of women who have sex with men only. In one study of patients at an STD clinic, 10% of women who had sex with only women in the previous 2 months had a prior male partner who was gay or bisexual, compared with 6% of women reporting sex with men only. Of women reporting sex with both men and women in the prior 2 months, 29% had a prior gay or bisexual male partner. Women who reported sex with both men and women in the previous 2 months were also more likely than women who had sex with only men or only women to have had more than four male sexual partners in a year, more likely to exchange sex for money or drugs, and more likely to have used intravenous drugs. In summary, lesbian and bisexual women may have past or current sex partners at high risk for HIV and other STDs.

Mosher WD, Chandra A, Jones J. Sexual behavior and selected health measures: Men and women 15–44 years of age, United States, 2002. *Adv Data* 2005;(362):1–55. [PMID: 16250464] (Among 12,571 respondents in this national sample, 11% of women reported having had a sexual experience with another woman. The proportion of women who had a female sex partner in the past year was 4.4%, representing approximately 2.71 million women in the United States.)

Scheer S, Peterson I, Page-Shafer K, et al; Young Women's Survey Team. Sexual and drug use behavior among women who have sex with both women and men: Results of a population-based survey. *Am J Public Health* 2002;92:1110–1112. [PMID: 12084692] (Population-based study in five northern California counties describing sexual risk behaviors, STDs, and HIV infection in women who have sex with women and men.)

Risk Reduction Counseling

No studies have directly addressed the acceptability or efficacy of STD risk reduction interventions among WSW. However, measures that reduce the potential for transmission of cervicovaginal secretions are likely to be effective in reducing STD transmission.

For women who practice digital-vaginal or digital-anal sex (hands or fingers in partner's vagina or anus), the risk is probably low unless secretions are actually transferred on the hands from the infected partner to the other. Interrupting this progression by avoiding the behavior or by using and removing gloves after contact is likely effective.

For minimizing transfer of infected secretions associated with insertive sex toys, several approaches are likely effective. These include minimizing sharing of unclean sex toys (either not sharing toys at all or cleaning them between use by one partner and the other), use of condoms on sex toys, and avoiding use of sex toys anally and vaginally in succession.

With regard to oral sex and STDs, WSW may be at increased risk of genital herpes infection with herpes simplex virus type 1 (HSV-1) due to a relatively higher frequency of orogenital sex. Serologic screening for HSV-1 is not useful to screen for potential infectiousness, because most adults are infected with HSV-1 orally, and serology does not distinguish between oral and genital infection. However, women should be counseled to avoid performing oral sex when lesions consistent with an oral herpes outbreak (eg, a cold sore, recurrent ulcer, or vesicle) are evident or if a recognizable prodrome (eg, ear pain or local lymphadenopathy) is underway.

Other important components of complete risk reduction counseling for all patients include a discussion of sex partner selection, sexual network assessment, and the patient's ability to negotiate safer sex practices. More detailed information can be found in Chapter 27.

Laboratory Studies

A. SCREENING OF ASYMPTOMATIC PATIENTS

Laboratory evaluation for STDs in WSW should closely mirror that for heterosexual women. With regard to STD screening of asymptomatic women without clinical findings, WSW should be screened for *Chlamydia trachomatis* as recommended by current screening guidelines (annually up to age 25 years or older, depending on risk). Although no data are available to estimate the risk of chlamydia transmission between women, chlamydial infection and pelvic inflammatory disease have been reported by WSW surveyed; further, WSW may engage in sexual networks that involve men, as previously noted, and may not be aware of their female partners' exposure to men. No cases of gonorrhea transmission between women have been documented; given the relatively low prevalence of this STD in many clinical settings, routine screening for gonorrhea in asymptomatic WSW without relevant clinical symptoms is not indicated.

Other STDs in WSW deserve comment, but should not be sought in asymptomatic women who report no contact with a male or female partner with an STD. Each should be considered in the relevant clinical setting (eg, complaint of abnormal vaginal discharge or of genital ulcers).

B. PATIENTS WITH ABNORMAL VAGINAL DISCHARGE

1. Bacterial vaginosis—Bacterial vaginosis is highly prevalent among WSW and has been the most common diagnosis in WSW evaluated at STD clinics (frequently, it is more common in WSW than in heterosexual women at those clinics). Risks for bacterial vaginosis among WSW include a higher number of lifetime female sex partners, having a female sex partner with bacterial vaginosis, use of a shared vaginally inserted sex toy, and receptive oral-anal sex. The exact cause of bacterial vaginosis is unknown, but these data suggest that some factor that promotes or causes this enigmatic condition may be transmissible between women during sex. Whether female partners of women diagnosed with bacterial vaginosis should be routinely tested and treated is not known. One reasonable approach is to test a woman's partner for bacterial vaginosis if she is symptomatic, or if the infection in the index case is recurrent, because treatment of the partner might theoretically effect a higher cure rate in the index case. However, the latter approach has not been studied.

2. Trichomoniasis—Other etiologies of abnormal vaginal discharge include infection with *Trichomonas vaginalis,* which has been self-reported in surveys by women with no history of prior sex with men and has also been reported as metronidazole-resistant trichomoniasis in both members of a monogamous lesbian couple. These data, along with the plausibility of transmitting vaginal fluid through the sexual practices of WSW, strongly support the conclusion that this infection can be transmitted in this manner.

C. PATIENTS WITH GENITAL LESIONS OR ULCERS

1. Human papillomavirus infection—HPV, a group of viruses that causes anogenital warts and cervical cancer, may be transmissible between women by skin-to-skin contact, digital-genital contact, and use of shared sex toys. Women who report never having sexual contact with men have been found to have vulvar warts, cervical neoplasia associated with HPV, and high-risk (associated with oncogenic risk) HPV DNA by genetic testing (polymerase chain reaction). In one study, HPV DNA was detected by genetic probe in 19% of women who had no prior sexual contact with men, and 14% had cervical dysplasia. Anogenital warts and abnormal Pap smears were also self-reported by women with no prior sexual contact with men.

Importantly, the finding that HPV is present in women whose sexual contact with men is either remote or nonexistent has important implications regarding Pap screening for these women. Such women may consider themselves at low risk for cervical cancer, and their health care providers may assume the same. Thus, routine screening for cervical dysplasia may be neglected in these women. WSW should receive Pap screening for cervical dysplasia according to the same guidelines as other sexually active women.

2. HIV infection—Case reports of sexual HIV transmission between women have been published, with a recent report substantiated by a finding of identical genotype of the HIV isolates from both women and a plausible clinical history. Oral-genital contact, mucosa-to-mucosa genital contact, sharing of blood or menstrual fluid, and contact with genital herpes lesions could facilitate transmission. Because the Centers for Disease Control and Prevention now recommends universal HIV screening in all primary care settings, WSW should be tested for HIV at least once, and retested depending on sexual risk behavior. Decisions to rescreen for HIV should be based on risk factors such as unprotected sex with men, particularly gay or bisexual men, number of recent female sex partners, and intravenous drug use.

3. Genital herpes infection—Genital herpes, usually caused by herpes simplex virus type 2 (HSV-2) but occasionally by HSV-1, can be transmitted by contact of mucous membrane to mucous membrane or vulnerable skin. Therefore, transmission between women is theoretically possible. Genital herpes has been reported in women who had no prior sexual contact with men. In a study of nearly 400 WSW in Seattle in 1998–2001, 2.6% of women who reported no male partners had antibodies to HSV-2. Likelihood of having HSV-2 antibodies increased with increasing lifetime number of male sex partners. The authors concluded that HSV-2 can be transmitted between women, although less efficiently than between men and women. Thus, routine screening for HSV-2 infection using type-specific serology is not recommended for WSW unless individual risk assessment indicates it should be performed (eg, history of unexplained genital lesions; recent multiple sex partners, especially men). In the Seattle study, the likelihood of WSW having antibodies to HSV-1, which typically causes oral herpes, increased with increasing number of lifetime female partners, suggesting a role for orogenital sex in facilitating transmission in this population. However, serologic screening is not indicated for this virus, because infection is widely prevalent, the test does not distinguish between oral and genital infection, and HSV-1 genital infection is associated with fewer recurrences and less subclinical shedding.

4. Syphilis—Although *Treponema pallidum*, the causative agent of syphilis, is relatively uncommon compared with the viral STDs discussed in the preceding paragraphs, sexual transmission between female partners has recently been reported. Because some WSW who choose to have sex with men may be more likely to choose bisexual men for partners, health care providers should bear in mind that recently the incidences of early syphilis and of fluoroquinolone-resistant *Neisseria gonorrhoeae* have markedly increased among men who have sex with men. Providers should thus screen and treat WSW appropriately based on STD risk assessment.

Kwakwa HA, Ghobrial MW. Female-to-female transmission of human immunodeficiency virus. *Clin Infect Dis* 2003;36: e40–41. [PMID: 12539088] (Although sexual transmission of HIV between women is probably relatively uncommon, this case report suggests that it can occur.)

Marrazzo JM, Stine K, Koutsky LA. Genital human papillomavirus infection in women who have sex with women: A review. *Am J Obstet Gynecol* 2000;183:770–774. [PMID: 10992207] (Summarizes the available data regarding infection with HPV among WSW.)

Marrazzo J, Koutsky LA, Eschenbach DA, et al. Characterization of vaginal flora and bacterial vaginosis in women who have sex with women. *J Infect Dis* 2002;185:1307–1313. [PMID: 12001048] (In this study of 329 self-referred WSW in Seattle, prevalence of bacterial vaginosis was 27%, and infection was more common among women who reported higher numbers of female partners, sharing of insertive sex toys, and receptive oral-anal sex. The likelihood of a woman having bacterial vaginosis was also greatly increased if her female partner had bacterial vaginosis, supporting the hypothesis that this infection may be sexually transmitted between women.)

RECOMMENDATIONS FOR SEXUAL HEALTH ASSESSMENT IN WOMEN WHO HAVE SEX WITH WOMEN

Available data strongly suggest that HPV, and probably other STDs (especially herpes simplex virus), are sexually transmitted between women. Thus, recommendations for Pap smear screening among lesbians should not differ from those for heterosexual women. Bacterial vaginosis may eventually be defined as an STD that is transmissible between women, but the exact etiology of the condition remains unknown. The recent increases in STDs among men who have sex with men but who do not identify as gay also emphasize that simply asking female patients their self-defined sexual orientation is not adequate. Assessment of specific sexual risk behaviors, and of previous sexual history, can provide a more complete tool for guiding the patient evaluation and counseling the patient about how to maintain sexual health.

PRACTICE POINTS

- *The finding that HPV is present in women whose sexual contact with men is either remote or nonexistent has important implications regarding Pap screening for WSW. WSW should receive Pap screening for cervical dysplasia according to the same guidelines as other sexually active women.*

Principles of Serologic Testing for Syphilis

26

Edward W. Hook III, MD

ESSENTIAL FEATURES

- *Serologic tests for syphilis are the most common means for diagnosis of syphilis and the best currently available tool for evaluating response to therapy.*
- *Serologic diagnosis of past or present syphilis infection is based on the results of two tests: a reactive nontreponemal serologic test for syphilis, confirmed by a test for syphilis based on unrelated treponemal antigens.*
- *Testing may be complicated by atypical immunologic responses by cross-reactive antibodies leading to false-positive test results, and by difficulties in distinguishing current from past infection.*

GENERAL CONSIDERATIONS

Syphilis is a chronic sexually transmitted disease (STD) with worldwide prevalence. From the time of acquisition of infection until diagnosis, the course of untreated infection may span decades. At any point in its natural history, a diagnosis of untreated syphilis warrants treatment. Although the causative organism, *Treponema pallidum,* may be demonstrated using darkfield microscopy during its earliest (primary and secondary) stages, this test is not useful for diagnosis except in the early stages of disease. Equally important, darkfield microscopy is often not performed even when lesions are present because a microscope equipped with a darkfield condenser is rarely available in the settings where patients with syphilis are seen. As a result, most syphilis diagnosis,

as well as follow-up to ascertain response to therapy, is carried out using serologic tests for syphilis. The practical utility of serologic testing may be complicated by atypical immunologic responses by cross-reactive antibodies leading to false-positive test results, and by difficulties in distinguishing current from past infection.

Serologic tests for syphilis become reactive early in the course of untreated infection as infected individuals begin to produce antibodies to *T pallidum*. It is estimated that up to 10% of patients with syphilitic chancres of primary syphilis will have nonreactive serologic tests for syphilis, most of which occur in the first few days following appearance of the lesion. After primary lesions have been present for several days, the likelihood of nonreactive serologic tests declines markedly. Over the course of untreated infection, serologic titers tend to rise and then may fall, reflecting disease activity and duration of infection. Nearly all patients with untreated secondary or early latent syphilis will have reactive serologic tests. With continuing infection and production of anti—*T pallidum* antibodies, serologic titers tend to increase. Thus, patients with primary syphilis tend to have somewhat lower serologic titers than those with secondary or early latent infection.

After rising over the first few years of untreated infection (ie, from primary through secondary and into the latent stage), serologic titers peak and then may decline gradually over time. Although serologic titers may roughly reflect duration of infection, there is far too much person-to-person variation in antitreponemal antibody production to allow currently available serologic test titers to be considered as precise reflections of duration of infection. Studies done more than 50 years ago suggested that a small (but poorly quantified) proportion of individuals with untreated late latent or late syphilis will have nonreactive serologic tests for syphilis, although the proportion of cases in which this occurs is unclear.

TYPES OF SEROLOGIC TESTS FOR SYPHILIS

At present, most syphilis diagnosis is based on a two-stage testing process. Patients are first tested using a "nontreponemal" serologic test that uses synthesized cardiolipin-lecithin-cholesterol antigens to detect cross-reacting antibodies to *T pallidum*. For purposes of confirmation, specimens that produce reactive nontreponemal results are subsequently tested with a second, "treponemal" test that uses *T pallidum* antigens. By utilizing this two-step algorithm to detect reactivity to two relevant, unrelated antigens, the proportion of false-positive test results is markedly reduced (see Table 26–1). Reactive nontreponemal tests that are not confirmed by reactive treponemal tests are typically considered to be false-positive serologic tests for syphilis.

Nontreponemal Tests

As mentioned, virtually all currently available nontreponemal tests currently utilized for syphilis testing are based on the reactivity of human immunoglobulin G (IgG) and immunoglobulin M (IgM) antibodies to *T pallidum* with a cardiolipin-lecithin-cholesterol antigen, typically performed as a flocculation test in which the antigen-antibody lattice formed by mixing patient plasma or serum with an antigen suspension is detected. The prototypic nontreponemal test for syphilis is the Venereal Disease Research Laboratory (VDRL) test. Other widely used nontreponemal tests include the rapid plasma reagin (RPR), automated reagin test (ART), and toluidine red unheated serum test (TRUST).

Table 26–1. Demonstration of why the sequence of two-step, confirmatory testing does not modify numbers of false-positive test results.

Assumptions: (1) no syphilis in this hypothetical population of 100,000; (2) false-positive rate within nontreponemal test is 1.5%; and (3) false-positive rate for treponemal test is 1%.

Step 1: Screening

Nontreponemal test (first)	Treponemal test (first)
100,000	100,000
× .015	× .01
1500	1000

Step 2: Confirmatory testing

Treponemal test (second)	Nontreponemal test (second)
1500	1000
×.01	×.015
15	15

An important characteristic of most nontreponemal tests is that they can be used both as qualitative tests, in which results are reported as either reactive or nonreactive, and as quantitative tests, in which the patient specimen is tested in a series of dilutions. The results are reported either as the minimum dilution of reactivity (ie, 1:1, 1:2, 1:4, 1:8, etc) or as the reciprocal of that dilution (ie, 1, 2, 4, 8, etc). The ability to provide a semiquantitative measure of antitreponemal serologic tests allows them to be used to evaluate response to therapy following treatment.

Treponemal Tests

This broad category of serologic tests for syphilis comprises those tests that use treponemal antigens as reagents. In the past these antigens were most often generated through purification of *T pallidum* that had been repeatedly passed in rabbits and then utilized to make tests in a number of different formats (immunofluorescence, hemagglutination, enzyme-linked immunosorbent assay [ELISA], etc). More recently, as information on the sequence of the *T pallidum* genome has become available, cloned treponemal antigens are increasingly being used for diagnostic syphilis testing. Among the advantages of these cloned antigens are that they can be produced in large quantities and that the antigens are not contaminated by potentially cross-reactive antigens, as is the case for antigen preparations generated from animal-passaged *T pallidum*.

Although investigators have periodically evaluated quantitative treponemal serologic tests for syphilis diagnosis, staging, or evaluation of response to therapy, the utility of these tests for these purposes is controversial. In most settings, treponemal tests are used qualitatively as confirmatory tests for patients with reactive nontreponemal serologic tests. In general, and unlike the nontreponemal tests, treponemal serologic test reactivity is life-long in the majority of persons with syphilis and is of little use for evaluating response to therapy. As for the nontreponemal tests, a small proportion of persons who are not infected with *T pallidum* or other pathogenic treponemes (see later discussion) will have reactive test results (ie, false positive). As a result, screening efforts that rely solely on treponemal tests—without confirmatory nontreponemal testing—are not recommended.

A recent development relating to treponemal serologic tests is the advent of ELISA screening assays, which can be used to efficiently test large numbers of specimens for *T pallidum* antibodies (ie, in blood banks or by some large commercial laboratories). Although ELISA test results are often presented in quantitative fashion, there is little experience in using these tests to evaluate response to therapy. Rather, persons identified as having syphilis using ELISA tests should then be tested using a quantitative nontreponemal assay for the purpose of evaluating response to therapy.

PITFALLS IN SEROLOGIC TESTING FOR SYPHILIS

Serologic tests for syphilis are utilized primarily for three purposes: (1) to screen populations for otherwise inapparent syphilis, (2) to confirm clinical diagnoses of patients with appropriate clinical manifestations or presentations, and (3) for evaluation of response to therapy. Theoretically, because each uses the serologic test for a different purpose, they should be considered separately. In practice, however, there is substantial overlap in the use of serologic tests for these purposes.

Screening

As screening tests, serologic tests for syphilis are used to identify individuals who may have infectious syphilis with the aim of either identifying disease that should be treated or of assuring the safety of blood and other tissues that might be transfused or transplanted to others. In the United States, all blood and blood products used for transfusion are routinely screened for syphilis. In the past, this screening typically utilized automated nontreponemal tests. However, the ease and lower costs of treponemal antigen-based ELISA tests has begun to supplant the use of the RPR test for this purpose in many settings. Individuals identified using ELISA assays for antitreponemal antibodies should be further evaluated using quantitative nontreponemal tests to confirm the diagnosis of syphilis. Those quantitative tests may then be used for follow-up of response to treatment.

Confirmation of Diagnosis

If patients have appropriate clinical manifestations of syphilis, serologic tests are used to confirm the diagnosis. At the same time there are occasions when these tests may be nonreactive despite the fact that a person truly has syphilis. One of the most common instances in which this occurs is in the early stages of infection, when patients may have a primary lesion (chancre) and yet have a nonreactive serologic test. The nonreactive test result is a consequence of the time required for the immune response to generate antibody concentrations sufficient to make the test reactive. This "window" period is relatively short lived and is almost rarely an issue for patients whose primary lesions have been present for more than 5–7 days.

A second reported, but uncommon, instance in which serologic tests for syphilis may be nonreactive in patients with untreated syphilis occurs in those with HIV infection, presumably because their underlying immune deficiency has failed to allow a typical serologic response to infection to occur. Several case reports have described HIV-infected individuals who presented with clinical manifestations of secondary syphilis as confirmed by demonstration of

T pallidum in biopsy specimens, yet who had nonreactive serologic tests. In the best described of these case reports, by Hicks and colleagues, the patient ultimately developed reactive serologic tests, thus his response was delayed rather than nonexistent. These occurrences are quite rare even in persons with HIV infection but are important for clinicians to consider when dealing with at-risk patients with appropriate clinical syndromes.

A final instance in which the serologic response may appear to be nonreactive is termed the *prozone reaction*. In this reaction, initial nontreponemal serologic testing at 1:1 dilution is nonreactive; however, upon further dilution the test becomes reactive. The prozone reaction occurs primarily in patients with secondary syphilis as a result of "antibody excess," which prevents the formation of the antigen-antibody lattice necessary for the serologic test to become positive. The prozone reaction should be considered in patients with nonreactive nontreponemal tests for syphilis who have clinical syndromes compatible with early, and particularly secondary, syphilis. Requesting that the laboratory evaluate the specimen for possible prozone reaction by diluting the serum specimen will address this potential problem.

Golden MR, Marra CM, Holmes KK. Update on syphilis: resurgence of an old problem. *JAMA* 2003;290:1510–1514. [PMID: 13129993] (Excellent review of syphilis management for the practicing clinician.)

Hart G. Syphilis tests in diagnosis and therapeutic decision making. *Ann Intern Med* 1986;104:368–376. [PMID: 3511822] (Practical review of the use and interpretation of syphilis tests.)

Hicks CB, Benson PM, Lupton GP, Tramont EC. Seronegative secondary syphilis in a patient infected with the human immunodeficiency virus (HIV) with Kaposi sarcoma. A diagnostic dilemma. *Ann Intern Med* 1987;107:492–495. [PMID: 3307583]

Evaluation of Response to Therapy

A third important use of serologic tests is for the evaluation of the response to syphilis therapy. For this purpose quantitative nontreponemal tests are most often used and are preferred. Because of day-to-day variability in test performance, when evaluating response to therapy, a two dilution (fourfold) or greater change in titers (or for specimens only reactive at a 1:1 dilution, a reversion to nonreactive status) is required to define an adequate patient treatment response. Thus, a person diagnosed with syphilis who has a titer of 1:16 on RPR testing could be considered to have responded appropriately to therapy if subsequent tests are found to have titers of 1:4 or less. In contrast, for the same patient, because a titer of 1:8 would represent only a one dilution (twofold) change, this result may not represent a meaningful change and therefore should not be considered evidence that the patient has responded appropriately to syphilis therapy.

The average time for the serologic response to syphilis therapy to be detectable also varies with the duration of infection; patients with more long-standing disease take longer to respond. Thus, serologic responses tend to occur more quickly in patients with primary syphilis than in those with secondary syphilis, who in turn respond more quickly than those with latent or late infection. An important further caveat for evaluating response to therapy using quantitative nontreponemal serologic tests is that titers generated with one type of test do not necessarily equate to titers as measured with a differently configured test. Thus, patients tested initially using the RPR test should be followed with RPR tests, whereas those initially diagnosed using VDRL tests should be followed with the VDRL.

In addition, large studies of patients with early (primary, secondary, early latent) syphilis have demonstrated that despite receipt of recommended doses of benzathine penicillin, nearly 20% of patients do not achieve a two dilution (fourfold) decline in serologic titers by 12 months following therapy. Most experts would classify the majority of such individuals as "nonresponders" rather than true treatment failures (or reinfections). In situations in which serologic titers have not declined two or more dilutions after recommended follow-up, in the absence of other indications of treatment failure or reinfection, whether such patients warrant retreatment, further evaluation (ie, lumbar puncture to assess for possible neurosyphilis), or continued follow-up is a clinical judgment that should consider factors such as continuing high-risk behavior, reliability, local disease epidemiology, and immune status.

There are several other situations in which patients with syphilis may have somewhat atypical serologic manifestations of infection. These include the challenge of interpreting changing serologic titers in patients with prior syphilis and evaluation of reactive serologic tests in pregnant women who may or may not have had syphilis in the past. There is thought to be a somewhat increased prevalence of biologic false-positive serologic tests for syphilis in pregnancy, and in women who have had prior syphilis it is believed that even without reinfection, nontreponemal serologic test titers may increase, possibly related to pregnancy-related immunologic changes. These phenomena are often talked about but have not been formally studied. False-positive serologic tests in pregnancy will be identified through the two-step testing procedure used to confirm serologic diagnoses of infection. In pregnant women who have had syphilis in the past and are found to have a fourfold or greater increase in serologic titers, because of the risks of syphilis for unborn children, most clinicians would favor erring on the side of caution and administration of retreatment.

Several carefully performed large studies have suggested that for patients with HIV infection, serologic tests may be changed in several ways. As previously mentioned, very rarely, HIV-infected individuals who acquire syphilis may have unusually delayed development of serologic test reactivity. In addition, in large studies of

patients with early syphilis and coexistent HIV infection, nontreponemal serologic titers tend to be somewhat higher than those in patients who do not have HIV. Although the tendency toward higher serologic titers in patients with coexistent HIV has been significant in some studies, the spectrum of serologic titers ranges from nonreactive to high-titer reactive specimens; thus, it is inappropriate to make assumptions regarding a person's HIV status on the basis of the magnitude of a nontreponemal serologic titer. In addition, with regard to patients with coexistent HIV infection and syphilis, there are no data to suggest that qualitative nontreponemal serologic tests are any less reliable for syphilis management than they are in those who do not have HIV infection.

Rolfs RT, Joesoef MR, Hendershot EF, et al. A randomized trial of enhanced therapy for early syphilis in patients with and without human immunodeficiency virus infection. The Syphilis and HIV Study Group. *N Engl J Med* 1997;337:307–314. [PMID: 9235493] (Most recent randomized clinical trial of syphilis treatment demonstrating that standard therapy with penicillin G benzathine was no worse than penicillin G benzathine plus high-dose amoxicillin orally. Although clinical failure was rare [<1%], about 15% of patients with early syphilis failed to show a fourfold decline in serologic titer at 12 months, and HIV-infected patients showed slower declines than HIV-uninfected patients.)

REACTIVE SEROLOGIC TESTS IN PATIENTS WITHOUT ACTIVE SYPHILIS

Several other pitfalls are regularly encountered in settings in which large numbers of serologic tests for syphilis are performed. These include the problem of biologic false-positive tests, evaluation of serologic tests in patients who have had prior syphilis, and the evaluation of serologic reactivity in patients from countries where other endemic treponematoses are prevalent. Each of these problems deserves brief comment.

Biologic false–positive results are a problem with virtually all serologic tests, including those for syphilis. Both nontreponemal and treponemal serologic tests for syphilis occasionally yield false-positive results. In general, false-positive results are slightly less common when treponemal tests are used rather than nontreponemal tests. However, the mathematics of the two-step sequential testing process for initial testing and subsequent confirmation is such that the number of false-positive reactions ultimately identified using the two-step testing algorithm is the same, irrespective of which test is used initially (see Table 26–1). To date, nontreponemal tests are preferred as the initial test because of their lower cost, ease of performance, and the fact that they provide the quantitative data that is widely used to evaluate response to therapy. Individuals whose immune system may be activated by other processes tend to have a somewhat higher rate of biologic false-positive serologic reactions than the general population. Thus, increased rates of reactive serologic tests for syphilis are more common in those who use intravenous drugs or have chronic infections such as malaria or HIV infection, and in those with underlying rheumatologic diseases, including rheumatoid arthritis and systemic lupus erythematosus.

In very rare instances, a person could, simply on the basis of statistical considerations, have a "double" biologic false-positive result (see Table 26–1). In such situations, careful counseling of the patient is warranted and in some instances, this unfortunate occurrence is best handled by documented administration of syphilis therapy despite the fact that infection may not be present.

Another commonly encountered conundrum for clinicians is the interpretation of reactive responses to serologic screening tests in people who have come to the United States from locations where the endemic treponematoses (yaws, pinta, endemic syphilis) are relatively common. Each of these diseases is, in fact, caused by either a *T pallidum* subspecies or, in the case of pinta, *Treponema carateum*, a closely related pathogenic spirochete. There are no currently available commercial tests to differentiate patients with endemic treponematoses from those with syphilis. At present, none of these diseases is endemic in North America and until recently they have been relatively uncommon worldwide. Despite the prior success of worldwide efforts to control yaws, over the past two decades the prevalence of this infection has again begun to increase in parts of Southeast Asia and the South Pacific. All of the endemic treponematoses are most common in younger individuals (infants, children, adolescents) and are manifested primarily as cutaneous disease.

Similar to syphilis, the endemic treponematoses are very susceptible to penicillin therapy. As a result, when the clinician encounters patients from countries where the endemic treponematoses are a possibility, if prior therapy for any treponemal disease cannot be documented, treatment should be administered. As a generalization, patients with reactive serologic tests due to long-standing or prior endemic treponematoses tend to have somewhat lower (1:4 or less) serologic titers and, following treatment, their titers tend to decline slowly, if at all. Thus, patients in whom long-standing latent syphilis or an untreated endemic treponematosis cannot be distinguished are perhaps best treated with three injections of benzathine penicillin, the recommended treatment for those with latent syphilis.

Antal GM, Lukehart SA, Meheus AZ. The endemic treponematoses. *Microbes Infect* 2002;4:83–94. [PMID: 11825779] (Comprehensive microbiologic review of endemic treponemal infections. The endemic treponematoses have not yet been eliminated and are currently thought to affect at least 2.5 million persons.)

EVALUATION OF ASYMPTOMATIC PERSONS NEWLY DISCOVERED TO HAVE REACTIVE SEROLOGIC TESTS

A commonly encountered clinical problem is how to best evaluate a patient who has been found to have a reactive serologic test for syphilis. In addition to the information provided in the preceding discussion, there are several potential sources of information to help clinicians in sorting out this problem (see Table 26–2).

The first step in such evaluations is to be sure the patient has a confirmed positive serologic test, not a biologic false-positive one. If testing confirms the diagnosis of syphilis, additional medical history is important for planning management.

Unfortunately, many patients in this situation give imprecise histories of prior illnesses, including whether or not they have been tested or treated for syphilis in the past and other historical elements that might help clinicians make management decisions. For patients who are uncertain about whether they have been tested for syphilis in the past, a history of past evaluation for STDs may allow the clinician to obtain records of whether a serologic test was performed in the past and, if so, the results. Similarly, if the person has donated blood or, for women, been pregnant, he or she is likely to have been tested for syphilis and records can be sought. Finally, the STD control programs of most state or local health departments keep "reactor files" in which helpful information, including serologic test titers and treatment histories, are recorded for most individuals with reactive serologic tests for syphilis. Contacting the local health department and requesting a syphilis record review can eliminate unnecessary diagnostic testing and treatment for some patients.

In addition to seeking information about prior tests and test results, despite reported "asymptomatic" status, clinicians evaluating patients who present with newly

Table 26–2. Steps in the evaluation of asymptomatic patients with newly recognized reactive serologic tests for syphilis.

1. Confirm that serologic confirmatory testing (ie, two-step) was performed
2. Obtain history to ascertain risk-taking behaviors and likelihood of follow-up
3. Obtain prior test results; possible sources include:
   • Pregnancy records
   • Blood or plasma donation
   • Prior STD evaluation or screening
   • Local health department
4. Perform physical examination with attention to possible cutaneous or mucosal lesions
5. Obtain available information regarding syphilis history in relevant sex partners

identified reactive serologic tests should carefully examine these patients for evidence of infection, including evaluation for skin or mucosal lesions occurring in the oropharynx, vagina, and anogenital region. Serologic evaluation of sex partners may also help to clarify management decisions in such patients.

Serologic tests represent powerful tools for diagnosis of syphilis and evaluation of treatment response. Although their interpretations occasionally are complicated by problems such as false-positive test results, difficulties in distinguishing current from past infections, and issues related to fluctuation in titers following therapy, used in combination with carefully obtained historical data and physical examination they provide important tools for control of this widespread and ancient disease.

PRACTICE POINTS

- Unlike the nontreponemal tests, treponemal serologic test reactivity is life-long in the majority of persons with syphilis and is of little use for evaluating response to therapy.
- Contacting the local health department and requesting a syphilis record review can eliminate unnecessary diagnostic testing and treatment for some patients.

Principles of Risk Reduction Counseling

27

Cornelis A. Rietmeijer, MD, PhD

ESSENTIAL FEATURES

- Effective counseling to prevent sexually transmitted diseases (STDs), including HIV, comprises the following elements:
- Conducting a thorough risk assessment using exploring, open-ended questions.
- Addressing barriers to risk reduction and supporting preventive actions already taken.
- Addressing misconceptions.
- Selecting with the patient a high-risk behavior he or she is most willing and able to change.
- Developing a step-wise risk reduction plan.
- Providing referrals if needed.

GENERAL CONSIDERATIONS

Education and counseling have historically played a role in STD prevention activities, usually as an adjunct to testing, treatment, and partner notification services. However, it was not until the advent of the HIV epidemic that behavioral interventions, including counseling, became the focus of systematic efficacy research. A detailed review of this research and its underlying theoretical considerations is outside the scope of this chapter. However, arguably the single most important study that put counseling to reduce sexual risk behaviors on the map as an effective and feasible intervention for use in a variety of settings was Project Respect. This randomized controlled trial demonstrated that a specific type of counseling (subsequently referred to as *prevention counseling*), comprising two 20-minute counseling sessions, was significantly more effective in preventing subsequent STDs when compared with standard prevention messages.

The findings of this study have important consequences for STD prevention, especially because the effects of prevention counseling were shown to be particularly favorable for populations at highest risk for STDs, including individuals younger than 20 years of age and those with a baseline STD. Thus, there is a strong rationale to include counseling to reduce sexual risk behaviors when providing care for persons at high risk for STDs—that is, as long as the counseling process adheres to a number of critical elements. Subsequent sections of this chapter describe these elements and suggest ways in which prevention counseling can be incorporated into a busy practice setting where time and resources are important limiting factors.

Kamb ML, Fishbein M, Douglas JM Jr, et al. Efficacy of risk reduction counseling to prevent human immunodeficiency virus and sexually transmitted diseases: A randomized controlled trial. Project RESPECT Study Group. *JAMA* 1998;280: 1161–1167. [PMID: 9777816] (Landmark randomized controlled trial demonstrating the superiority of counseling over brief educational messages in the reduction of sexual risk behavior and subsequent STDs in persons attending STD clinics.)

PRINCIPLES OF PREVENTION COUNSELING

Guidelines for HIV prevention counseling have been put forth by the Centers for Disease Control and Prevention (CDC) since 1986. Prevention counseling as evaluated in Project Respect (sometimes also referred to as *client-centered counseling*) was first described in 1993 and updated most recently in 2001. An adapted summary of these guidelines appears in Table 27–1, and a more detailed description follows.

Centers for Disease Control and Prevention. Revised guidelines for HIV counseling, testing, and referral. *MMWR Recomm Rep* 2001;50(RR-19):1–53. [PMID: 11718472] (Standard reference providing guidelines for risk reduction counseling.)

Table 27–1. Principles of prevention counseling.

Principle	Comment
Keep session focused on HIV or STD risk reduction	Counseling should be tailored to address personal risk of the patient rather than provision of predetermined counseling messages Counselors should not be distracted by the patientís additional, unrelated problems
Use open-ended questions, role-play scenarios, attentive listening, and a nonjudgmental and supportive approach	Encourages the patient to remain focused on personal risk reduction
Conduct an in-depth, personalized risk assessment, exploring previous risk reduction efforts and identifying successes and challenges	Assists the patient in identifying concrete, acceptable measures of risk reduction
Acknowledge and support positive changes already made	Enhances the patient's belief that change is possible
Clarify critical misconceptions	Focus on misconceptions verbalized by the patient and avoid general discussions
Negotiate a concrete, achievable behavior-change step that will reduce HIV or STD risk	Risk reduction steps must be acceptable to the patient
In patients with multiple risks, focus on the behavior the patient is most willing to change	Risk reduction does not always involve a personal risk behavior (eg, talking with a partner about his or her HIV serostatus or motivating the partner to be tested)
Identify barriers and facilitators in achieving the behavioral goal	Referral to additional prevention and support services may be necessary
Provide skill-building opportunities (eg, role play, condom demonstration)	Builds patient self-efficacy and confidence in his or her ability to complete the action
Use explicit language in providing test results	Avoid in-depth technical discussions that may diffuse prevention message
Develop and implement a written counseling protocol that should be part of clinic standing orders	Providing a written protocol, which may include examples of open-ended questions and risk-reduction steps, keeps clinicians or counselors and supervisors on task
Ensure support by supervisors and administrators	Provide ongoing training opportunities to staff Include counseling skills in performance evaluations
Avoid using counseling sessions for data collection	If possible, complete paperwork at the end of the counseling session Checklist risk assessments are detrimental to effective counseling; relevance of routinely collected data should be periodically assessed
Avoid the provision of unnecessary information	Discussion of theoretical risks may shift focus away from patientís risk situation and may cause him or her to lose interest

Adapted from Centers for Disease Control and Prevention (CDC). Revised guidelines for HIV counseling, testing, and referral. *MMWR Recomm Rep* 2001;50(RR-19):1–53

General Counseling Guidelines

For prevention counseling to be most effective, an environment must be created that is conducive to an open dialog about the patient's sexual risk behavior and ways to reduce these risks. A nonjudgmental attitude on the part of the provider is essential to avoid impediments to this process, including feelings of shame, guilt, and stigma by the patient. An open and inviting attitude and attentive listening will be perceived by patients as permission and encouragement to talk about these private issues. For example, an opening statement might be: "I realize that it may be difficult for you to discuss sexual matters, but it is important that I understand a bit better what's going on in your life so that I can best help you." The use of open-ended questions, discussed in greater detail below, is very helpful in the process of encouraging patients to talk freely about their sexual behavior. This is not to say that the provider should not be directive. Indeed, it is very important that counseling address personal risk behaviors of the patient and not be distracted by unrelated problems or theoretical discussions (eg, how likely it is that a certain STD will be transmitted from one person to another, or how long a person can remain infectious).

Risk Assessment

A thorough risk assessment is the first and most important step in the prevention counseling process, because all subsequent counseling actions naturally flow from it. Traditionally, risk assessments have followed a more or less standardized checklist approach, including questions on numbers of partners, gender of partners, types of sexual intercourse (vaginal, anal, oral), and condom use. Although such an approach may provide a quick gauge of the patient's risk and repertoire of behavior, there are several important caveats when limiting the risk assessment to such "closed-ended" questions. Given the inherent sensitivity of questions related to sexual behavior, a patient may downplay or deny behaviors when these questions are not followed by further exploration. More importantly, these questions will not give answers to why this person is at risk or what the specific circumstances are that may lead to risky situations.

To explore these circumstances, and subsequently identify a specific risk behavior on which to focus the risk reduction phase of the counseling process, open-ended questions are very useful. For example, a provider may ask a female patient who has been diagnosed with chlamydia: "What do you think happened that put you at risk for this infection?" Answers to these questions generally determine the direction of the next steps of the counseling process. For instance, the patient just diagnosed with chlamydia may respond: "Well, usually I'm very careful and I always use condoms." In fact, she tells her provider that she relies on condoms for both birth

control and STD prevention. Further prompting ("So, what happened?"—another open-ended question), may reveal that she was in a bar and "got drunk and slept with a guy I didn't know and we didn't use a condom." Alternatively, the patient may tell her provider that she is in a steady relationship with a man who has other partners but refuses to use condoms. Clearly, the circumstances in these two cases are very different. In the first example, the STD may be seen as the result of an isolated event, whereas the second example may indicate a more structural problem with a higher likelihood of recurrence. Thus, each of these cases represents its own particular issues and, consequently, risk reduction counseling should follow a different course for each.

During the risk assessment, the provider should carefully avoid making assumptions and coming to judgments based on partial information, a common caveat in prevention counseling. Consider, for example, a 30-year-old man who requests an HIV test. Standard risk screening indicates that he is in a long-standing sexual relationship with his wife, but that he has had an "outside partner" a month prior. He is very concerned about HIV and is worried about transmission to his wife, who is 6 months pregnant. Based on this information, the provider does not believe that a single sexual event with another woman will put the man at high risk for HIV and proceeds with the counseling process along this path. However, a more inquisitive assessment ("Tell me what happened with your outside partner") would have resulted in some noticeable hesitation by the patient, who, after further encouragement and prompting would have told his provider that the outside partner was, in fact, another man with whom he had had unprotected intercourse in a local bathhouse.

Several other factors need special attention during the risk assessment phase. First, as has been shown in the preceding example, many patients have already taken measures to reduce risks, such as condom use or by practicing sexual behaviors that are perceived to have lower risk (eg, oral, rather than vaginal or anal sex). It is important throughout the counseling process to acknowledge and support positive efforts, because this enhances the patient's belief that change is possible. In more technical terms, it serves to empower the patient to make healthy sexual decisions, which, in a theoretical sense, forms the foundation of the prevention counseling process.

Second, the risk assessment may also indicate barriers to the adoption of risk reduction behaviors. For example, the woman with the partner who refuses to use condoms may be in an abusive relationship and fear for her safety if she insists on the use of condoms. The bisexual man requesting the HIV test may still be closeted, and disclosure of his orientation to his wife may not (yet) be a realistic expectation. It is important to keep these barriers in mind when discussing the risk reduction plan to assure that such a plan is realistic.

Third, the care provider or counselor needs to be aware of the patient's misconceptions that may form a barrier to the adoption of preventive behaviors. For example, a patient may believe that condoms are ineffective because they have holes large enough to allow passage of most bacteria and viruses. An HIV-infected patient may believe that his sex partners are not at risk because he has an undetectable viral load. As previously indicated, addressing such misconceptions should not lead to general discussions that take away the focus of the counseling session. It is often better to keep these issues in mind and address them at the end of the session.

Selecting a Risk Behavior for Change

The next step in the prevention counseling process is the identification of behavior the patient is willing (and able) to change or an action the patient can take to reduce the risk of future STD exposure. Not all these behaviors or actions necessarily involve changes in behavior by the patient. For example, insisting on condom use may not be feasible (or safe) for the woman with the partner who refuses to use condoms. However, notifying him of the fact that he may have an STD and that he needs to be evaluated and treated may be acceptable for her. Likewise, should patient-delivered partner therapy be available, she may be willing to give her partner antibiotics. To the extent that many STD reinfections are the result of exposure to untreated partners, this may be a very effective approach to prevent future infections. The bisexual man in the earlier scenario may choose to focus his prevention efforts on the sexual relations he has with other men and using condoms with them consistently while continuing to have unprotected intercourse with his wife.

This last example illustrates another point. As providers, we may not agree with the types of behaviors our patients engage in and we may find it immoral that the man in this example keeps his pregnant wife in the dark about his visits to the bathhouse. However, judging patients will not help them reduce high-risk behaviors and may disturb the patient-provider relationship. On the other hand, encouraging a small step in the change process, as imperfect as this may feel to us as providers, could be the beginning of further and more profound change down the road.

Negotiating a Step-wise Risk Reduction Plan

Many providers tend to be very directive and absolute in giving prevention messages: "You must stop smoking"; "You will have to lose 20 pounds and exercise more to take care of your diabetes"; "You must drink less alcohol"; and, in the realm of STD prevention, "You must reduce the number of partners you have sex with" and "You must use condoms correctly and consistently." However, as was demonstrated in Project Respect, these types of counseling messages are not very effective and have proved inferior to the development of a step-wise plan negotiated and developed in collaboration with the patient.

The first step in this process, selecting a behavior a patient is willing to address, has already been described. The next step is to define what immediate action the patient is willing to take to achieve risk reduction. This step should be feasible and realistic and should have the full commitment of the patient. Importantly, rather than being global, such as "always using condoms," these action steps should be very specific, such as, "carrying a condom the next time I go to the bar or club," or "starting tonight I will require my partner to use a condom or I will not have vaginal or anal sex."

Although the action plan is often identified by the patient, the provider can and should play a very active role in this process. For instance, in the second scenario described earlier, the woman has indicated that she wants to talk to her partner and have him evaluated and treated. However, she has trepidations as she anticipates a hostile reaction from him. Here the provider could educate the patient about the nature of chlamydial infections: that her partner may be infected and not know it, that she may experience complications, including the risk for infertility should she become reinfected, and, importantly, that she may have been infected for a long time, even prior to her current relationship. This knowledge makes it easier for the patient to come to the decision "to speak to my partner as soon as I get home and urge him to go to the clinic."

The woman in the first scenario, whose risk was precipitated by alcohol use, may decide to avoid such situations in the future. As a longer term goal, she may also decide to use an alternate form of birth control that is not dependent on spur-of-the-moment decisions, such as a depot or oral contraceptive, or an intrauterine device.

The provider could also suggest action steps the patient may not have considered. For example, the man in the third scenario, who plans to use condoms all the time with his male partners when he engages in anal sex, should also consider regular STD testing or discussing HIV status with his male partners and selecting partners whose status is negative. Of course, the protective benefit from the selected action is not absolute, but the goal is not risk avoidance but risk reduction. The objective is harm reduction, helping the patient move along the spectrum from higher to lower risk sexual behavior.

Again, as previously mentioned, these action steps may appear inadequate to the provider and many providers may feel better about themselves having spoken the hard truth that only abstinence or engaging in a mutually monogamous relationship with an uninfected partner will prevent STDs. Still, for many patients this is not a feasible, achievable alternative and for some, feelings of shame and rejection may lead to a return to past unhealthy behaviors rather than forming a motivation for behavior change. By contrast, engaging the patient in planning for a small step in the change process, followed by a small success, will do much more to empower this person for future changes than failing an unachievable goal.

Useful Adjuncts to the Counseling Process

Of several additional tools that can be used in the patient-provider interaction to help in the development of behavioral goals and action steps, two will be briefly mentioned here: stage-based counseling and motivational interviewing. Both are fully compatible with prevention counseling as outlined in this chapter, and some providers may find the more proscriptive approach of these models useful in their daily practice.

A. STAGE-BASED COUNSELING

In the stage-based model, the risk assessment phase is used to "stage" a patient for a certain behavior (eg, condom use for vaginal sex with a casual partner) using the transtheoretical model, which identifies the following five stages of behavior change: (1) precontemplation, (2) contemplation, (3) preparation, (4) action, and (5) maintenance. The clinician then uses the corresponding processes of change in an effort to move the patient to the next stage.

Although the concept of a step-wise approach is similar to the prevention counseling model, the stage-based model is more directive. For example, to move a patient along the earlier stages of change, the focus of counseling may be on the perception of risk and susceptibility to a health problem (eg, HIV infection) and its perceived consequences, whereas in later stages it is more important to focus on self-efficacy and social norms.

B. MOTIVATIONAL INTERVIEWING

According to the second model (the information, motivation, and behavior skills model), individuals are more likely to adopt STD preventive behaviors to the extent that they are well informed, motivated to act, and possess the required skills to act effectively. In counseling interventions based on this model, the technique of motivational interviewing is used to assess the importance individuals assign to changing a certain behavior (often rated on a scale from 1 to 10) as well as the confidence they have that such change is possible (also rated on a scale from 1 to 10). The clinician then explores with the patient what it would take to increase these ratings and thereby determine the deficits in information, motivation, and behavioral skills that can be addressed and modified in the intervention.

Additional Tools

Finally, to the extent possible, skill-building opportunities, such as role play around negotiating safer sex, or practicing the use of condoms on a penis model, are useful adjuncts to the counseling process because they increase self-efficacy for the patient.

Coury-Doniger P, Levenkron JC, Knox KL, et al. Use of stage of change (SOC) to develop an STD/HIV behavioral intervention: Phase 1. A system to classify SOC for STD/HIV sexual risk behaviors—development and reliability in an STD clinic. *AIDS Patient Care STDs* 1999;13:493–502. [PMID: 10800528] (The authors report their experience demonstrating that it is possible to develop, implement, and sustain an integrated provider-delivered STD/HIV behavioral intervention based on a stage-based model in a busy urban STD clinic.)

Fisher JD, Cornman DH, Osborn CY, et al. Clinician-initiated HIV risk reduction intervention for HIV-positive persons: Formative Research, Acceptability, and Fidelity of the Options Project. *J Acquir Immune Defic Syndr* 2004;37:S78–S87. [PMID: 15385903] (Study demonstrating that HIV prevention interventions by clinicians treating HIV-positive patients were acceptable and easily implemented in routine clinical care.)

WHEN TO REFER TO A SPECIALIST

Prevention counseling is intended to be a brief intervention that can be easily integrated in the care setting. However, as shown by the earlier scenarios, situations may be revealed during counseling that require more specific and longer term interventions. For example, the woman in the first scenario may have a substance abuse problem, the second scenario may represent a woman experiencing spousal abuse, and the man in the third scenario may have problems with sexual addiction. Dependent on the underlying problems, these patients could benefit from referral to appropriate services, including specialized medical care and treatment, mental health services, reproductive health services, drug and alcohol prevention and treatment, partner counseling and referral services, and prevention case management.

PREVENTION COUNSELING FOR SPECIFIC PATIENT GROUPS

For patients requesting HIV or STD testing, risk assessment and subsequent prevention counseling do not present many problems because patients expect that the provider will ask questions related to sexual risk behaviors for STDs. For patients who present with other health problems or concerns, asking questions about sexual behavior may be perceived as awkward by both providers and patients. Nonetheless, screening for sexual risk behaviors is considered to be included in the standard of preventive health care, and the US Preventive Services Task Force recommends inclusion of sexual health screening for all persons aged 13–65 years of age.

Most providers who have included sexual health screening in their preventive health repertoire do not find it particularly difficult to broach the subject, for example, through a question such as: "I routinely ask my patients if they have concerns about their sexual behavior or sexually transmitted diseases so that we can decide if they need to be checked for any of these diseases. Do you have concerns like this that you want to tell me about?" Such a (closed-ended) question, if answered affirmatively, could be followed by an open-ended one: "Could you tell me more about that?" The clinician should probe a bit further with certain patients who may be at higher risk if they deny any concerns; these patients include adolescents and young adults, men who have sex with men, and men and women who have been recently divorced or widowed. In these instances, a more pointed question may be, "Do you have a regular (steady) sex partner (boyfriend, girlfriend)?"; "Other sex partners?"; followed by further exploratory questions.

Patients with HIV infection comprise another group requiring additional attention. Advances in HIV treatment have led to longer and healthier lives for many patients with HIV infection. Most are enjoying sexual activity again, and some are engaging in sexual risk behavior that could lead to HIV transmission to others. This concern has led to a shift in public health policy, placing a greater emphasis on ongoing prevention efforts among individuals living with HIV infection.

Given the often long-standing relationship between HIV-infected patients and their care providers, these providers may be particularly effective in addressing ongoing risk behaviors in this group of patients. However, many HIV care providers feel uncomfortable engaging their HIV-infected patients in ongoing risk assessments or believe this will be antagonistic to the patient-physician relationship. Clinic logistics and lack of financial reimbursement, discussed in the next section, may form other barriers to the provision of this service. Yet most patients with HIV infection have concerns about their sexual relationships, including the potential transmission to others, and appreciate the opportunity to discuss these concerns with their care providers. The prevention counseling approach outlined in this chapter lends itself very well to being adapted to this special circumstance, and curricula to train HIV care providers in the provision of this prevention service have been put forth by the CDC and Health Resources and Services Administration. A detailed description of these curricula falls outside the scope of this chapter. Those interested are referred to the training web sites of these agencies, which are listed at the end of this chapter.

Centers for Disease Control and Prevention; Workowski KA, Berman SM. Sexually transmitted diseases treatment guidelines, 2006. *MMWR Recomm Rep* 2006;55(RR-11):1–94. [PMID: 16888612] (The most recent guidelines on STD treatment from the CDC.)

Centers for Disease Control and Prevention (CDC). Advancing HIV prevention: New strategies for a changing epidemic—United States, 2003. *MMWR Morbid Mortal Wkly Rep* 2003;52:329–332. [PMID: 12733863] (Guidance from the

CDC emphasizing an increased focus on prevention for HIV-infected persons, often called "prevention with positives.")

BARRIERS TO COUNSELING & WAYS TO OVERCOME THEM

As previously noted, there are several barriers to consistent inclusion of prevention counseling in many clinical settings. This is particularly true of primary care settings, where a large proportion of all STDs are diagnosed and treated. Logistical constraints—specifically, the limited amount of time than can be devoted to each patient—and the general lack of reimbursement for counseling services are among the most important barriers that prevent the adoption of more widespread prevention counseling in these settings.

Without trivializing this problem, there may be ways to address this issue from a different perspective. Prevention counseling in the primary care setting should not be seen as a categorical problem, but rather as part of the spectrum of health risk behaviors that primary care clinicians encounter on a daily basis; among many others, these include smoking and other substance abuse, lack of exercise, and eating disorders. The advantage of the prevention counseling models detailed in this chapter is that they are not necessarily behavior specific. Indeed, the theories that underlie these models were in large part developed for other behavioral problems, including smoking cessation, weight control, and psychological distress, long before the onset of the AIDS epidemic made them relevant for HIV and STD prevention. Prevention counseling as discussed in this chapter thus finds an interesting corollary in the primary care literature in the concept of patient-centered care, which operates along very similar lines to work with patients to agree on their most salient health problems and to take an incremental approach to setting attainable (behavioral) goals. In that sense, the nature of the health problem is secondary to the patient-centered approach taken by the care provider. Thus, in a patient with significant risks of STD or HIV acquisition, prevention counseling to reduce high-risk sexual behavior is no longer an alien, time-consuming add-on for the overburdened primary care provider, but rather a natural outflow of a generic patient-provider interaction model. Moreover, most providers find that with adequate practice, prevention counseling, on average, takes no more than 5–10 minutes of their time.

Although a personal interaction between the patient and care provider is arguably the most effective mode of delivery for prevention counseling, there are ways to make the process more efficient and less time-consuming. First a screening question could be added to the previsit patient questionnaire (eg, "Are there any concerns related to your sexual behavior or sexually transmitted diseases that you want to discuss with your care provider today?")

that may facilitate the introduction of the topic matter during the visit. Second, prevention counseling could be delegated to a designated clinic staff member, such as a prevention case manager or social worker. This may be particularly useful when complex issues are involved, as previously discussed. Third, several recent developments that take advantage of computer technologies could be used to develop tailored interventions, mimicking the in-person prevention counseling model (see the web site at the end of this chapter). Finally, video-based waiting room interventions may be effective as stand-alone interventions or may be linked to other prevention activities in the clinic.

In certain clinical settings, it may be useful to develop a written prevention counseling protocol. This serves to remind clinicians that sexual risk counseling is part of the standard of care. The protocol should list the necessary steps of prevention counseling, provide examples of open-ended questions, and outline the difference between patient-specific risk reduction steps versus less desirable global prevention messages. Finally, and importantly, a clinic protocol indicates the commitment and support for counseling by clinic supervisors and administrators. This support could be further demonstrated by providing clinicians with training in patient-centered counseling techniques, by assessing counseling skills as part of performance evaluations, and through ongoing modeling of effective counseling by the clinic leadership.

PRACTICE POINTS

- *An open and inviting attitude and attentive listening will be perceived by patients as permission and encouragement to talk about private issues, such as sexual activity and risk behaviors.*
- *It is important throughout the counseling process to acknowledge and support positive efforts, because this enhances the patient's belief that change is possible.*

Relevant Web Sites

[Health Resources and Services Administration. Special initiatives: Prevention with HIV infected persons in primary care settings:]

http://hab.hrsa.gov/special/pop_overview.htm.

[Resources Online CARE for HIV/STDs:]

http://www.ronline.com/care/

Partner Notification & Management · 28

Thomas A. Peterman, MD, MSc, & Richard H. Kahn, MS

ESSENTIAL FEATURES

- *Partner notification is an important component of treating patients for most sexually transmitted diseases (STDs).*
- *Partner notification for syphilis, HIV, and possibly hepatitis B is usually best done by collaborating with experts from the local health department.*
- *Partner notification is also a priority for gonorrhea, chlamydia, trichomoniasis, nongonococcal urethritis, and pelvic inflammatory disease, although patients will usually need to notify partners themselves after appropriate coaching.*
- *Some patients resist notification out of fear of losing a relationship or because a relationship has already ended.*
- *Emphasizing the health benefits helps patients initiate and successfully complete notification, thereby improving their own health, the health of partners, and the health of the community.*

GENERAL CONSIDERATIONS

Tracing partners of patients with STDs has been done for centuries but was first introduced on a national scale by Surgeon General Thomas Parran as part of his five-point plan to control syphilis in 1937. At the time, syphilis was killing about 20,000 people per year in the United States. Parran's campaign, and the subsequent discovery of penicillin, led to a nadir in syphilis rates in 1956. As rates dropped, health department efforts expanded beyond partners to test other people in the patient's social network, but decreases in funding were followed by increasing rates of syphilis and periodic epidemics. Meanwhile a gonorrhea control campaign began in the 1970s, a chlamydia campaign began in the 1990s,

genital herpes was increasingly diagnosed, human papillomavirus was linked to cervical cancer, and HIV infection appeared.

With an estimated 19 million new STDs each year in the United States, the most common approach to partner notification has become denial. Patients and clinicians who know the importance of treating partners may ignore it because they are uncomfortable or unfamiliar with the process. Becoming familiar with the partner notification process can help overcome this denial and improve the patient's health.

Partner notification involves talking to patients with STDs about approaches to testing and treating their partners. Ideally, exposed partners can be cured before they develop complications or become infectious and transmit disease to others. Health department assistance with notification is not available for all STDs. Health departments seek active involvement in addressing syphilis and, to a slightly lesser extent, HIV. Some health departments will try to notify some partners of people with hepatitis B, gonorrhea, or chlamydia. For many STDs, however, patients are responsible for notifying their own partners. Most patients wonder what to do about their partners and appreciate advice from their physicians.

BENEFITS OF PARTNER NOTIFICATION

Patients benefit when their partners are notified. Patients who have been cured are susceptible to reinfection; untreated partners pose a risk to patients who have been treated for syphilis, gonorrhea, chlamydia, or trichomoniasis. Patients with chronic infections such as HIV can obtain social support from partners who become aware of their infection. Finally, most infected persons want what is best for their partners, and thus want them to be aware of their exposure because it is important for the partner's health.

Partners benefit if notification occurs early enough to prevent or cure an infection that would otherwise have caused illness. Infections that lead to serious illness (eg, HIV) are more important than infections that less often cause disease (eg, herpes simplex virus or human papillomavirus). Partners benefit more when notified about bacterial infections, which usually are curable, in contrast to viral infections, which usually are not. However, treatment of HIV infection, while not curative, provides significant benefits to partners who might otherwise remain untreated. Partners who have acquired incurable infections also benefit from knowing about their infection because they can avoid transmitting it to other partners. Uninfected partners who are notified can take steps to avoid infection. Vaccination can prevent acquisition of infection by partners of hepatitis B carriers. Uninfected partners of HIV-infected patients can question their contacts about the infection or will need to change sex practices with all of their partners to reduce risk of infection, because health departments do not disclose the identity of the infected person. Changing high-risk behavior could reduce risk of infection for all persons notified about an STD.

Communities benefit when partner notification reduces the likelihood of infection in the community. Health department personnel can identify potential avenues for intervention in a community by interviewing patients and their partners about how and where they met, and what their sexual practices were. This information can lead to screening programs at high-risk venues, focused prevention campaigns (eg, posters showing syphilis ulcers), or informing persons in high-risk areas that syphilis is being transmitted via oral sex.

Yet another benefit of partner notification is that it fulfills the ethical obligation to share with individuals information that may be important to their health. This obligation extends to both the patient, who has a duty to disclose, and the health care provider, who has a duty to warn. This obligation is most compelling for serious curable infections or in situations where exposure is likely to be ongoing. However, even when there is not much to be done about it, partners have a right to know important information about their health.

WHO SHOULD BE NOTIFIED

The potential benefits of notification for the patient, partners, and community depend on the particular infection and what can be done following notification. The greatest benefits are for serious but easily curable infections that have a long incubation period (see Table 28–1). The potential to interrupt transmission is greater for syphilis and hepatitis B, in which there is a relatively long time between infection and infectiousness (3–4 weeks), compared with other infections (several days or less). The cost of finding new infections via partner notification compares favorably with screening campaigns when the infection is rare.

Currently, in the United States, partner notification offers the greatest benefit for syphilis. Syphilis can progress to fatal disease or result in stillbirth, it is easily cured, it is not transmissible until about 3 weeks after infection, and many infected persons are otherwise unaware of their infection. Other infections are good candidates for partner notification in some respects, but not in others. For example, HIV is a serious infection, but treatment does not eliminate infection, and preventing transmission depends primarily on behavior change. Thus, for HIV, partner notification, counseling, testing, and early treatment of infected partners may produce substantial prevention and clinical benefits for a very serious condition, but these benefits require additional interventions beyond notification and may not be realized in all cases. For human papillomavirus infection, there is no evidence that treatment affects elimination of infection, and infection is very common, often transient, less serious, and difficult to diagnose, so partners are not usually rigorously sought for notification.

Rapid notification of partners increases the chance of preventing further transmission and decreases the risk of serious complications among persons who are already infected. Usually partner notification is discussed when patients are told about their diagnosis and treatment. When HIV is diagnosed, patients may need time to react to their diagnosis, and it may be better to discuss the details of partner notification at a second visit a few days later. Because HIV is a chronic infection, patients may need to be reinterviewed for HIV partner notification if they acquire a new STD or if they have new partners who were not informed about the patient's infection.

Partner notification aims to reach the partner who transmitted infection to the infected patient (the source) as well as any subsequent partners who may have acquired infection from the patient ("spread contacts"). The infecting organism and clinical findings provide clues about when the patient acquired the infection.

For syphilis, the interval for notifying partners varies by stage of disease: for primary syphilis, 3 months prior to the onset of symptoms; for secondary syphilis, 6 months prior to the onset of symptoms; for early latent syphilis, 1 year prior to the time of diagnosis.

For HIV infection, partners to be notified include all partners since 3 months before the last negative serologic test or 3 months before presentation with acute retroviral syndrome. When there is no previous HIV test, or when infection could have been acquired several years before the diagnosis, health departments often limit searches to partners from the year prior to the positive test because of difficulties in locating earlier partners. The US Congress has mandated that, for HIV infections, STD control programs notify all marital partners from the preceding 10 years.

Table 28–1. Priority for partner notification in cases of sexually transmitted diseases.

Priority, Infection[a]	Seriousness	Intervention for Partners	Notification Period
1 Syphilis	Stillbirth, congenital syphilis, neurosyphilis, tertiary syphilis	Prevention and cure	Primary: 3 mo before symptom onset Secondary: 6 mo before symptom onset Early latent: 12 mo before diagnosis
1 HIV	Usually fatal if untreated	Treatment Counseling to avoid infection, transmission	3 mo before previous negative HIV test, sometimes limited to 1 y
? 1 Hepatitis B	Hepatitis, chronic liver disease, hepatic carcinoma	Vaccination	Not established (see text)
2 Gonorrhea	Pelvic inflammatory disease, infertility, ectopic pregnancy	Cure	60 d before symptom onset (or diagnosis)
2 Chlamydia	Pelvic inflammatory disease, infertility, ectopic pregnancy	Cure	60 d before symptom onset (or diagnosis)
2 Trichomoniasis	Vaginitis, cervicitis	Cure	60 d before symptom onset (or diagnosis)
3 Herpes simplex virus	Neonatal infection (can be fatal)	Symptom relief Counseling to avoid infection and transmission	—
3 Human papillomavirus	Some types cause cervical and other genitoanal cancers	Wart removal or treatment of cervical dysplasia do not necessarily clear infection Counseling	—

[a]Priority is a function of the seriousness of the disease and the potential interventions for partners.

Hepatitis B notification intervals have not been established. The greatest benefits from hepatitis B notification would be from vaccinating partners who may be exposed again, and from administering hepatitis B immune globulin to partners exposed in the preceding 14 days.

Gonorrhea, chlamydia, and trichomoniasis partner investigations generally go back 60 days prior to the onset of symptoms or the date of the positive test.

TYPES OF PARTNER NOTIFICATION

There are two basic approaches to notifying partners. In provider notification, trained health department employees (often called disease intervention specialists) gather information about partners from the patient and then notify the partners without revealing the identity of the patient. In patient notification, patients notify their partners after coaching by their physician.

Advantages of provider referral include verification that notification took place; protection of the patient's confidentiality because no information about the patient is disclosed to partners; help with diffusion of any partner anger or blame; on-the-spot information about the disease and appropriate counseling; and possible collection of specimens for testing. Advantages of patient referral include lower cost and the potential for more rapid referral because the patient is more familiar with the identity and location of the partner.

Provider Referral

This method of notification is usually used for syphilis, HIV, and, sometimes, hepatitis B. The provider, usually a health department employee but sometimes a physician, performs partner notification.

Years of experience, and two randomized controlled trials have shown that patients are not as successful at notifying their partners as trained professionals from the health department. This may be surprising to patients and providers. However, well-intentioned patients often find it more difficult than anticipated to broach the subject to their partners. They may also rationalize that certain partners are not infected because the partners are asymptomatic or too "nice," another partner gave it to them, they fear reprisal, or they do not really care about the partners. Sometimes patients drop subtle hints and think that they have notified their partners, but their partners miss the hints. Moreover, notified partners may deny their own risk and not seek treatment. Most of these issues do not apply to health department professionals who have the advantage of training in finding partners, responding to their reactions, and answering questions about the infection.

To be effective, partner notification must be voluntary and conducted in a confidential environment that fosters mutual trust. Patients are more likely to name partners when they are assured that their information is confidential and that their names will not be revealed to their partners. Health departments seek to maintain partner notification staff that is confident, knowledgeable, caring, motivated, discreet, and has a genuine interest in people.

Clinicians can facilitate successful provider notification by telling their patients that they will be contacted by the health department and encouraging them to work together to assure that partners are notified. As with any other referral, the attitude of the referring physician is important. Patients may benefit from being told the rationale for partner notification and how it benefits them, their partners, and the control of infection in their community (see Table 28–2). They should also be assured that the information will remain confidential. Clinicians who have met with their health department colleagues will be in a better position to recommend them. Thus, clinicians who diagnose patients with syphilis or HIV should consider contacting the health department to arrange a meeting with a disease intervention specialist.

Table 28–2. Select strategies to increase the acceptance and practice of partner notification in patients with STDs.

Strategy	Comment
Empathize with patient and display compassion	Patients often wonder what to do about partners and appreciate advice and support from their physician
Promote discussion that is open, honest, and clear	Talking with patients about their sex lives is similar to talking with them about any other health issue except that some patients (and providers) are more uncomfortable talking about sex than about diet, exercise, or other behaviors To be effective, this communication requires assertiveness, which is facilitated by a health care provider who has confidence, believes in the activity, and believes the activity will achieve the desired goals Patients do not resent invasive questions, they resent a judgmental approach
Stress benefits of treatment and rationale for notifying partners	Points to emphasize: Reduces spread and reinfection Prevents complications in patient and partner Reexposure would require returning for retreatment Responsibility to others and to public health in general Eliminates future problems by handling them now: • Partner treated before infecting another person • Partner treated before suffering complications and becoming angry • Partner treated before pregnancy and childbirth • Treatment provided before infection spreads to others in the social group Asymptomatic nature of the infection (eg, unknown infection) Possibility of exposure to other infections

If the health department first learns of a potential new infection from a reporting laboratory, the investigation begins by searching past serologic information on file at the health department to determine if it is indeed likely to be a new infection. Health department databases are usually limited to past positive syphilis or HIV serologic results. For syphilis, comparison of current and past nontreponemal test titers can help distinguish old infection from reinfection. Unless a record search determines that an infection is old and previously treated, the investigator will contact the physician's office to determine the diagnosis, treatment, and any clues to when the infection was acquired. When physicians report a case of syphilis to the health department, the case is rapidly assigned to a disease intervention specialist, thus eliminating some of the delays involved in laboratory-based reporting. This increases the chance of reaching partners before they develop the disease or transmit infection to others.

Patient interviews usually take place at the health department but can take place anywhere and at any time that is convenient, confidential, and safe. After reaching and assuring the identity of the patient, the investigators go to a private place to talk, introduce themselves, establish rapport, express concern, and explain the confidential nature of their discussions. They then discuss the infection and the importance of notifying partners. Patients are asked about their understanding of disease, past diagnoses, signs and symptoms, and laboratory tests to help determine the likely date of infection. After framing the interview interval using a calendar and anchoring events, they discuss how many partners the patient has had during that interval. Each partner is discussed in turn to outline the first and most recent sexual encounter, frequency and type of sexual contact, and to obtain the partner's name, description, and locating information.

When partners are not known by name, disease intervention specialists seek any information that might enable confidential notification such as places frequented, physical description, or Internet chat name. In some cases, the interview is followed by a reinterview, because patients often remember partners or information that was omitted at the initial interview. In some cases, patients may be told that their partner was "taken care of," but patients are not told their partner's test results. That information, like the information about the patient, is not disclosed.

Disease intervention specialists attempt to contact partners at their homes. If no one is home, the specialist may leave his or her name and phone number in a plain envelope with the partner's name on it. If someone else is there, the specialist asks that person to give the partner the envelope. After contacting and confirming the identity of the partner, the specialist finds a private place and identifies himself or herself as being from the health department. Partners often want to know who gave the disease intervention specialist their name. The usual response to is "I cannot tell you because that information is confidential, but I can tell you it was someone who was concerned about you and your health. They want to make sure that if you have this infection you get treated." The specialist provides information about the infection. Partners are advised about places where they can obtain free or low-cost evaluation and may be offered assistance in getting to a clinic, or specimens may be collected on the spot for transport to the laboratory. In some instances, treatment may be offered by the disease intervention specialist as well.

Patient Referral

In patient referral, the patient performs partner notification. Some patients with STDs state a preference for notifying their own partners; however, notifying partners is often more difficult for patients than they anticipate. Thus, patients with HIV or syphilis who say that they will notify their own partners should still be encouraged to talk with someone from the health department. Medical providers and health departments sometimes use "contract referral" in which patients are given an agreed upon period (eg, a few days) to refer their partners. If partners are not brought in by the patient, the process reverts to provider referral. In practice, contract referral for syphilis has been similar to provider referral because very few syphilis patients bring in their own partners.

Health department assistance with partner notification is generally not available for patients with gonorrhea, chlamydia, or trichomoniasis, yet partner treatment is essential to prevent reinfection of the patient, prevent complications from the disease in partners, and reduce the prevalence of disease in the community. Patients should be convinced to notify their partners (see Tables 28–3 and 28–4) and given tips on how to do so. Patients with multiple partners often forget some of their partners during the interview. In a trial of various cues for patients who initially reported more than one partner, the number of partners recalled increased by 3–5% following nonspecific prompting or simply reading back the list of partners already named. Spending an additional 5–10 minutes reading a list of common names or a list of common locations for meeting partners increased the list by an additional 21%. These additional partners were nearly as easy to find and equally likely to be infected as the partners named without prompting.

Patients are more successful at notifying their partners when they have had some opportunity to discuss and practice their approach. Items to discuss include when, where, and how to notify, and possible reactions the partner may have (see Table 28–5). Patients should be encouraged to notify their partners promptly, in a private setting, and to avoid blame by stating that "because my test was positive, I am worried about your health

Table 28–3. Techniques to use (or avoid) in communication with patients about partner notification.

Use	Avoid
Open-ended questions: "Who ...?"; "What ... ?"; "When ...?"; "Where ... ?"; "Why ...?"; or "How can I contact you if you are not at home?"	**Closed-ended questions:** "Are there ...?"; "Is there ...?"; "Do you ... ?"; "Will you ... ?"; "Did you ... ?"; "Can you remember their names?"—It is too easy to just say "no" and end the conversation.
Polite imperatives: "Tell me ... "; "Show me ..."; "Explain to me ... "; "Give me your boyfriend's address."	**Negative questions:** "You don't know your partners' names, do you?"
Suggest answers in a nonjudgmental way: "Do you have sex with men, women, or both?"; "How many different people have you had sex with in the past year—2, 5, 20, more?"	**Labels:** "Are you gay or homosexual?"; "Do you have a lot of sex partners?"
Explanations: "You know firsthand about the complications of this infection. I want to talk with you about how not to become infected again. Unless your partners are confidentially informed, they may get very sick and have to go to the hospital. They might also give the infection back to you. So, who needs an exam?"	**Language that is not understood by the patient:** "{...} the B cells start antibody production" **Moralizing:** "I can't believe you have unsafe sex"
Communication facilitators: Appropriate eye contact Supportive facial expressions Interested posture with body oriented toward the patient Feedback to show that you are listening to the content and the emotion	**Communication barriers:** Distractions in the environment Apathetic demeanor Failure to listen Interrupting Lecturing or preaching

and want to encourage you to get tested and treated." Anticipating partner reactions will facilitate appropriate responses. Patients can be asked how they think their partner will react, how their partner has reacted to difficult news in the past, and what might be done to deal with that reaction. Written information helps reinforce messages, provides an opportunity for the patient to review what was discussed, and can be used by patients when they talk to their partners.

Although there have been few studies of patient referral, some strategies have been shown to improve its effectiveness. Perhaps the cheapest and most effective way to improve patient referral is to call the patient to check on progress with notification. In one study this resulted in one more partner presenting for care for every three patients called. Pamphlets with information about the disease are helpful supplements to a thorough

partner interview, but when used alone they are not as effective as a thorough interview for getting partners in for testing. Educational videos have increased patients' knowledge about their disease but did not necessarily translate into more partners undergoing examination. Verbal, nurse-given health education together with patient-centered counseling by lay workers has increased the rate of partners treated compared with standard care. Another approach that increased partner testing was giving patients a kit that their partners could use to mail in specimens for testing. More partners were tested when patients were given a collection kit (0.98 per patient) compared with giving them a slip telling them to go to their physician (0.37 per patient).

Giving patients medication to bring to their partners may be more effective than just asking them to refer their partners for treatment. In one study, women diagnosed

Table 28–4. Communication tips for difficult patient interactions.

Situation	Sample Dialog to Facilitate Communication
Poor memory or recall of partners	Patient: "I don't have any other partners." Clinician: "Remember that I mentioned before how serious this disease can be if someone who has it does not get treated. Think a minute about anyone you had sex with around the 4th of July. Who comes to mind?" Patient: "No one." Clinician: "Well, what did you do that day? Did you go to a party?"

Reluctance to discuss a partner	Clinician:
	"What are you worried (angry, scared) about?"
	"What problems will this cause for you?"
	"What do you think will happen if we discuss this?"
	"What will you lose?"
	Patient: "I have not had sex for over a year."
	Clinician approaches:
	  Present information: "Sex means different things to different people. When was the last time you had oral sex?"
	  Direct challenge: "Since you have a sore, we know it has been no more than a few months. What is your concern in talking about this?"
	  Withdrawal of prior reinforcement: "Before I told you that I thought you acted responsibly by coming in today. However, by saying that you don't care about your partner's treatment, I'm not sure you really understand the seriousness of this disease."
	Patient: "They have already been taken care of?"
	Clinician: "How do you know that?"
	Patient: "No one told me so they can find out for themselves too"
	Clinician: "Why do you think your partner knew about this disease? It sounds as if you think someone did this to hurt you…"

Relationship issues	Patient: "It will ruin my relationship." Clinician: "Sounds like you care a lot for this person. How might letting your partner go untreated benefit the relationship?"

with chlamydia were, at random, either given azithromycin to bring to their partners or told to refer their partners for treatment. When the women were retested 1 and 4 months later, persistent or recurrent infection was detected in 12% of the patient-delivered partner treatment arm and 15% of the patient referral arm ($P = .1$). A second study that included male and female patients with gonorrhea or chlamydia found persistent or recurrent infection in 10% of the patient-delivered partner therapy arm and 13% in the patient referral arm ($P < .05$). This high rate of persistent or recurrent infections has been found in many studies, suggesting that persons who are diagnosed with those STDs should be tested again in 3 months because many will have a new asymptomatic infection.

Effectiveness of Provider versus Patient Referral

The effectiveness of partner notification is difficult to evaluate because there are many potential benefits and outcomes to consider. Although some reports show that disease rates fell in communities following intensive partner notification efforts by the health department, there have been no randomized community trials. Critical reviews of the literature have identified only a handful of studies with solid methodology that compared provider and patient notification. These studies usually compare effectiveness at testing partners or identifying infected partners. A study of HIV-infected persons diagnosed in North Carolina randomized 157 subjects to provider referral and 153 to patient referral. Providers notified 78 partners, tested 36, and identified 9 as being newly identified infected. Patients notified 10 partners, tested 5, and identified 1 as newly identified infected. Based on these numbers, provider notification was about seven times as effective as patient referral in reaching partners for testing, or finding infected partners.

In a second study, in Indianapolis, men with nongonococcal urethritis were randomized to provider referral or two different types of patient referral. The 221 men in the provider group led to treatment of

Table 28–5. Topics to review with patients who will notify their own partners.

Topic	Comment
Notification of exposure	When and where notification will occur What will be said How it will be brought up
Disease comprehension	What will be said about the disease, symptoms, complications Pamphlets are often helpful and are available from the health department, on-line, or from the American Social Health Association (*http://www.ashastd.org*)
Referral	Where and when the partner should go for testing Whom to call if questions (give appointment card)
Reactions	Prepare for anger, denial, sadness, disbelief, or confusion
Follow-up	Set a time frame for completion of referral Tell patient you will call to check progress

159 partners while the 457 in the other groups led to treatment of 91 partners. In this study, provider notification was 3.6 times as effective as patient notification in reaching partners for testing and treatment.

Most other studies did not use randomized controls and only reported the number of persons tested and treated due to the partner notification efforts. Partner notification for syphilis, gonorrhea, and chlamydia generally leads to one partner with newly diagnosed and treated infection for every four to five patients interviewed. HIV partner notification, on average, leads to one new infection identified for every seven to eight patients interviewed. The contribution of these additional cases to disease control in the community is difficult to estimate. Without notification, some partners may have been particularly likely to transmit disease because they were unaware of their infections. Others may be part of the core group of high-efficiency transmitters who are responsible for maintaining disease in the community. An investigation of a patient's partners is unlikely to reach all of them. However, when many infected persons are interviewed in a community, the important partners often are named by

multiple individuals and thus are likely eventually to be reached.

The cost of notifying partners varies widely and has not been well characterized. Estimates of the cost of finding a partner with a newly identified HIV infection range from $810 to $3205. Finding and treating a new syphilis infection has cost $300–$500.

Based on these costs, and the potential benefits of partner notification (see Table 28–2) health department provider notification efforts are usually limited to syphilis and HIV. A survey of health departments found they more often performed partner notification interviews for syphilis (89%) than for HIV (52%), gonorrhea (17%), or chlamydia (12%). The areas with the most disease had health departments that were least likely to interview persons with gonorrhea or chlamydia.

Brewer DD. Case-finding effectiveness of partner notification and cluster investigation for sexually transmitted diseases/HIV. *Sex Transm Dis* 2005;32:78–83. [PMID: 15668612] (Well-written, comprehensive review that includes references to a broad range of studies.)

Brewer DD, Potterat JJ, Muth SQ, et al. Randomized trial of supplementary interviewing techniques to enhance recall of sexual partners in contact interviews. *Sex Transm Dis* 2005;32: 189–193. [PMID: 15729158] (Interesting trial of practical ways to enhance recall.)

Golden MR, Whittington WL, Handfield HH, et al. Effect of expedited treatment of sex partners on recurrent or persistent gonorrhea or chlamydial infection. *N Engl J Med* 2005;352: 676–685. [PMID: 15716561] (In this large trial, involving practitioners and pharmacies throughout the community reduced persistent or recurrent infection.)

Landis SE, Schoenbach VJ, Weber DJ, et al. Results of a randomized trial of partner notification in cases of HIV infection in North Carolina. *N Engl J Med* 1992;326:101–106. [PMID: 1445500] (Probably the best partner notification study ever performed.)

Mathews C, Coetzee N, Zwarenstein M, et al. A systematic review of strategies for partner notification for sexually transmitted diseases, including HIV/AIDS. *Int J STD AIDS* 2002;13: 285–300. [PMID: 11972932] (This review found moderately strong evidence that provider referral, when compared with patient referral, increases the rate of partners presenting for medical evaluation; contract referral, when compared with patient referral, results in more partners presenting for medical evaluation; and verbal, nurse-given health education together with patient-centered counselling, when compared with standard care, results in small increases in the rate of partners treated.)

Passin WF, Kim AS, Hutchinson AB, et al; HIV/AIDS Prevention Research Synthesis Project Team. A systematic review of HIV partner counseling and referral services: Client and provider attitudes, preferences, practices, and experiences. *Sex Transm Dis* 2006;33:320–328. [PMID: 16505750} (Review of US HIV partner notification programs confirming that patients were willing to self-notify partners and participate in provider notification, with few reported negative effects. The majority of health care providers were in favor of HIV partner notification; however, they did not consistently refer index clients to HIV partner notification programs.)

ISSUES IN TREATING PARTNERS

Partners should be tested for the infection the patient had as well as for other STDs. Partners of patients with gonorrhea, chlamydia, or trichomoniasis should be treated without waiting for their test results. This stops any possible transmission back to the patient or to the other partners. Partners exposed to syphilis can be managed based on test results if their last contact was at least 90 days before the test, they have no signs or symptoms of syphilis, and they can be reached when test results are available. Partners exposed to syphilis within 90 days of their examination should be treated immediately regardless of their test results, because they may have an infection that is too early to detect. Partners who have positive tests should be interviewed and their partners should be notified.

RISKS OF PARTNER NOTIFICATION

Individuals who acquire an STD or HIV are often at increased risk for partner violence even without partner notification. Partner notification has apparently provoked domestic violence in some situations, but it appears to be rare. One study of 201 HIV-infected women who notified their partners found one had been assaulted by her partner and one had assaulted her partner. Disease intervention specialists often assess the risk of violence by asking patients how their partners will react when notified. The risk of violence appears to be lower if partners are notified by a qualified public health worker rather than the patients themselves, because the health worker can diffuse some of the anger and convince the partner that the decision to reveal his or her name was based on genuine concern for the partner's health. In some instances, concerns over violence may be great enough to preclude notification, but in most instances the benefits of notifying and treating the partner exceed the risk from potential violence.

Although HIV partner notification could increase transmission in a community by breaking up partnerships and increasing mixing, two studies found that a patient's number of partners and new partnerships decreased after partner notification compared with before notification. Patients tend to notify the partners they are most concerned about and are therefore more likely to stay in a relationship with a partner who is notified compared with a partner who does not receive notification.

LEGAL CONSIDERATIONS

Health care providers have conflicting obligations to protect the patient's confidentiality and to warn partners of a potential danger. Most states have statutes that address this specifically for HIV infection by limiting the obligation, yet providing total immunity for disclosure if physicians notify a partner. This has been termed the *privilege to warn*. Health care providers can ask the health department about the relevant laws in their states. At a minimum, health care providers should warn patients of their potential to infect others, recommend that they disclose their infectious status to partners before any future sexual contact, and recommend they also take steps to reduce transmission during future sexual contact.

Gostin LO, Hodge JG. Piercing the veil of secrecy in HIV/AIDS and other sexually transmitted diseases: Theories of privacy and disclosure in partner notification. *Duke J Gend Law Policy* 1998;5:9–88. [PMID: 11979604] (Comprehensive review of the history, effectiveness, and legal aspects of partner notification.)

NETWORK ANALYSIS

Public health workers have always used information from partner notification activities to inform them of the networks of people acquiring and transmitting infection in communities. Syphilis and gonorrhea appear to be maintained in a community by a small "core group" of high-frequency transmitters. STD control programs might be able to control or limit transmission in the community by limiting disease occurrence in core group members.

Frequently, a public health worker will ask patients if they can identify others who are not sex partners but might benefit from testing for the infection either because they have symptoms or because the patient suspects they might be infected ("suspects"). Uninfected persons may also be asked to identify persons they think might have lesions or contact with infected partners, or otherwise might benefit from an examination ("associates"). Research studies have shown that in some situations evaluation of suspects and associates and evaluation of social rather than strictly sexual networks can identify a substantial number of persons with syphilis or HIV infection.

Analyses of the networks involved in different epidemics have shown how some individuals are key to transmission in their communities because they are linked to many other cases or because they form a bridge between two networks. Other analyses suggest that the type of network connections are different for some infections versus others. For example, gonorrhea may be more common in networks where people mix with partners like themselves (assortative mixing) whereas chlamydia may be more common in networks where people mix with partners who are different from themselves (disassortative mixing). Identifying where people have met their sex partners can also help the health department offer screening in areas where multiple patients reported meeting their partners. At present it is not clear how to move from these academic findings to practical interventions, but as disease investigators have known for years, some individuals are more important to reach than others.

Centers for Disease Control and Prevention. Using the Internet for partner notification of sexually transmitted diseases—Los Angeles County, California, 2003. *MMWR Morb Mortal Wkly Rep* 2004;53:129–131. [PMID: 14981362.] (Describes two cases in which public health officials used the Internet to notify partners who were otherwise anonymous.)

Rothenberg R. The transformation of partner notification. *Clin Infect Dis* 2002;35(suppl 2):S138–145. [PMID: 12353200] (A leading partner notification theorist describes the evolution of partner notification and network considerations.)

extends to both the patient, who has a duty to disclose, and the health care provider, who has a duty to warn.

• Patients are more likely to name partners when they are assured that their information is confidential and that their names will not be revealed to their partners.

PRACTICE POINTS

• Partner notification fulfills the ethical obligation to share with individuals information that may be important to their health. This obligation

Relevant Web Sites

[American Social Health Association
http://ashastd.org
[Internet-based system for patient referral partner notification:]
http://www.InSpot.org

Management of Abnormal Pap Smears

29

Michael E. Hagensee, MD, PhD

ESSENTIAL FEATURES

- *Starting at age 21 or no more than 3 years after becoming sexually active, women should have a Papanicolaou (Pap) smear on a yearly basis until they have had three consecutive normal tests, after which the screening interval can be increased to every 3 years.*
- *All women whose test samples show cellular abnormalities, persistent atypical squamous cells, or atypical squamous cells of unclear significance that test positive for high-oncogenic-risk human papillomavirus (HPV) require referral for colposcopy and biopsy.*

GENERAL CONSIDERATIONS

Cervical cancer is the second most common cancer in women worldwide. An estimated 466,000 new cases of cervical cancer are diagnosed each year, resulting in 231,000 deaths. The majority of these cases occur in countries that have limited or no effective screening programs. In the United States and other developed countries, rates of cervical cancer have markedly diminished over the past 30 years as a result of Pap smear screening. Despite this, more than 10,000 cases of cervical cancer are diagnosed in the United States each year, leading to almost 4000 deaths. Countries that initiate Pap screening experience decreases in cancer rates compared with countries that do not. For example, in the mid-1960s, Finland, Sweden, and Iceland all initiated Pap smear screening whereas Norway did not. In the subsequent 20 years, the incidence of cervical cancer did not change in Norway but dropped 50% in the other countries.

Despite widespread screening in the United States, about 50% of all women with cervical cancer have not had a Pap smear in the preceding 3 years and another 10% have not been screened in the past 5 years. Over 50 million Pap smears are obtained each year in the United States, and 7% (3.5 million) of these are abnormal. A woman who never has a Pap smear has a 3.5% risk for developing cervical cancer; this is reduced to 0.8% with Pap smear screening. Infection with high-oncogenic-risk HPV is found in most, if not all, cervical cancers. Detection of high-oncogenic-risk HPV types from cervical samples is now a part of routine clinical management to identify women with abnormal Pap smears who need further treatment

DEVELOPMENT OF THE PAP SMEAR

In 1928 George Papanicolaou initiated the sampling of vaginal cells, speculating that these cells would predict which women would develop cervical cancer. His initial findings were not appreciated by the general medical community, but he persevered and, together with Dr Herbert Traut, published a monograph in 1943 that eventually resulted in Pap smears becoming the standard of care in cervical cancer screening. The procedure they outlined was modified in 1947 by Ayre, who collected cervical cells directly using a wooden spatula.

Although the Pap smear (also called the Pap test) has reduced the incidence of cervical cancer by almost 75%, it is difficult to collect and read a Pap smear in a uniform manner. This lack of uniformity led to widespread confusion about what constituted an abnormal test result. The development of common terminology was essential to standardize the interpretation of this cancer prevention test. In 1988, a workshop was held in Bethesda, Maryland, that provided a general consensus on how to read Pap smears and initial guidelines designed to decrease the variability among laboratories in reporting of results.

A second workshop in 1991 modified these guidelines based on actual practice and clinical experience. The Bethesda 1988 and 1991 guidelines both emphasized delineating squamous intraepithelial lesions—low grade (LSIL) and high grade (HSIL)—from atypical squamous cells of unclear significance (ASC-US) and normal Pap smears.

A decade later, numerous questions about Pap smear interpretation had arisen from clinical practice, necessitating another consensus panel, Bethesda 2001. Some of the issues addressed by this panel included ensuring the adequacy of samples, determining the significance of both atypical squamous cells and atypical glandular cells, and assessing the impact of liquid-based technology on reading of a Pap smear. The Bethesda 2001 consensus panel resulted in the following revisions in the terminology used to report Pap smear results, and in management recommendations for women with abnormal results:

1. Significant changes were made in the management of atypical squamous cells. The guidelines retained the ASC-US designation and added the subcategory of "atypical squamous cells favoring HSIL" (ASC-H). ASC-US carries a moderately low incidence of CIN 2 or 3 (10%) and very low incidence of cancer (0.1%), whereas ASC-H is associated with a much higher incidence of CIN 2 or 3.

2. The Bethesda 2001 guidelines also eliminated the categories of "reactive change Pap smear" and "atypical squamous cells of unclear significance favoring reactive change Pap smear."

3. The category of "atypical glandular cells of unclear significance" (AGC-US) was eliminated, primarily to avoid confusion with that of ASC-US. On average 44% of women with AGC-US have a subsequent tissue examination that yields a diagnosis of cervical dysplasia, and cancer is diagnosed in 8%.

4. The finding of AGC was made more specific in the 2001 guidelines with the inclusion of two categories: "AGC favoring neoplasia" and "adenocarcinoma in situ" (AIS).

In the United States, the Bethesda guidelines are used by the vast majority of laboratories. The standard set of terms currently used for reporting test results is summarized in Table 29–1.

Cannistra SA, Niloff JM. Cancer of the uterine cervix. *N Engl J Med* 1996;334:1030–1038. [PMID: 8598842] (A classic review of Pap smear diagnosis, cervical biopsy, and treatment.)

Solomon D, Davey D, Kurgan R, et al. The 2001 Bethesda System: Terminology for reporting results of cervical cytology. *JAMA* 2002;287:2114–2119. [PMID: 11966386] (Overall review of the current guidelines for reporting of Pap smear results and definitions of all conditions.)

Table 29–1. Reporting terminology and management of Pap smear results.

Abbreviation	Pap Smear Result	Follow-up Tests and Treatment
NILM	Negative for intraepithelial lesion or malignancy	None
ASC		
• ASC-US	Atypical squamous cells—undetermined significance	HPV testing Repeat Pap smear Colposcopy and biopsy Estrogen cream
• ASC-H	Atypical squamous cells—cannot exclude HSIL	Colposcopy and biopsy
AGC[a]	Atypical glandular cells	Colposcopy and biopsy Endocervical curettage
LSIL	Low-grade squamous intraepithelial lesion	Colposcopy and biopsy
HSIL[b]	High-grade squamous intraepithelial lesion	Colposcopy and biopsy, endocervical curettage Further treatment with LEEP, cryotherapy, laser therapy, conization, or hysterectomy

[a]The Bethesda guidelines identify 3 subcategories: "AGC—not otherwise specified," "AGC favoring neoplasia," and "adenocarcinoma in situ" (AIS).
[b]The guidelines further specify "with features suspicious of invasion" when evidence supporting cancer is present.
HPV, human papillomavirus; LEEP, electrosurgical excision procedure.

INITIAL CLINICAL EVALUATION

Symptoms & Signs

Few, if any, symptoms or signs usually point to the likelihood that a woman will have an abnormal Pap smear result. This is the underlying justification for performing routine, preventative Pap smear screening. Symptoms when present can include abnormal vaginal bleeding, irregular menses, and weight loss.

Pap Smear Technique & Interpretation

A. FREQUENCY OF SCREENING

The age at which Pap smear screening should be initiated has led to much debate and, in fact, varies in different locations around the world. In the United States, the most recent recommendation is to screen for the first time 3 years after onset of sexual activity or before age 21, whichever comes first. This is likely a very conservative initiation point, because it appears to take at least 10–20 years for cervical cancer to develop. In some European countries, initial Pap smear screening is performed at age 30.

The optimal screening frequency is also debatable and varies greatly. The initial recommendation that women should undergo annual Pap smear screening was based more on convenience for medical providers and patients than on any scientific data. However, this recommendation is supported by the American College of Obstetricians and Gynecologists (ACOG). The American Cancer Society (ACS) recommends every-other-year screening when using liquid-based cytology (see later discussion). After age 30, the interval between screenings can be increased to 2–3 years. More frequent (ie, annual) Pap smears are recommended for women exposed to diethylstilbestrol (DES), women who are immunocompromised (eg, HIV-infected women), and women with a previous history of stage 2 or 3 cervical intraepithelial neoplasia (CIN).

Although Pap smear screening can be performed on a greater-than-1-year basis, a basic gynecologic examination is a recommended component of a yearly medical checkup. The need for yearly gynecologic examinations is strongly supported by ACOG, particularly for the detection of vaginal, vulvar, uterine, and ovarian cancers. It is also important for women to have prompt repeat Pap smear testing, usually within 3–6 months, for inadequately collected or processed samples. Similarly, follow-up colposcopy for abnormal Pap smear results should also be performed within a 3- to 6-month time interval.

Women who have a hysterectomy for nonmalignant reasons do not need Pap smears. Although vaginal Pap smears can be used to follow women posthysterectomy, vaginal cancers are much less common (0.3 per 100,000 women) than cervical cancer. Furthermore, vaginal intraepithelial neoplasia progresses much more slowly than cervical lesions, and there is a high false-positive rate of Pap smears from vaginal tissue. Generally speaking, women older than 65 years of age can stop undergoing screening if they have had three negative Pap smears in the past 10 years, or if other medical conditions predict a short life expectancy.

B. SAMPLE COLLECTION

The optimal method of collection is one that obtains samples of endocervical cells. The woman is placed in the lithotomy position, a speculum is inserted, and the cervix is brought into view and effaced so that the os can be clearly visualized. Adequate visualization can sometimes be difficult, because the position of the cervix is highly variable. Once an optimal view of the cervix is achieved, the squamocolumnar junction is sampled. The location of this junction varies between women and also changes during the lifetime of a single woman. Before the onset of sexual maturity, the junction is located far lateral to the os. As the woman enters the reproductive years, the junction shifts medially, and with advancing age, it moves up into the endocervical canal.

The sampling device must collect cells from the area surrounding and extending into the os. The extended-tip spatula and cervical broom are more effective sampling devices than the traditional Ayre spatula. Combining a brush with the spatula is a more effective collection method than spatula alone, as well.

Several studies have been performed using a self-sampling technique to provide cells for cytologic evaluation. Self-sampling devices include self-cervical lavages, swabs, cytobrushes, brooms, and tampons that would be inserted into the vagina as far as possible, rotated or left in place for a short period of time, and then removed. In general, these techniques have shown inferior sensitivity (55–94%) but comparable specificity (>80%) to conventional collection devices. Numerous self-sampling techniques to detect HPV viral DNA have also been tested, and these have compared favorably with provider-obtained cervical samples. These methods include cervical swabs, conical brush, tampons, and urine-based testing. Methods to improve further the accuracy of self-collecting tests, using either multiple sampling devices or the same device on multiple occasions, are in development.

C. LIQUID VERSUS CONVENTIONAL PAP SMEAR TECHNIQUE AND AUTOMATED READING

The conventional Pap smear technique consists of obtaining a sample of the cervical transition zone (as outlined earlier), applying the cells to a glass microscope slide, fixing the cells, and then sending the specimen (or "smear") to a pathology laboratory for interpretation. Among the many difficulties with this technique are low sensitivity (50–75%) for all cervical abnormalities; inability to standardize how many cells are applied to the glass slide; uneven distribution of cells; obscuring of cervical epithelial cells by blood, mucus, or inflammatory immune cells; and incomplete fixation due to inadequate air drying or application of fixative. Liquid-based Pap screening solves many of these problems.

With the liquid-based Pap smear technique, the collected cells are placed in a liquid medium and then read in the same medium, allowing for improved visualization of morphologic characteristics. To date, two liquid-based cytology systems have been cleared by the Food and Drug Administration (FDA): the SurePath system (Tri Path Imaging, Burlington, NC) and the ThinPrep system (Cytyc, Boxborough, MA).

Using the SurePath system, collected fluid is density centrifuged to remove debris, and the remaining cells are allowed to attach to a glass side. This technique has been shown to be equivalent to conventional testing. In the ThinPrep system, the fluid is passed through a filter, which removes debris and creates a thin even layer of cellular material on the slide. Using the ThinPrep system, ASC-US, LSIL, and HSIL were all detected more readily than with a conventional smear. One of the main advantages of liquid-based systems is that they allow for HPV DNA testing on the residual fluid.

Automatic reading devices were invented and are FDA-cleared for quality-control purposes in the repeat evaluation of Pap smear results. Test systems include the PAPNET, which uses a neural network, and AutoPap, which is a computerized high-speed video microscope. The AutoPap system has also been cleared for the primary screening of Pap smears and has generally shown an increased sensitivity for all grades of Pap smear. This system has shown statistically significant improvements on sensitivity for ASC-US and LSIL but not for HSIL compared with technician-read smears.

D. INTERPRETATION

Adequacy of the sample is paramount in the interpretation of a Pap smear. The Bethesda guidelines recommend that 8000–12,000 squamous cells be obtained for a conventional Pap smear but only 5000 cells for a liquid-based sample. For both sample types, 10 high-powered fields should be read. Cells can be obscured by blood, mucus, and inflammatory cells. If more than 75% of the cells are obscured, the sample is inadequate and a new sample must be tested. If 50–75% of the cells are obscured, the sample is adequate but partially obscured. The presence of endocervical cells (at least 10) is recommended but not required in samples from women younger than 40 years of age but is required from women older than 40.

It is essential that women with an inadequate Pap smear sample have a repeat examination within 3–6 months. It cannot be overemphasized that an inadequate sample provides absolutely no clinical information. In some clinical settings, such as teaching hospitals, high rates of inadequate sampling (>10%) must be anticipated, detected, and corrected by improved supervision or in-service training of staff.

The results are reported by the laboratory using the standard terms outlined in Table 29–1. These results are described in more detail below.

1. Negative result—A negative Pap smear result is stated as such: "negative for intraepithelial lesion or malignancy" (NILM). It is optional for the pathologist to add information about other infections such as candida, trichomoniasis, bacterial vaginosis, or herpes simplex virus. Normal mature cells are polygonal in shape, with abundant cytoplasm and a small nucleus with granular chromatin.

2. ASC—The category of "atypical squamous cells" (ASC) has been used in the past to define changes more marked than the range of normal, suggestive of a squamous intraepithelial lesion but lacking the formal criteria, qualitatively or quantitatively, for LSIL. This has been a diagnosis of exclusion in the past, commonly referred to as the "wastebasket." It has been the largest category of abnormal Pap smears in the United States, and more than 300,000 women receive this result each year.

The Bethesda guidelines regarding atypical squamous cells emphasize the ability to distinguish between HSIL and LSIL. Overall, it is thought that 10–30% of women with a finding of ASC on a Pap smear have underlying CIN grade 2 or 3, and 0.1% may have invasive cancer. These atypical cells have an enlarged nucleus 2.5–3 times normal size, variation in nuclear shape, and nuclei that are mildly hyperchromatic, but with chromatin that is finely granular.

a. ASC-US—It is estimated that 90–95% of all findings of ASC fall into the category of ASC-US. Women with a Pap smear result of ASC-US have a 5–17% chance of having CIN 2 or 3. Furthermore, 39% of women with CIN 2 or 3 have a previous finding of ASC-US on Pap smear. In addition, ASC-US is associated with HPV in about 33–67% of cases.

b. ASC-H—The category of ASC-H describes atypical cells that are morphologically suspicious of HSIL but too few in number to qualify as HSIL. ASC-H is more highly associated with HSIL than ASC-US and is the most common precursor lesion for CIN. Follow-up of women with a finding of ASC-H leads to diagnosis of CIN 2 or 3 in 68% (range, 24–94%) of these women. However, this category is fraught with lack of reproducibility among pathologists. It is hoped that with time, the lesions suggested by this finding can be more accurately and quickly identified, because they often progress to CIN 2 and 3 lesions that will require therapy.

3. AGC—The category of "atypical glandular cells" (AGC) is further differentiated according to whether the cells are endocervical, endometrial, or not otherwise specified. These cells occur in sheets or strips and have minimal nuclear overlap, only slight hyperchromasia, and distinct cell borders. This finding is relatively rare, occurring in 0.17–1.8% of all Pap smears; however, the presence of these cells has serious medical implications because women with a finding of AGC have a 9.7 times higher risk of progressing to CIN 2.

a. AGC favoring neoplasia—This finding on Pap smear may correspond with high-grade lesions on tissue examination (27–96% of the time). The atypical cells so identified may have rosettes, nuclear crowding and overlap, and diminished cytoplasm, with occasional mitotic figures.

b. Adenocarcinoma in situ (AIS)—The atypical cells of AIS are notable for increased nuclear enlargement to at least three times normal size, less cytoplasm and more hyperchromasia than normal cells, and mitotic figures. A finding of AIS corresponds with high rates of advanced lesions on tissue examination. However, the fact that AIS is of relative low prevalence has led to serious problems with poor interobserver variability. Use of the liquid-based Pap smear technique has not improved the ability to identify this cytologic abnormality.

4. LSIL and HSIL—The ability to distinguish between LSIL and HSIL findings is of utmost importance. Studies have shown that the finding of LSIL is more variable and less reproducible than HSIL, and repeatable in only 80% of smears. The Bethesda guidelines further specify "with features suspicious of invasion" when histologic evidence supporting cancer is present.

E. Counseling Women Who Have an Abnormal Pap Smear Result

An abnormal Pap smear result can be emotionally devastating for women because of the implications regarding sexual activity, concern about the likelihood of progression to cervical cancer, and possible associations with other sexually transmitted diseases (STDs). Women with abnormal Pap smear findings should be counseled that HPV infection has been linked with the development of cervical cancer, and that HPV is the most common viral STD, affecting up to 70% of the sexually active population. In contrast to other STDs, the source of transmission of the virus is often difficult to identify, and the infection may have been acquired years prior to the current abnormal Pap smear. Thus, the patient's current sex partner may not be responsible for changes observed in the abnormal Pap smear. Furthermore, because of potential coexposures in patients diagnosed with an STD, testing for HIV infection and other STDs is warranted. Finally, it should be understood by both patient and provider that Pap smears are only effective when appropriate referrals are made and attended for the follow-up of an abnormal test.

Additional Tests & Examinations

A. Human Papillomavirus DNA Testing

The detection of HPV DNA can assist in the management of women with indeterminate Pap smear results. Appropriate management of women with a Pap smear finding of ASC-US can be selected based on the presence or absence of high-risk HPV DNA types. Several large studies, most of which used the FDA-cleared Hybrid Capture II (Digene) test, have shown that treatment selection based on the result of this test is cost-effective. For example, in the ASCUS LSIL trial study (ALTS), the use of the HPV DNA test resulted in a sensitivity of 96% and a colposcopy rate of 56%, the best outcomes studied. The sensitivity of the HPV DNA assay for detecting HSIL is 83–100% and is greater than repeat Pap smear testing in all of the reported studies. In addition, the negative predictive value of a HPV DNA test is also reported to be quite high (>98%).

The most efficient way to perform HPV DNA testing is through "reflex" testing. At the time of Pap smear, either a liquid-based Pap smear is obtained or, if conventional Pap smear technique is utilized, an additional cervical swab is collected. The residual fluid from the liquid-based Pap test or the additional cervical swab is saved for potential HPV DNA testing. If a woman's Pap smear result identifies ASC-US, her stored sample can then be tested for HPV DNA. In this reflex manner, women can be identified who require either colposcopy (ie, the DNA test result is positive for high-oncogenic-risk HPV) or follow-up and management with annual Pap tests (ie, the DNA test result is negative).

Recent recommendations are that women older than 30 years of age have an HPV DNA test as well as a Pap smear. If results of both tests are negative, the ACS and ACOG recommend that screening then occur every 3 years. The recommendations also specify that a positive HPV DNA test in a women older than 30 years of age should be followed up by repeat HPV DNA and Pap smear testing in 6–12 months. If the retest is again positive for high-risk HPV DNA, then colposcopy is indicated. HPV DNA testing would cease at the same time as Pap smear testing. A final recommendation proposes that there is no need for HPV DNA testing beyond the age of 30 years in immunosuppressed HIV-infected women, who would require colposcopy regardless of the result, or in women who have had a hysterectomy for benign reasons, because these women have virtually no risk of cancer, no matter what the result of the HPV DNA test.

It is important to note that these recommendations are based on few published studies, and do not include data from women in the United States. Several studies currently underway must be completed and reviewed before practitioners can be assured that this is a well-founded cancer screening protocol. Several reservations have also been raised regarding these recommendations.

Some experts have expressed concern that women may not return for their next Pap smear in 3 years. Scheduling of an annual Pap smear, it is thought, may be easier to remember, in addition to being linked to acquisition of interventions for birth control. Furthermore, even if an annual Pap smear is not recommended, ACOG guidelines call for all women to have an annual gynecologic evaluation. It should be noted that the US Preventative Services Task Force has stated that there is insufficient evidence to support these recommendations at this time.

B. COLPOSCOPY

Women with an abnormal Pap smear should undergo colposcopy to visualize epithelial defects, along with biopsy to obtain tissue specimens for laboratory examination. First used by Hinselman in 1925, the colposcope in modern times is stereoscopic and magnifies the cervix 4–40 times. The goal of colposcopy is to identify areas of epithelial defects that may reflect preneoplastic changes, which are then targeted for biopsy. The cervix is initially viewed with the colposcope. A dilute solution of 3–5% acetic acid is then applied, which removes mucus and tends to dry out the surface, highlighting the epithelial defects as acetowhite lesions. These lesions are not specific to cervical dysplasia caused by HPV but

help to identify potential areas from which to obtain biopsy specimens. Some experts recommend applying Lugol iodine solution, which stains normal but not abnormal cells. This technique can be useful to identify abnormal epithelial cells, but it is not clear if it increases diagnostic sensitivity.

Treatment

Treatment of women with abnormal Pap smear results is dependent on the pathologic findings, as illustrated by the treatment algorithm in Figure 29–1.

Based on Pap Smear Result

A. ASC-US

Women with a finding of ASC-US are now managed in private practice, and increasingly in the public sector, primarily through reflex HPV DNA testing (see Figure 29–1). This approach leads to overall cost savings and fewer referrals for colposcopy. More specifically, 72% of women with CIN 3 are diagnosed by DNA testing, which is superior to colposcopy or Pap smear alone. DNA testing also results in 50% fewer referrals for colposcopy. Women with a positive HPV DNA test result are referred for colposcopy, and those with a negative result, for a repeat Pap smear in 12 months. Alternatively, ASC-US

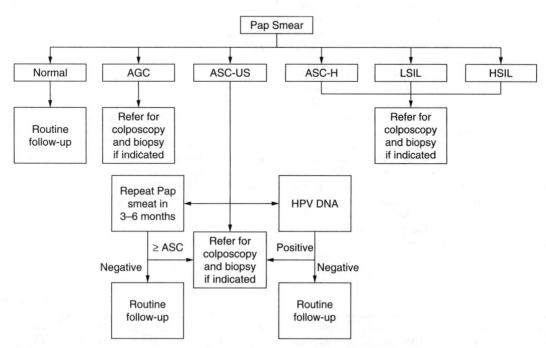

Figure 29–1. Algorithm for the workup of women with abnormal Pap smears. AGC, atypical glandular cells; ASC-US, atypical squamous cells of unclear significance; ≥ASC, Pap smear grade of ASC or higher; ASC-H, atypical squamous cells favoring HSIL; LSIL, low-grade squamous intraepithelial lesion; HSIL, high-grade squamous intraepithelial lesion.

can be managed by either immediate referral for colposcopy or by repeat Pap smear testing in 3–6 months (see Figure 29–1). If colposcopy is used and CIN is not found on examination of a biopsy specimen, the woman can resume routine screening at 12-month intervals. If CIN is found, it is managed as described below.

B. ASC-H

Women whose Pap smear result shows ASC-H should be referred for immediate colposcopy and biopsy. Women in whom tissue examination confirms the presence of abnormal cells are managed according to guidelines for squamous intraepithelial lesions and CIN. Those with normal findings on tissue examination should be closely followed; in these women, the finding of ASC-H needs to be reassessed. If the original finding is deemed correct, follow-up in 6 months with repeat Pap smear testing is advisable, as well as HPV DNA testing in 12 months.

C. AGC

As previously noted, a Pap smear result showing AGC carries a substantially higher risk of cervical abnormalities than ASC, and management of women with this result can be quite difficult and challenging. For "atypical cells—not otherwise specified" (AGC-NOS), the risk of a high-grade lesion (CIN 2 and above) is between 9% and 41%; for "AGC favoring neoplasia," 27–96%, and for AIS, 48–69%. Women with all three of these Pap smear findings should be managed initially by colposcopy and endocervical sampling (see Figure 29–1). The endometrium should also be sampled in patients with abnormal endometrial cells on Pap smear who are aged 35 years or older or have a history of abnormal vaginal bleeding.

Women with abnormal tissue findings require a definitive therapeutic intervention. Those with normal tissue findings and a Pap smear result of AGC-NOS should have Pap smears every 6 months until four consecutive smears are normal, at which point they can resume annual follow-up. Because of the increased rate of higher grade disease in women with AGC favoring neoplasia or AIS, patients with these results should have definitive therapy even if the tissue examination does not show abnormal cells. The therapy recommended by the consensus panel is cold-knife conization. HPV DNA testing has not been studied extensively enough to know if it will aid in the management of these women; however, a negative HPV DNA test should provide reassurance, because all women with AIS would test positive for HPV DNA.

D. LSIL

LSIL is noted in 1.6% of all Pap smears. Between 15% and 30% of women with a finding of LSIL on Pap smear have CIN 2 or 3 on subsequent examination of a cervical biopsy specimen. In addition, 12% of women with LSIL and CIN 1 on tissue examination progress to CIN 2 or 3 over the next 2 years. All women with LSIL should

therefore be referred for colposcopy and biopsy (see Figure 29–1). If the tissue examination is positive for CIN 2 or 3, the woman should be managed as outlined below; if negative, follow-up Pap smears at 6 and 12 months and HPV DNA testing at 12 months are recommended. Women with a grade of ASC-US or higher on follow-up Pap smears or a positive HPV DNA test should be referred again for colposcopy. The routine use of HPV DNA testing for LSIL is not indicated, because more than 80% of women with this finding on Pap smear have a positive HPV DNA test.

E. HSIL

All women with HSIL should undergo prompt colposcopic evaluation and biopsy (see Figure 29–1). HSIL accounts for only 0.45% of all Pap smear results, but CIN 2 or 3 is seen in 70% of women with this finding, and 3% have invasive cancer. Women with a CIN 2, CIN 3, or a higher-grade lesion should be managed as outlined below. For those with CIN 1 or no lesion on tissue examination, a careful review of the Pap smear and biopsy results is warranted. If HSIL remains the cytologic diagnosis, an excision procedure is recommended, preferably a loop electrosurgical excision procedure (LEEP). Collection of the biopsy specimen may be omitted if LEEP is planned, but this applies only to patients who might not return for definitive therapy or for older women in whom the risk of infertility from the excision procedure is not an issue. Similarly to LSIL, the routine use of HPV DNA testing is not recommended, because more than 95% of women with this finding are HPV DNA-positive.

Based on Biopsy Result

The use of Pap smear screening is extremely useful in identifying women at high risk for the development of cervical cancer. However, to prevent cancer, additional information is needed; namely, histologic confirmation of premalignant lesions from cervical biopsy specimens. The additional information provided by examination of these specimens results in often curative treatment of these lesions, which is reflected in the dramatic decrease in the incidence of cervical cancer seen over the past 30 years.

A. CIN 1

It is estimated that one million women each year are diagnosed with CIN 1 in the United States. The recommended treatment of this stage of cervical neoplasia is close observation, because only 11% of women with CIN 1 progress to CIN 2 and 3, and only 0.3% progress to cervical cancer. Most cases regress spontaneously. Many experts believe that evidence of LSIL and CIN 1 is part of the natural history of HPV infection and that no specific intervention is necessary other than to follow the patient closely to ensure that progressive pathologic changes do not occur. Numerous research studies have been performed to identify risk factors that can distinguish women who will progress to more advanced stages of cervical cancer from those who will regress. Among these are HPV genotype and variant identification, p16INK4a detection, telomere activity, and Ki-67 expression. These markers are similar to those studied to determine the management of an abnormal Pap smear. They have not yet been shown to significantly improve clinical care.

Follow-up consists of Pap smear screening at 6 and 12 months and HPV DNA testing at 12 months. A woman with a Pap smear grade of ASC-US or higher or a positive HPV DNA test requires colposcopic evaluation. After two negative Pap smears or a negative DNA test, the woman can be managed with routine annual follow-up. Women with persistent LSIL should also be followed annually. Those with persistent or incident CIN 1 can be treated with ablative (cryotherapy or laser ablation) or excisional therapy (LEEP, laser and cold knife conization). Women with recurrent CIN 1 or those who have had an inadequate colposcopic examination should undergo a diagnostic excision procedure. The selection of the procedure to be performed is based on the reason for treatment, the skills of the gynecologist, and the preference of the patient.

B. CIN 2 AND 3

CIN 2 and 3 are more worrisome pathologic entities than CIN 1 and require definitive therapy. Because these lesions can progress more readily to invasive cervical cancer, observation alone is not recommended. The rates of progression are somewhat similar, which allows for similar management of these two entities. For example, CIN 2 that is not treated will regress 43% of the time, progress in 22% of patients, and persist in 35%. CIN 3 will regress in 32% of patients, progress in 14%, and persist in 56%.

For women with histologic confirmation of CIN 2 or 3 that rules out invasive disease, the treatment can be ablation or excision of the entire transformation zone. Women with recurrent CIN 2 or 3 should undergo an excision procedure, and those with an unsatisfactory colposcopic examination should have a diagnostic excision procedure. In general, the cold-knife conization procedure produces the same results as LEEP; however, some studies have shown that the margins are easier to interpret when conization is used. Finally, for women with recurrent CIN 2 or 3, hysterectomy is a treatment option.

After treatment, women with CIN 2 or 3 should be followed closely. At least three negative Pap smears obtained 4–6 months apart are needed before the patient resumes annual screening. Numerous studies have also shown that a negative HPV DNA test after a definitive procedure predicts those who can be managed with annual follow-up. If a Pap smear grade of ASC-US or higher is reported or the HPV DNA test is positive, colposcopic examination and endocervical biopsy should be performed.

C. INVASIVE DISEASE

Invasive lesions should be managed by a skilled gynecologist-oncologist. Microinvasive disease can be managed using cone biopsy and close follow-up or simple hysterectomy. Full invasive lesions require staging to determine the treatment (ie, surgery and x-ray therapy for lower stages, and chemotherapy with or without x-ray therapy for more extensive disease).

Apgar BS, Brotzman G. Management of cervical cytologic abnormalities. *Am Fam Physician* 2004;70:1905–1016. [PMID: 15571057] (Readable review with nicely displayed algorithms outlining management for the common Pap smear abnormalities.)

Wright TC, Cox JT, Massad LS, et al. 2001 Consensus Guidelines for the management of women with cervical cytological abnormalities. *JAMA* 2002;287:2120–2129. [PMID: 11966387]

SPECIAL MANAGEMENT CONSIDERATIONS

Adolescents

The nature of the maturing cervix and its predominant columnar epithelium place adolescents at higher risk for HPV infection and dysplasia than older women. However, adolescents have very low rates of cervical cancer, because these cytologic abnormalities regress in the vast majority of cases. For example, regression of LSIL occurs in 60% of older women compared with over 90% of adolescents. In addition, most patients with a HSIL on Pap smear are found to have CIN 2 on tissue examination, and this also tends to regress on its own. Finally, cervical cancer rates from the National Cancer Institute database yield no cases per 100,0000 for adolescents aged 10–14 and 15–19 years.

Adolescents with HSIL and no evidence of CIN or with only CIN 1 on tissue examination can be followed with repeat colposcopy and cytology at 4- to 6-month intervals for 1 year. Because the rate of cancer is so low in this age group, adolescents in whom CIN 2 is identified on tissue examination can also be followed conservatively. If the tissue findings progress to CIN 3, definitive care (ablation or excision) would then be recommended. Adolescents with an unsatisfactory colposcopic examination may be followed closely rather than undergoing further diagnostic or therapeutic procedures.

Postmenopausal & Elderly Women

A few reports have noted increased rates of ASC-US in the Pap smears of elderly women associated with more benign findings on tissue examination. Among women older than 50 years of age, 12.8% of those with ASC-US had dysplasia compared with 29.5% of women younger than 50 years. For women with a Pap smear result of LSIL, management should consist of repeat Pap smear evaluation at 6 and 12 months and HPV DNA testing at 12 months. If a grade of ASC-US or higher is detected on Pap smear or an HPV DNA test is positive for high-oncogenic-risk types, then the woman should be referred for colposcopy. For both ASC-US and LSIL, if atrophic cells are present, intravaginal estrogen (if not contraindicated) can be prescribed, followed by a repeat Pap smear 1 week after treatment. If a negative result is obtained, then repeat testing in 6 months is advised. If the test is again negative, the woman can resume annual screening.

Pregnant Women

Cervical cancer is the most common malignancy of pregnancy, with an incidence of 1.2–4.5 cases per 10,000 pregnancies, and abnormal cytology in noted in 0.5–3% of all pregnant women. A contributing factor in the high rate of abnormal Pap smears is the presence of placental cells, which can mimic cervical abnormalities. For example, the appearance of degenerating decidual cells or cytotrophoblasts may be similar to HSIL, and syncytiotrophoblasts can be confused with dysplastic cervical cells. Another factor contributing to the high reported rate may be inadequate cervical sampling by clinicians who may fear possible adverse affects to the fetus with the use of a cervical brush. However, several studies have demonstrated that use of a brush carries no higher risk to the fetus than use of a spatula.

Colposcopy and punch biopsies are safe and reliable in pregnant women. The hypervascularity of the cervix during pregnancy must be distinguished from that associated with cancers and premalignant lesions. Physiologic eversion of the cervix may increase the area of squamous metaplasia, whereas vaginal laxity may obscure the cervical os.

Management of pregnant women with a Pap smear result of ASC-US is similar to that of nonpregnant women. For higher grade lesions, it is recommended that biopsies be performed by obstetricians-gynecologists experienced in the management of cervical disease in pregnant women.

The regression rate in pregnant women for cytologic abnormalities identified on Pap smear is as follows: for ASC-US and LSIL, 60–65%, and for HSIL, about 50%. Women with biopsy findings of CIN 2 or 3 can be followed closely, because about 70% of these lesions regress postpartum. AGS can be difficult to manage in pregnant women, and close follow-up with colposcopy and biopsy is indicated. Other cytologic results should be reevaluated no sooner than 6 weeks postpartum. If colposcopic examination is unsatisfactory, the clinician should repeat the procedure in 6–12 weeks, because these examinations are easier to perform as pregnancy advances.

Because procedures involving excision can lead to excessive bleeding and preterm labor, only cancer should be treated.

HIV-Infected & Other Immunosuppressed Women

Women who are immunosuppressed are thought to be at higher risk for invasive cervical cancer. Indeed, HIV-infected women have between a fivefold and ninefold increased risk of this cancer. This is also manifested by a fourfold increase in squamous intraepithelial lesions on Pap smear, and an increased incidence of LSIL (15%) and HSIL (8%). Women with lower CD4 cell counts, in general, have increased rates of HPV infection and cervical dysplasia.

Women with Hodgkin disease and those who are organ transplant recipients are also at higher risk for cervical dysplasia. Women with Hodgkin disease have a fourfold higher incidence of squamous intraepithelial lesions compared with normal women. Even more dramatic are the findings in renal transplant recipients; these patients have a 17-fold increased incidence of squamous intraepithelial lesions, and even higher rates of dysplasia, linked to the high doses of immune suppressive drugs required to counteract rejection. All of these women require close follow-up.

Pap smears are equally sensitive in HIV-infected and HIV-uninfected women. It is recommended that HIV-infected women have a Pap smear every 6 months until they have had two consecutive negative results, at which time they can resume annual screening. There are no clear guidelines for women with Hodgkin disease or transplant recipients, but examination and Pap smear every 6 months is a management approach consistent with recommendations for other immunosuppressed women.

All immunosuppressed women with a Pap smear finding of ASC-US should be referred for colposcopy and endocervical biopsy, because studies show that only 34% of women with this finding revert to normal and 21% go on to develop HSIL. Higher regression rates are seen in women receiving treatment for HIV infection; however, the majority of cervical lesions fail to resolve in these women, as well. Use of HIV antiretroviral therapy may decrease dysplasia by improving immune function and overall health; conversely, by allowing HIV-infected women to live longer, this therapy may increase their risk of eventually developing cervical cancer. In addition, the improvement in overall health in patients receiving HIV antiretroviral therapy may lead to a return to high-risk sexual behavior and further exposure to HPV infection.

HIV-infected women have a higher rate of recurrence after treatment for cervical dysplasia and should be followed carefully. Indeed, in one study recurrence was observed in 62% of HIV-infected women compared with only 18% of HIV-uninfected women. In the same study, 50% of those with one recurrence had a second recurrence. Topical 5-fluorocytosine, imiquimod, and retinoids have been used in these women and may decrease recurrence rates.

HPV Prophylactic Vaccines & the Use of Pap Smear Screening

HPV prophylactic vaccines have been developed based on the immunogenicity of virus-like particles consisting of the L1 protein. These vaccines have been shown to prevent infection with the HPV types contained in the vaccine (usually HPV low-risk types 6 and 11 and high-risk types 16 and 18). In June 2006 the FDA approved one such vaccine for the prevention of cervical cancer in women and girls aged 9–26 years. Expert groups recommend vaccination at ages 11–12 years, before the onset of sexual activity. It is possible that widespread use of these vaccines will reduce the incidence of cervical cancer and perhaps allow for less-aggressive Pap smear screening strategies. Although use of the vaccine will still necessitate routine Pap smear screening, management models have been proposed that initiate screening at a later age (25 years) and include a longer screening interval (3 years). It is too early to recommend changes in Pap smear screening initiation or intervals at this time.

Goldie SJ, Kohli M, Grima D, et al. Projected clinical benefits and cost-effectiveness of a human papillomavirus 16/18 vaccine. *J Natl Cancer Inst* 2004;96:601–615. [PMID: 15100338] (Models showing the benefit of vaccination and less-frequent Pap smear screening.)

FUTURE DIRECTIONS

Pap smear screening has led to a marked decrease in cervical cancer in the developed world and is a mainstay of cancer preventative methods. These methods need to be applied in the developing world so that the worldwide incidence of cervical cancer can continue to decline. Women who do not participate in screening efforts are at higher risk of invasive disease. The detection of HPV DNA from self-sampling methods could lead to even better prevention of disease than current screening measures and should be investigated as a means of screening women who are reluctant to seek medical care.

Immunosuppressed women, such as transplant recipients and those with HIV infection, are at higher risk for cervical cancer than immunocompetent women. Treatment advances in the care of immunosuppressed women may, conversely, lead to future increases in the incidence of cervical cancer.

PRACTICE POINTS

• The extended-tip spatula and cervical broom are more effective sampling devices than the traditional Ayre spatula. Combining a brush with the spatula is a more effective collection method than spatula alone, as well.

Relevant Web Sites

[American Cancer Society:]
http://www.cancer.org
[American College of Obstetricians and Gynecology:]
http://www.acog.org
[Centers for Disease Control and Prevention:]
http://www.cdc.gov/std/hpv/default.htm#cancer
[National Cancer Institute fact sheet on Pap smear testing:]
http://www.cancer.gov/cancertopics/factsheet/Detection/Pap-test
[US Department of Health and Human Services web site on management of initial abnormal Pap smear (regularly updated):]
http://www.guideline.gov/summary/summary.aspx?doc_id=8327

Commonly Encountered Genital Dermatoses

30

Laura Hinkle Bachmann, MD, MPH

Patients may seek a sexually transmitted disease (STD) evaluation for essentially anything they perceive as abnormal and that is located "below the belt." Although the presence of an STD should always be considered and ruled out, many patients who seek care for a suspected STD have nonsexually transmitted genital conditions. For this reason, clinicians should have a basic understanding of the spectrum of both normal skin findings and common dermatologic conditions that arise in the genitalia so they can prescribe appropriate therapy, refer the patient to a dermatologist for additional evaluation and management when necessary, or provide reassurance.

This chapter discusses the nonsexually transmitted dermatologic conditions most commonly encountered in the STD clinic setting, as well as normal variants. The discussion of pathologic lesions that follows is organized by morphology and color of lesion. A review of definitions employed to describe skin lesions is found in Table 30–1. A section on ectoparasites concludes the chapter. For a more comprehensive review of genital dermatology, the reader is referred to the text references listed below.

Edwards L. *Genital Dermatology Atlas.* Lippincott Williams & Wilkins, 2004.

Fisher BK, Margesson LJ. *Genital Skin Disorders: Diagnosis and Treatment.* Mosby, 1998.

Habif TB. *Clinical Dermatology,* 4th ed. Mosby, 2004.

Wolff K, Johnson RA, Summond D. *Fitzpatrick's Color Atlas & Synopsis of Clinical Dermatology,* 5th ed. McGraw-Hill, 2005.

■ HISTORY

A thorough history is an essential component in the evaluation of an individual presenting with genital lesions or rash. Useful questions to ask include the following:

(1) How long has the lesion or rash been present? The duration of a genital lesion is important for directing evaluation. For example, a genital ulcer or atypical lesion that has been slowly growing over the course of months to years implies the need for immediate biopsy, whereas an ulcer of shorter duration (that does not appear atypical) may warrant a workup for common infectious etiologies, and perhaps empiric therapy, with biopsy reserved for situations in which the workup is negative and the lesion fails to resolve.

(2) Does the lesion look the same now as it did when it first appeared? If not, how is it different? Understanding the evolution of a lesion or rash may assist the clinician in narrowing the differential diagnosis. For example, a patient may have self-treated a herpes simplex virus infection, resulting in a contact dermatitis. Only a thorough history will allow the clinician to sift through the details and put the story together.

(3) What other areas are involved? Are the abnormalities confined to the genital region or widespread? In general, disseminated rashes require more urgent evaluation than localized rashes, particularly if accompanied by systemic signs and symptoms. In addition, syphilis should always be considered in the evaluation of a disseminated rash (see Chapter 19).

(4) What are the characteristics of the rash or lesion? Was the onset of the rash or lesion associated with anything in particular? A pruritic rash may imply an ectoparasitic infection or a drug reaction, whereas a genital rash that stings and burns may be a result of contact dermatitis. In the case of irritant contact dermatitis, the patient may recall the close temporal relationship between application of an offending product and symptom onset.

(5) Has this ever happened to you before? If so, what was determined to be the cause that time? Fixed drug eruption, a lesion that occurs at the same anatomic site (and worsens) with each exposure to the drug, would often

Table 30–1. Terminology used to describe skin lesions.

Term	Description
Macule	Area of color change <1.5 cm and smooth
Patch	Area of color change >1.5 cm and smooth
Papule	Palpable lesion <1 cm
Plaque	Palpable lesion >1 cm
Nodule	Papule or plaque with deeper extension into the skin
Scale	Abnormal shedding or accumulation of cornified cells
Vesicle	Blister <1 cm
Bulla	Blister >1 cm
Pustule	Pus-filled vesicle
Erosion	Shallow skin defect
Ulcer	Deep skin defect
Crust	Amorphous accumulation of dried serum, pus, or blood

escape diagnosis unless the clinician elicited a previous history. Likewise, a patient with a widespread dermatosis, such as psoriasis, may have experienced genital lesions in the past.

(6) What are your hygiene habits? What products does your partner use? Do you use condoms, lubricants, or spermicides when you have sex? It is often helpful to address issues of personal hygiene and sexual practice in an open-ended fashion, followed by more pointed questions. At times it may be necessary to ask patients to review their daily hygiene routine with the clinician as this may jog their memories.

■ NORMAL ANATOMIC VARIANTS

When a patient presents for initial evaluation of a genital condition, one of the first issues to consider is whether or not the abnormality in question is pathologic or simply a normal variant. This distinction is important, because intervention involving a normal anatomic variant often is not in the best interest of the patient. Among the commonly encountered normal variants are pearly penile papules, vestibular papillae, and Fordyce spots.

PEARLY PENILE PAPULES

ESSENTIALS OF DIAGNOSIS

- *Skin-colored papules most commonly located in the coronal sulcus of the penis.*
- *Asymptomatic papules with rounded tips and discrete bases.*

One of the most commonly encountered dermatologic conditions in male patients who seek care at STD clinics, pearly penile papules are usually brought to the attention of the clinician when the patient presents for evaluation of possible condylomata acuminata. The papules are found more commonly in uncircumcised men and are located primarily around the coronal sulcus. They may also be found on the distal penile shaft, near the frenulum, or on the posterior part of the glans penis. These asymptomatic lesions are usually flesh-colored or pink and rounded with discrete bases. They may be elongated into papillae (see Figure 30–1).

The primary entity with which pearly penile papules are confused is condylomata acuminata. Unlike pearly penile papules, however, condylomata acuminata often have spiked tips or are contiguous at the base.

The diagnosis of pearly penile papules is based on the clinical appearance. Biopsy is usually not necessary but, if performed, would reveal a benign angiofibroma. Reassurance is the only treatment necessary.

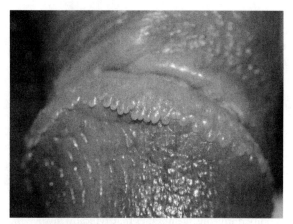

Figure 30–1. Pearly penile papules. Note the homogeneous appearance of the lesions as well as the typical location. (Courtesy of Jay Sizemore, MD.)

VESTIBULAR PAPILLAE

ESSENTIALS OF DIAGNOSIS

- *Asymptomatic, small, monomorphous, symmetric tubular papillae located within the vaginal vestibule.*
- *Often confused with condylomata acuminata.*

Vestibular papillae occur in one third to one half of women and are a normal anatomic variant distinguished by monomorphic appearance, rounded tips, discrete nature of the base of the lesions, and symmetric distribution. Some variants of vestibular papillae are short and confluent, giving a cobblestone texture to the skin. These lesions are typically found in the vaginal vestibule and are asymptomatic. Although there is some debate as to the role of human papillomavirus (HPV) in the development of vestibular papillae, the current consensus is that HPV is not related to these lesions.

The primary entity with which vestibular papillae are confused is condylomata acuminata. The two conditions can usually be distinguished from one another based on the appearance of the lesions.

The diagnosis of vestibular papillae is based on the appearance and distribution of the lesions. Application of acetic acid 5% does not reliably distinguish these lesions from genital warts. Other than reassuring the patient, no treatment is necessary.

FORDYCE SPOTS

ESSENTIALS OF DIAGNOSIS

- *Flesh-colored to yellowish, small, smooth papules.*
- *Most commonly located on the medial aspect of the labia minora or the proximal quarter of the penile shaft.*

Fordyce spots are enlarged sebaceous glands located on modified mucous membranes that typically involve the medial aspect of the labia minora in women and the proximal quarter of the penile shaft in men. They are asymptomatic, papular, and flesh-colored to yellow in appearance (see Figure 30–2). They may be discrete and multilobular or confluent.

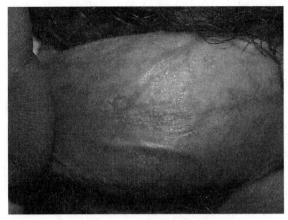

Figure 30–2. Fordyce spots involving the penile shaft. Note the yellowish color typical of these lesions. (Courtesy of Jay Sizemore, MD.)

No laboratory studies are necessary; diagnosis is based on clinical appearance. Although the appearance of Fordyce spots is characteristic, it may be possible to confuse them with small condylomata acuminata. No treatment is necessary.

■ PATHOLOGIC LESIONS

FLESH-COLORED PAPULES

1. Molluscum Contagiosum

ESSENTIALS OF DIAGNOSIS

- *Common viral infection characterized by flesh-colored, pearly papules with central umbilication.*
- *Self-limited in immunocompetent hosts.*

General Considerations

Molluscum contagiosum is caused by the molluscum contagiosum virus, a member of the DNA poxvirus group, and is common in children and young adults. It is usually transmitted through sexual and other close contact.

Clinical Findings

The infection is characterized by firm, dome-shaped, flesh-colored, "pearly" papules with central umbilication

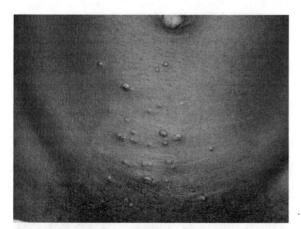

Figure 30–3. Pearly papular lesions of molluscum contagiosum. Central umbilication is present on some, but not all, of the lesions. (Courtesy of Jay Sizemore, MD.)

(see Figure 30–3). Although the classic central umbilication may not be present on all lesions, usually there are several on which this depression may be found. If the lesion of molluscum contagiosum is incised, a central core, usually waxy, can be expressed. The central umbilication and waxy core help differentiate molluscum contagiosum from other diseases. Lesions are most often asymptomatic but may be described as pruritic. They are most often located in the pubic area, proximal and medial thighs, and penile shaft. Lesions are larger and more numerous in immunosuppressed patients.

Biopsy is rarely required to diagnose molluscum contagiosum. If performed, histologic examination will reveal large eosinophilic inclusion bodies within epidermal cells.

Differential Diagnosis

Molluscum contagiosum may be confused with condylomata acuminata, and molluscum lesions that are more vesicular in appearance may be confused with herpes simplex virus. Sebaceous gland hyperplasia, basal cell carcinoma, and, in immunosuppressed individuals, fungal infections such as cryptococcosis and histoplasmosis should also be considered. If the patient presents with molluscum-like lesions in the setting of systemic symptoms, evaluation should proceed quickly to rule out disseminated fungal infection.

Treatment

Although the course of infection in the immunocompetent host is usually self-limited, generally resolving over months, patients may desire treatment for cosmetic purposes. In contrast, molluscum contagiosum in the immunocompromised host is often persistent, larger, and more distressing to the patient in terms of appearance and often requires treatment.

Treatment requires either destructive or immunomodulatory modalities. Molluscum contagiosum can be effectively treated with curettage or incision followed by expression of the central white core of the lesion, also known as the "molluscum body." Other therapeutic modalities include electrosurgery and cryotherapy. Cantharidin may be used for lesions found outside the genital region but, because of painful blisters and erythema that result from therapy, should be avoided in sensitive areas of the body. Recent studies have found variable success with imiquimod, applied three times a week overnight for up to 16 weeks; clearance rates have ranged from 33% to 100%, depending on the population studied. Finally, podophyllin, podofilox 0.5%, laser therapy, and trichloroacetic acid may be used.

Molluscum contagiosum is usually not eliminated in one treatment and lesions may continue to occur for a time after treatment. Relapse is particularly frequent in immunocompromised hosts.

Barba AR, Kapoor S, Berman B. An open label safety study of topical imiquimod 5% cream in the treatment of Molluscum contagiosum in children. *Dermatol Online J* 2001;7:20. [PMID: 11328641] (This small study [n = 12] found imiquimod 5% cream nightly for 4 weeks to be a safe treatment in children with molluscum contagiosum.)

Liota E, Smith KJ, Buckley R, et al. Imiquimod therapy for molluscum contagiosum. *J Cutan Med Surg* 2000;4:76–82. [PMID: 11179929] (In this study, molluscum contagiosum lesions in 14 of 19 immunocompetent adults, 4 of 4 adults with HIV type 1 disease, and 6 of 13 children resolved in less than 16 weeks with imiquimod therapy.)

Ting PT, Dytoc MT. Therapy of external anogenital warts and molluscum contagiosum: A literature review. *Dermatol Ther* 2004;17:68–101. [PMID: 14756893] (Recent comprehensive review of wart and molluscum contagiosum treatments, including physical and chemical destruction, surgical removal, and biologic response modifiers to enhance the natural immune response.)

2. Squamous Intraepithelial Neoplasia & Squamous Cell Carcinoma

ESSENTIALS OF DIAGNOSIS

- Lesions are characterized by skin-colored, pink or white, flat-topped papules or plaques that may ulcerate over time.
- Lesions typically are present for a year or longer.

General Considerations

The terminology describing squamous intraepithelial neoplasia has proved to be confusing at times to the non-dermatologist. The histology of intraepithelial neoplasia is described using terminology similar to that used to describe Papanicolaou (Pap) smears and represents a spectrum from mild dysplasia of the epithelium to severe dysplasia (carcinoma in situ). The final step in this pathway is frankly invasive squamous cell carcinoma, which has metastatic capability. Vulvar involvement with intraepithelial neoplasia is referred to as vulvar intraepithelial neoplasia, and penile involvement as penile intraepithelial neoplasia. There is currently a move to use this more general terminology and steer away from the terms used to describe various types of intraepithelial neoplasia that were used in the past that included, but were not limited to, Bowen's disease, bowenoid papulosis, keratotic balanitis, and erythroplasia of Queyrat.

Multifocal intraepithelial neoplasia has been documented to occur in a slightly younger age group (20–40 years) than unifocal disease (typically >50 years) and is more likely to be linked to high-risk HPV types, primarily 16 and 18. Multifocal intraepithelial neoplasia is less likely to progress to frankly invasive squamous cell carcinoma, as compared with single lesion intraepithelial neoplasia.

Risk factors for the development of intraepithelial neoplasia include advanced age, smoking, and compromised immune status. The presence of a long-standing inflammatory dermatologic condition such as lichen sclerosis is a risk factor for the development of squamous cell carcinoma.

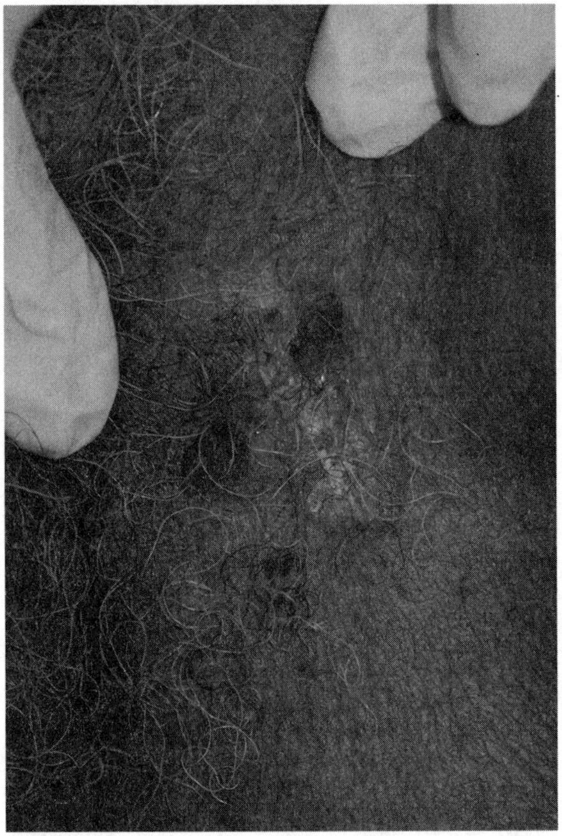

Figure 30–4. Squamous cell carcinoma in situ (vulva). (Courtesy of Lauren Hughey, MD.)

Clinical Findings

The appearance of intraepithelial neoplasia is variable, and lesions may be flesh-colored, red, or white. Multifocal intraepithelial neoplasia (formerly known as bowenoid papulosis) usually appears as multiple discrete flat-topped papules or plaques on the glans, prepuce, and penile shaft in men or the vestibule and outer labia minora in women. Single lesion intraepithelial neoplasia is usually a larger, well-defined patch or plaque with scale that may ulcerate over time. Some forms of intraepithelial neoplasia, especially after progression to squamous cell carcinoma, may appear more verrucous, become friable, and bleed easily (see Figure 30–4). Long-standing squamous cell carcinoma may result in destruction of the genitalia (see Figure 30–5).

The history is the key to the correct evaluation and diagnosis of patients with intraepithelial neoplasia and squamous cell carcinoma. The time course of the lesion is long, often on order of years. The lesions are usually asymptomatic, although some patients may complain of pruritus, with growth so slow as to often be imperceptible.

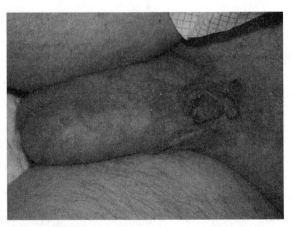

Figure 30-5. Squamous cell carcinoma resulting in destruction of the penis. (Courtesy of Jay Sizemore, MD.)

The diagnosis of intraepithelial neoplasia and squamous cell carcinoma should be confirmed by biopsy.

Differential Diagnosis

Vulvar intraepithelial neoplasia and penile intraepithelial neoplasia may be confused with condylomata acuminata. Some forms of squamous cell carcinoma may be confused with granuloma inguinale (donovanosis). Biopsy can distinguish between these etiologies.

Treatment

Treatment of vulvar intraepithelial neoplasia, penile intraepithelial neoplasia, and squamous cell carcinoma involves local destruction or removal of lesions. Patients should be referred to a dermatologist and may require referral to a gynecologist or urologist if the disease process is advanced.

INFLAMMATORY PAPULES & PLAQUES

1. Pityriasis Rosea

ESSENTIALS OF DIAGNOSIS

- *Characterized by often widespread papulosquamous, hyperpigmented, scaling lesions that develop a "Christmas tree" pattern on the back.*
- *Widespread rash is often preceded by a "herald lesion."*

General Considerations

A common rash affecting children and young adults, pityriasis rosea is often asymptomatic but distressing due to its generalized nature. The etiology is unclear but is thought to be a postviral exanthema, a hypothesis supported by the self-limited nature of the rash and the fact that cases often appear in clusters.

Clinical Findings

The first symptoms of pityriasis rosea frequently include nonspecific viral respiratory tract symptoms followed by the development of the herald patch, usually located on the trunk. The herald patch is usually 2–10 cm in diameter, ovoid, erythematous, and slightly raised with a collarette of scale at the margin.

Several days to weeks after the appearance of the herald patch, a widespread rash appears, with lesions typically

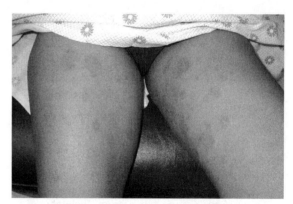

Figure 30–6. Pityriasis rosea. (Courtesy of Lauren Hughey, MD.)

concentrated on the trunk. The extremities may become involved and, rarely, the palms and soles. Genital involvement may also occur, leading the patient to present to an STD clinician for care. The generalized rash is salmon-colored and, like the herald patch, ovoid with a collarette of scale (see Figure 30–6). Lesions follow Langer lines (cleavage lines) and, when they occur on the back, result in a "Christmas tree" pattern. Pityriasis rosea may occur in an inverse form, in which the rash is concentrated on the extremities and the trunk is spared. The rash also may be localized.

Although classic pityriasis rosea is readily recognized, less typical patterns of rash distributions often present diagnostic challenges. The most common symptom reported in patients with pityriasis is pruritus. Otherwise, no systemic symptoms occur at the time the rash is present.

The diagnosis of pityriasis rosea is usually based on the clinical appearance of the rash. Biopsy is rarely necessary to make the diagnosis.

Differential Diagnosis

The herald lesion may be confused with tinea corporis, especially in the absence of the generalized rash. Secondary syphilis is an important consideration in the differential diagnosis, and a nontreponemal serologic test (eg, rapid plasma reagin [RPR] or Venereal Disease Research Laboratories [VDRL]) should be performed to rule out this etiology in sexually active individuals. (See Chapter 19 for discussion of the presentation of secondary syphilis.)

Treatment

The rash usually lasts 5–8 weeks, and the control of pruritus is the primary goal of therapy. Topical or systemic corticosteroids and a commonly used antihistamine such as hydroxyzine, 25 mg orally up to four times daily, may be used to provide symptom relief.

Stulberg DL, Wolfrey J. Pityriasis rosea. *Am Fam Physician* 2004;69:87–91. [PMID: 14727822] (General review of the diagnosis and management of this common condition.)

2. Tinea Cruris

ESSENTIALS OF DIAGNOSIS

- *Superficial dermatophyte infection most commonly caused by* Trichophyton rubrum, Trichophyton mentagrophytes, *and* Microsporum canis.
- *Rash often has a leading edge and scale.*

General Considerations

Tinea cruris is a common dermatologic condition encountered by primary care providers and STD clinicians. The condition is most commonly caused by the dermatophytes *T rubrum, T mentagrophytes,* and *M canis* and is transmitted by transfer of arthroconidia-laden scales through direct contact with an infected individual or through contact with objects that carry the infected scales. Autoinfection may also play a role.

Clinical Findings

Once infection occurs, the organism invades the stratum corneum and the terminal hair of the affected area, resulting in a rash that frequently extends from the groin to the inner thighs and perineal or perianal areas. The rash often has a leading edge and scale with central clearing, giving it an annular appearance. The primary symptom is pruritus.

The diagnosis may be confirmed by scraping the leading edge of the affected skin and adding 10–15% potassium hydroxide to the specimen. Examination under a microscope often reveals septate hyphae coursing through the squamous cells. A culture of skin scrapings, plated on Sabouraud agar media and incubated at room temperature, typically yields an organism within 2 weeks.

Differential Diagnosis

Seborrheic dermatitis, psoriasis, candidiasis, eczema, and lichen simplex chronicus are the primary dermatoses to be differentiated from tinea cruris. Eczema, unlike tinea cruris, more commonly involves the labia majora and scrotum. Psoriasis can usually be differentiated based on the presence of typical psoriatic lesions elsewhere on the body.

Treatment

Treatment of tinea cruris most often involves topical therapy with an antifungal agent such as an azole (miconazole, clotrimazole, etc), an allylamine (naftifine, terbinafine), benzylamine derivatives (butenafine), and hydroxypyridones (ciclopirox olamine). Occasionally, oral therapy may be required. Possible oral therapeutic agents include fluconazole, 150–300 mg weekly for 2–4 weeks; itraconazole, 200 mg/day for 1 week; terbinafine, 250 mg/day for 2–4 weeks; ketoconazole, 200 mg/day for 4–8 weeks; and griseofulvin, 250 mg twice daily until cured.

Gupta AK, Chaudhry M, Elewski B. Tinea corporis, tinea cruris, tinea nigra, and piedra. *Dermatol Clin* 2003;21:395–400, v. [PMID: 12956194] (Review of the diagnosis, management, and prevention of tinea infections with special attention to differential diagnosis.)

3. Contact Dermatitis

ESSENTIALS OF DIAGNOSIS

- *May be caused by allergic response to an agent or the direct irritant effect of an agent.*
- *Acute inflammation manifests as erythema, edema, vesicles, bullae, or superficial erosions with exudation.*
- *Chronic inflammation is characterized by lichenification, scaling, fissures, and hypo- or hyperpigmentation.*

General Considerations

Contact dermatitis is one of the most common non-STD genital dermatoses encountered in a patient presenting for STD evaluation. It is characterized by an inflammatory response mediated by a specific immunologic response (type IV) to an allergen (allergic contact dermatitis), or occurring as the result of a direct irritant effect of an agent on the skin (irritant contact dermatitis).

Clinical Findings

The inflammatory process may be acute or chronic at the time the patient presents for care. The acute phase of a contact reaction is often characterized by erythema, edema, vesicles, and bullae, with progression to erosions and exudation in some cases (see Figure 30–7). The

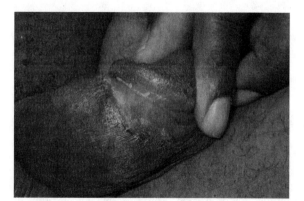

Figure 30–7. Contact dermatitis secondary to neomycin cream. (Courtesy of Lauren Hughey, MD.)

Table 30–2. Common causes of contact dermatitis affecting the genital area.

Allergic
Topical medications (eg, benzocaine, nupercaine, diphenhydramine, neomycin)
Latex (condoms, diaphragms, elastic bands)
Pessaries
Spermicides
Personal hygiene products
Nail polish
Fragrances
Irritant
Wart medications (eg, trichloroacetic acid, podophyllin, liquid nitrogen, fluorouracil, cantharidin)
Extreme heat
Bleach
Feces or urine
Water
Deodorant
Alcohol

patient may complain about irritation, itching, and burning at this time. The onset of symptoms may provide a clue to the pathophysiology of the response, because allergic contact dermatitis classically presents within 12–48 hours of antigen exposure and persists for 3–4 weeks, whereas irritant contactants may elicit symptoms within minutes to hours. However, this is not a hard and fast rule, and the differentiation between potential pathophysiologies (allergic versus irritant) involved in the process is not important in terms of determining the treatment regimen.

Although the distribution and location of a contact dermatitis rash can give important clues as to the offending agent when located in other areas of the body, the warmth and dampness that is inherently present in the genital area often lead to the contactant being spread around and the subsequent loss of any defined pattern. If the etiology of the allergic or irritative response is not elicited and the response becomes chronic, the skin often becomes lichenified and scaly, and fissures may develop. In addition, postinflammatory hyper- or hypopigmentation may result, leading to additional cosmetic concerns. Table 30–2 lists some common causes of contact dermatitis affecting the genital region.

The diagnosis of contact dermatitis is dependent on a thorough history and examination of the patient. It is important to ask about sexual and grooming habits of both the patient and his or her sex partners, because the patient's dermatologic condition may be a manifestation of a response to something the partner is using (ie, condoms or spermicide). Examining the skin outside the genital area may yield important clues as well.

Patients in whom a specific contactant cannot be implicated or who fail to respond to appropriate treatment may require referral to a dermatologist for patch testing. Patch testing is not a useful diagnostic test for irritant contact dermatitis, which is not an immunologically mediated response.

Differential Diagnosis

The differential diagnosis of contact dermatitis is broad. For chronic contact dermatitis it includes atopic dermatitis, seborrheic dermatitis, psoriasis, and fungal infections such as tinea cruris. Acute contact dermatitis may be confused with herpes simplex virus infection, pemphigus vulgaris, candidiasis, and other blistering or erosive diseases. The differentiation between these diseases may be made on the basis of history and the distribution of lesions, especially when other areas of the body are involved.

Treatment

The cornerstone of treatment of contact dermatitis is identification and removal of the offending agent. Unfortunately, the longer the process continues, the more difficult it can be to determine the etiology of the initial insult, especially as patients often self-treat and thereby may confuse the picture. If the specific contactant cannot be identified, the patient should be instructed to avoid all topical agents in the genital area except clear water and petrolatum. Unscented, mild soaps may be used in moderation if the patient feels the need to cleanse the area with something besides water.

Acute contact dermatitis may be improved through the use of cool soaks and sitz baths. Oral prednisone may speed recovery of acute allergic dermatitis at doses of 40–60 mg/day and should be tapered rapidly over 5–10 days. Topical low- and mid-potency corticosteroids, such as 1% hydrocortisone ointment twice daily or tri-amcinolone 0.1% twice daily, respectively, may be used as well, especially if inflammation is not severe. Topical corticosteroid creams and ointments may be used for chronic contact dermatitis, although long-term use of these products may lead to steroid atrophy. Finally, nighttime sedation (eg, with an antihistamine) should be employed to prevent symptoms of irritation and itching that are often noticed more at night.

McKenna JK, Leiferman KM. Dermatologic drug reactions. *Immunol Allergy Clin North Am* 2004;24:399–423, vi. [PMID: 15242718] (This review focuses on the most common or severe cutaneous drug reaction patterns. Knowledge of the clinical morphology and the most commonly associated medication aids in rapid diagnosis and institution of the appropriate therapy.)

4. Psoriasis

ESSENTIALS OF DIAGNOSIS

- *Common dermatologic condition that frequently affects the genitalia.*
- *Skin findings outside the genital region are often the key to the diagnosis.*

General Considerations

Psoriasis is a relatively common dermatologic disorder caused by an unusually rapid proliferation of the epidermis. Although the cause is unknown, there is a strong hereditary component to the disease, and approximately one third of patients report a family history. Psoriasis also is seen more frequently in HIV-infected individuals. For example, preexisting psoriasis may worsen in an individual who becomes HIV-infected or, conversely, an HIV-infected individual with a genetic predisposition may present with psoriasis for the first time. Therefore, psoriasis may be one of the first signs of HIV infection and should lead the clinician to consider HIV testing of the individual, especially when the onset of disease is rapid and the case is severe.

Clinical Findings

Psoriasis is classically manifested as red, sharply demarcated plaques with silvery scale and frequently involves the scalp, elbows, knees, gluteal cleft, and umbilicus. Approximately 50% of patients with psoriasis have typical nail findings including, but not limited, to nail pitting. Genital lesions, when present, are often not as thick as those found on other areas of the body and typically have less scale. Pruritus may or may not be present.

Inverse psoriasis, a variant with prominent genital involvement, may predominantly involve the skinfolds such as the axilla, gluteal fold, inframammary skin, umbilicus, and crural creases. The lesions of inverse psoriasis may not be as thick and well marginated, and the classic silvery scale is often less apparent. Although inverse psoriasis may be seen in immunocompetent hosts, immunodeficient individuals, particularly those who are HIV-infected, are more likely to present with this form of psoriasis.

Psoriasis often has nail manifestations, including nail pitting, "oil-drop spots" (brownish-red discoloration of the nail bed), and onycholysis. Nail findings should be sought during the clinical evaluation of the patient, because they may provide helpful diagnostic clues, especially given the often less characteristic qualities of the genital rash.

The diagnosis is often made on the basis of a consistent genital rash in the setting of characteristic lesions present elsewhere on the body. Biopsy may be necessary to confirm the diagnosis in the absence of extragenital involvement or when the genital lesions are not characteristic.

Differential Diagnosis

The differential diagnosis of genital psoriasis includes lichen simplex chronicus, vulvar intraepithelial neoplasia or penile intraepithelial neoplasia, tinea cruris, and seborrheic dermatitis. Inverse psoriasis, in particular, may be confused with a fungal infection and should be considered in the differential diagnosis when a patient has a refractory yeast infection.

Treatment

A full discussion of the treatment of psoriasis is outside the scope of this chapter. Although topical corticosteroids are first-line therapy, potent and ultrapotent formulations usually are necessary, and long-term corticosteroid use is likely. Patients should be referred to a dermatologist for management.

5. Lichen Planus

ESSENTIALS OF DIAGNOSIS

- *Disease of cell-mediated immunity characterized by many different morphologic appearances.*
- *Lesion characteristics depend on the type of epithelium involved.*

Clinical Findings

Lichen planus is a disease of cell-mediated immunity characterized by well-circumscribed violaceous or brown flat-topped papules with white striae (Wickham striae) and scale, when keratinized epithelium is involved. The glans penis or keratinized surfaces of the vulva may be involved, and lesions may have a polyhedral or an annular configuration. Mucous membrane involvement with lichen planus is marked by the presence of a fernlike or lacy reticular pattern on the vulvar vestibule, vagina, or, in instances when the mouth is involved, the buccal mucosa. Severe mucous membrane involvement, known as erosive lichen planus, may result in denudation of the epithelium and a malodorous, profuse vaginal discharge. The papular and mucous membrane variants of lichen planus may coexist in one patient.

Severe itching may be present, especially with the papular variant, whereas burning, irritation, and dyspareunia are more common with erosive lichen planus, particularly when the vaginal area is involved. Characteristic areas of involvement in lichen planus that may yield diagnostic clues during the examination include the ventral aspect of the wrist (papular lichen planus) and the buccal mucosa (fernlike white papules).

The clinical diagnosis of lichen planus is made by finding typical fernlike white papules on the mucous membranes or modified mucous membranes of the buccal mucosa or vagina. A biopsy may be necessary to confirm the diagnosis.

Differential Diagnosis

The differential diagnosis of papular genital lichen planus includes a host of dermatologic conditions, including Bowen disease (vulvar intraepithelial neoplasia or penile intraepithelial neoplasia), psoriasis, and candidiasis. Erosive lichen planus may be mistaken for lichen sclerosus, cicatricial or bullous pemphigoid, or pemphigus.

Treatment

Papular lichen planus usually resolves over the course of years. Erosive lichen planus, especially severe forms, may lead to genital scarring, obliteration of the vaginal vault, or resorption of the genitalia. Topical, and occasionally oral, corticosteroids are often necessary to control disease. The patient should be referred to a dermatologist or gynecologist for optimal management.

VESICLES, BULLAE, & EROSIONS

1. Erythema Multiforme, Stevens-Johnson Syndrome, & Toxic Epidermal Necrolysis

ESSENTIALS OF DIAGNOSIS

- *Rash characterized by targetoid lesions, with or without blisters, and frequent mucous membrane involvement.*
- *Often associated with specific medications and herpesvirus infections.*

Clinical Findings

Erythema multiforme is a dermatologic disease frequently encountered during the practice of medicine. It is characterized by targetoid lesions, with or without blisters, that tend to be in an acral distribution. Oral lesions and mucosal involvement may also be present, and it is possible for the rash to be confined to the palms, soles, and mucous membranes alone. Blisters located on mucosal surfaces erode quickly to form ulcers. Although lesions heal relatively quickly, scarring may result, especially when involvement is severe, as in Stevens-Johnson syndrome and toxic epidermal necrolysis.

Erythema multiforme may be associated with various medications and infectious processes. Recurrent erythema multiforme, for instance, is commonly associated with herpes simplex virus infections. Many experts think that erythema multiforme is on one end of a clinical spectrum, followed by Stevens-Johnson syndrome and toxic epidermal necrolysis, but this idea is controversial. Stevens-Johnson syndrome and toxic epidermal necrolysis are characterized by progressively increased mucosal involvement, widespread full-thickness epidermal necrosis and detachment (<10% for Stevens-Johnson syndrome and >30% for toxic epidermal necrolysis), and increasing mortality rates ranging from 5% for Stevens-Johnson syndrome to 40% for toxic epidermal necrolysis.

The diagnosis of erythema multiforme, Stevens-Johnson syndrome, or toxic epidermal necrolysis is made on the basis of the characteristic skin lesions, the extent of cutaneous and mucous membrane involvement, and the medication history. In the case of recurrent erythema multiforme, a history of recurrent herpes simplex virus infection is helpful. A biopsy may be necessary to confirm the diagnosis and rule out other etiologies.

Differential Diagnosis

Pemphigus vulgaris and bullous pemphigoid may be difficult to differentiate from blistering forms of erythema multiforme. Fixed drug eruption should also be considered in the differential diagnosis, although the number of lesions seen in a fixed drug eruption is usually far fewer than the number seen in erythema multiforme.

Treatment

Evaluation of patients presenting with symptoms consistent with these entities is urgent, because withdrawal of the offending drug is the most important aspect of treatment of drug-induced disease. In cases of recurrent erythema multiforme, suppression of herpes simplex virus is helpful, although the acute treatment of the virus is not as beneficial. Local care is important to prevent bacterial superinfection. The use of intravenous immune globulin has been reported to be helpful in more severe, blistering forms of erythema multiforme whereas corticosteroid use continues to be controversial.

2. Fixed Drug Eruption

ESSENTIALS OF DIAGNOSIS

- *Skin and mucous membrane lesions may be present.*
- *Lesions recur at the same sites following rechallenge with the implicated drug.*

Fixed drug eruption is a hypersensitivity reaction to a specific medication. Commonly implicated medications are listed in Table 30–3. Lesions vary in appearance depending on the type of epithelium involved. Lesions involving keratinized epithelium, for instance, appear as a well-demarcated, round, erythematous plaque whereas mucous membrane lesions blister and erode quickly. The glans penis is the most commonly involved genital site. Patients may complain of burning in the area of involvement. Rechallenge with the offending medication results in a recurrence of the lesions in the same places. The lesions frequently become more severe and

Table 30–3. Drugs commonly implicated in fixed drug eruptions.

Tetracyclines
Sulfonamides
Barbiturates
Phenolphthalein
Nonsteroidal anti-inflammatory drugs
Metronidazole
Oral contraceptives
Penicillins
Salicylates
Furosemide
Acetaminophen

result in more pronounced postinflammatory hyperpigmentation with each rechallenge.

Diagnosis is usually based on the appropriate clinical appearance in the setting of a consistent medication history. Biopsy is rarely needed but the histologic findings are characteristic. Recurrent herpes simplex virus, erosive lichen planus, and trauma are the primary etiologies to be considered in the differential diagnosis.

Withdrawal of the offending agent is the primary treatment, and lesions usually resolve within 7–10 days after removal of the agent. Local care may be necessary.

WHITE PATCHES & PLAQUES

3. Lichen Sclerosus

ESSENTIALS OF DIAGNOSIS

- *The most common genital dermatosis characterized by white or hypopigmented lesions.*
- *Women are affected more often than men.*

Lichen sclerosus is a relatively common, often asymptomatic disorder that results in hypopigmentation, thinning of the skin, and increased tissue fragility. It most commonly affects the genitalia although other sites may be involved, including the trunk and arms. The etiology is unknown, but it has been associated with autoimmune diseases.

Findings on physical examination include white papules and plaques that are covered by atrophic skin having the consistency of cigarette paper. The lesions may become confluent, and the periclitoral area, labia minora, interlabial sulcus, perineum, and perianal area may become involved (see Figure 30–8). When all of these areas are involved, a classic figure-of-eight pattern may result. In men, involvement of the prepuce and glans are most common. Pruritus is the most common symptom. Due to tissue fragility, secondary changes may occur, including ecchymoses, erosions, and excoriations—findings that may be confused with sexual abuse, especially in children. Long-standing, poorly controlled lichen sclerosus is associated with genital scarring as well as an increased risk for squamous cell carcinoma.

The differential diagnosis of lichen sclerosus includes vitiligo, postinflammatory hypopigmentation, and the end stage of other poorly controlled genital dermatoses, including lichen planus and cicatricial pemphigoid.

The diagnosis may be made on a clinical basis but should be confirmed by biopsy. Patients should be referred to a dermatologist for management.

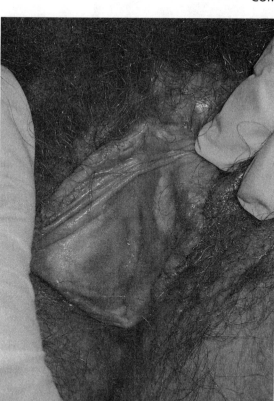

Figure 30–8. Classic hypopigmented lesions of lichen sclerosis. (Courtesy of Lauren Hughey, MD.)

ECTOPARASITIC INFECTIONS

SCABIES

ESSENTIALS OF DIAGNOSIS

- *Infestation caused by the mite* Sarcoptes scabiei, *with pruritus as its chief manifestation.*
- *Frequent involvement of the genitalia, especially the glans penis and scrotum in men.*

General Considerations

Scabies is a common dermatologic condition caused by the arthropod *Sarcoptes scabiei* and characterized by

erythematous papular skin lesions accompanied by severe pruritus. Two primary types of skin eruptions are seen: (1) erythematous papular or vesicular lesions that are associated with burrows, and (2) a more generalized papular rash.

Clinical Findings

A. SYMPTOMS AND SIGNS

The eruption from scabies is most frequently observed in the interdigital web spaces, and on the wrists, anterior axillary folds, periareolar area in women, periumbilical skin, groin, pelvic girdle, and the glans penis in men (see Figure 30–9). The head and neck are typically spared. Although the etiology is the same, scabies affecting the glans penis and scrotum may appear more nodular (ie, nodular scabies) than eruptions elsewhere on the body.

The distribution of the rash, along with a history of pruritus that is more severe at night, serve as diagnostic clues. The burrow, made by the female mite, is the most classic diagnostic sign of scabies and appears as a grayish serpiginous line that may be difficult to visualize with the unaided eye. The severe pruritus is due to hypersensitivity to *S scabiei* and, therefore, although scabies may take 4–6 weeks to become symptomatic in individuals experiencing infestation for the first time, symptom onset occurs within 24 hours during subsequent infestations. The average burden on an immunocompetent host is approximately 10–12 mites and, once removed from the host, *S scabiei* is able to survive 24–36 hours at room temperature.

The appearance of scabies in an immunocompromised host may be atypical. Crusted or "Norwegian" scabies is a variant seen more frequently in patients with advanced HIV infection, human T-lymphotrophic virus type 1 infection, various hematologic malignancies, and organ transplant recipients, as well as in those who are malnourished, mentally retarded, or receive systemic or

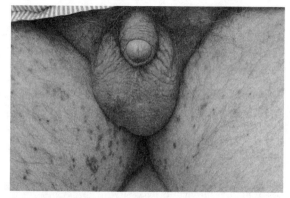

Figure 30–9. Scabies infestation involving the genitalia and upper thighs. (Courtesy of Lauren Hughey, MD.)

potent topical corticosteroids. Crusted scabies is characterized by thickened skin and hyperkeratotic warty crusts that are most predominant on the hands, feet, trunk, and scalp. However, the lesions may appear anywhere on the body. Sometimes the lesions of crusted scabies bear a resemblance to psoriasis. For this reason, new-onset psoriasis in an immunocompromised patient deserves a second look. Patients with crusted scabies may harbor millions of mites and are very infectious. Pruritus may be minimal or absent. Bacterial superinfection with typical skin pathogens (eg, *Staphylococcus aureus* and *Streptococcus pyogenes*) is a common complication of untreated scabies and, due to the compromised epidermal barrier, may lead to subsequent bacteremia and death.

B. LABORATORY FINDINGS

The diagnosis of scabies is based on a combination of clinical and laboratory findings. A presumptive diagnosis may be made based on the presence of a papular rash in the typical distribution, accompanied by pruritus that is worse at night. Parasitologic confirmation of the diagnosis may be made by removing the top of the burrow with a scalpel, placing the material on a slide containing 10% potassium hydroxide or mineral oil, and examining it under a low-power microscope for mites, eggs, egg cases, or fecal pellets.

Differential Diagnosis

Atopic dermatitis and seborrheic dermatitis are the primary conditions that may be confused with scabies. Crusted scabies may be confused with psoriasis, and insect bites may appear similar to nodular scabies.

Treatment

A. PHARMACOTHERAPY

Options for the treatment of scabies include several topical medications and one oral agent. The current treatment of choice in the United States is permethrin cream 5%. A well-tolerated pyrethroid insecticide derived from chrysanthemums, permethrin is poorly absorbed across the skin and has a low toxicity profile. Permethrin is a pregnancy category B drug and can be used in pregnant women as well as in children and infants older than 2 months of age. In adults, permethrin cream should be applied from the neck down and washed off after 8–14 hours. In children younger than 5 years of age and the elderly, scabies infestation may involve the head; therefore, topical treatment should be applied to the entire skin surface except the eyes. Patients may experience mild itching and stinging on application. At present, permethrin resistance is not commonly encountered in the *S scabiei* mite, although continued surveillance for this potential problem is necessary.

Lindane (gamma benzene hexachloride 1%), an organochloride insecticide, has fallen out of favor because of problems with resistance and toxicity. Unlike permethrin, lindane is easily systemically absorbed when topically applied, especially in patients with widespread dermatologic conditions and in infants and children. Neurotoxicity (predominantly seizures) has occurred when lindane was applied following a bath, as well as in infants, children, the elderly, patients weighing less than 50 kg, and those with widespread skin damage. In addition, rare cases of aplastic anemia have been associated with lindane use. Lindane resistance has been well-documented; however, the drug is effective in most areas of the world. In adults, 1 oz of lindane 1% lotion or 30 g of cream should be applied in a thin layer to all areas of the body from the neck down and thoroughly washed off after 8 hours. Lindane should not be used immediately after a bath or shower and should be avoided in individuals with extensive dermatitis, pregnant or lactating women, and children younger than 2 years of age.

Ivermectin, a macrocyclic lactone antibiotic, is the only oral treatment option for scabies. Ivermectin has broad-spectrum activity against both nematodes and arthropods and results in a cure rate approaching 100% when given in two doses separated by 2 weeks. The currently recommended regimen is 200 mcg/kg orally, repeated in 2 weeks. Additional doses or a combination of oral and topical treatment may be necessary to control crusted scabies. Although one study demonstrated increased mortality among elderly patients who received ivermectin, this finding has not been confirmed by subsequent reports. Ivermectin is a pregnancy class C drug and is secreted in low concentrations in breast milk; it is therefore not currently recommended for use in pregnant and lactating women. The Food and Drug Administration has not labeled this drug for use in children weighing less than 15 kg.

Patients may continue to experience symptoms for up to 2 weeks after therapy. The primary reasons for persistent symptoms include incorrect initial diagnosis, ongoing hypersensitivity to the mite antigen, sensitization to the topical medication, reinfection from untreated contacts or contaminated fomites, treatment failure due to incorrect application of the medication or inadequate penetration of the topical medication into crusted areas, and drug resistance.

When symptoms continue 2 weeks after treatment, it is often unclear what should be done. If live mites are present, the need for retreatment is straightforward. Some clinicians proceed with retreatment in the absence of live mites, as reinfection is relatively common. The drug used for retreatment should be different than the drug used for initial therapy.

B. OTHER MEASURES

Because mites may survive up to 72 hours away from the human host, environmental measures are an important adjunctive to medical therapy. Therefore, bedding and clothing should be decontaminated, either through machine washing and drying using a hot cycle or by dry-cleaning. An alternative is to remove the clothing from body contact for at least 72 hours. It is unnecessary to fumigate living areas. In addition, because scabies is transmitted through close personal contact, including sexual contact, both sexual and close personal or household contacts within the preceding 30 days should be examined and treated.

Centers for Disease Control and Prevention; Workowski KA, Berman SM. Sexually transmitted diseases guidelines, 2006. *MMWR Recomm Rep* 2006;55(RR-11):1–94. [PMID: 1688612]

Chosidow O. Clinical practices. Scabies. *N Engl J Med* 2006;354:1718–1727. [PMID: 16625010] (Up-to-date review of scabies diagnosis and management, including recommendations for the use of ivermectin.)

Flinders DC, De Schweinitz P. Pediculosis and scabies. *Am Fam Physician* 2004;69:341–348. [PMID: 147654774] (Practical review of the diagnosis and management of those infections.)

PUBIC LICE

ESSENTIALS OF DIAGNOSIS

- *An infestation caused by the crab louse,* Phthirus pubis.
- *Pubic hair is the most common hair type involved.*

Clinical Findings

Pubic lice, a common condition caused by the crab louse, *Phthirus pubis,* may lead patients to present for the evaluation of genital pruritus. The pubic louse, which is distinct from lice that infest the scalp (*Pediculus humanus capitis*) and the body (*Pediculus humanus humanus*), is 0.8–1.2 mm in length and can be seen with the naked eye (see Figure 30–10). The louse primarily infests pubic hair but may attach to adjacent hair of the chest, abdomen, legs, and buttocks. Eyelashes may also become infested.

Phthirus pubis lives for approximately 2 weeks, during which females produce about 25 ova. The nits incubate for 1 week, and the nymphs mature to adults over the subsequent 2 weeks. Because the accompanying pruritus results from hypersensitivity to louse saliva, it may be 2 or more weeks before symptoms develop following initial infestation. Bluish-gray macular lesions secondary to deep dermal hemosiderin deposition from the bites of the louse, known as *maculae cerulean,* may be noted in patients with established infestation.

Crab lice and nits may be seen with the naked eye; therefore, the presence of one or both of these forms in the hair is diagnostic. The presence of maculae cerulean may also provide a diagnostic clue.

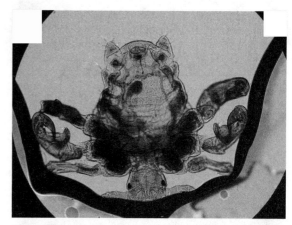

Figure 30–10. Phthirus pubis, also known as the "crab" or pubic louse. (Courtesy of Jay Sizemore, MD.)

Differential Diagnosis

Nits may be mistaken for white piedra and trichomycosis pubis. Pubic lice may cause a perifolliculitis that may be confused with bacterial folliculitis.

Treatment

Permethrin 1% cream rinse and pyrethrins with piperonyl butoxide are the primary agents recommended for the treatment of pubic lice and are the drugs of choice for pregnant or lactating women. These agents should be applied to the affected areas and washed off after 10 minutes. Resistance to pyrethrins has been documented, and the use of permethrin 5% may be necessary to overcome this problem, although experience with this higher concentration is largely anecdotal. Malathion 0.5% lotion is an alternative when treatment failure is thought to be secondary to drug resistance. The agent should be applied to the affected area for 8–12 hours and rinsed off. As noted earlier, lindane has fallen out of favor due to toxicity issues and should be used only as an alternative agent. If it is to be used, the 1% shampoo formulation should be applied for 4 minutes to the affected area and then thoroughly rinsed off. Lindane should not be used in children younger than 2 years of age or in pregnant or lactating women. Finally, ivermectin (200 mcg/kg as a single dose, repeated in 2 weeks), provides an oral alternative for therapy. When eyelash infestation is present, an occlusive agent such as petroleum jelly should be applied twice daily for 10 days. If symptoms persist after 1 week of treatment, the patient should be evaluated. If lice are found or nits are present at the hair-skin junction, retreatment should be initiated with an alternative agent.

Pubic lice are primarily spread through sexual contact. Therefore, all partners with whom the patient has had sexual contact within the previous 30 days should be evaluated and treated, and sexual contact should be avoided until all partners have successfully completed treatment and are thought to be cured. Because of the strong association between the presence of pubic lice and classic STDs, patients diagnosed with pubic lice should undergo evaluation for other STDs. Bedding and clothing should be decontaminated or removed from body contact for at least 72 hours.

Ko CJ, Elston DM. Pediculosis. *J Am Acad Dermatol* 2004;50:1–12. [PMID: 14699358] (Detailed review of the diagnosis and management of human lice infestations.)

 PRACTICE POINTS

- *Pearly penile papules are sometimes confused with condylomata acuminata. Unlike pearly penile papules, however, condylomata acuminata often have spiked tips or are contiguous at the base.*

- *If the lesion of molluscum contagiosum is incised, a central core, usually waxy, can be expressed. The central umbilication and waxy core help differentiate molluscum contagiosum from other diseases.*

- *Nail findings should be sought during the clinical evaluation of the patient with suspected genital psoriasis, because they may provide helpful diagnostic clues, especially given the often less characteristic qualities of the genital rash.*

- *Characteristic areas of involvement in lichen planus that may yield diagnostic clues during the examination include the ventral aspect of the wrist (papular lichen planus) and the buccal mucosa (fernlike white papules).*

Relevant Web Sites

[Online atlas of dermatologic lesions hosted by Johns Hopkins University; regularly updated:]
http://www.dermatlas.org

The Sexual History

31

Jeffrey D. Klausner, MD, MPH

ESSENTIAL FEATURES

- *Sexual history taking should be routine, nonjudgmental, and comprehensive.*
- *Patients should understand how an assessment of sexual behavior will help the clinician take care of the patient.*

Collecting an accurate sexual history from patients is essential to the effective clinical management of patients with sexually transmitted diseases (STDs). Many clinicians, however, do not feel comfortable or well-trained in sexual history taking. A useful sexual history is collected in a nonjudgmental manner in which the patient shares personal information about sexual behaviors that might put him or her at risk for STDs. Such information not only guides further evaluation of patients but also may provide opportunities to introduce consideration or reflection about risk-reduction measures into the provider-patient discourse. Key aspects of obtaining a sexual history are summarized in Table 31–1.

The Setting

The initiation of a sexual history requires that the patient feel comfortable and empowered. The interview should be in a private space with the patient in street clothes sitting at a level equal to or higher than the clinician. There should be no physical barrier (eg, table or desk) between the patient and clinician. The body language of the clinician should suggest openness and acceptance, with hands and legs uncrossed. The clinician should look directly at the patient, nodding encouragement, prompting, and offering periods of silence and reflection of statements.

Early in the session, the clinician should remind the patient that all the information collected during the interview is confidential and cannot be shared with others without the expressed permission of the patient. The clinician should articulate why the sexual history is valuable in a direct and noncondescending manner, using a statement such as the following: "In order for me to take better care of you, I need to ask a few personal questions about your history of sexually transmitted diseases and sexual behavior. Some of these questions may make you feel uncomfortable or may be embarrassing. That is normal and I assure you everything you tell me will stay in this room." Similarly, many patients find it reassuring to be encouraged to ask questions if they do not understand why some elements of the sexual history are being asked.

ASCERTAINMENT OF SEXUALLY TRANSMITTED DISEASE HISTORY

Many clinicians often begin by eliciting a history of STDs, because they have more experience with collecting information about a patient's medical history and believe this meets the more immediate expectations of the patient. Unfortunately, many patients assume that they have been tested for "everything" in the course of usual care. Although questions such as "In the past have you ever had a sexually transmitted disease or STD?" are typically too general for an accurate sexually history, they may be a useful introduction to the topic. Such an opening should be followed by specific questions regarding each STD: "Were you ever told by a doctor or nurse that you had or were you ever treated for syphilis? Gonorrhea? Chlamydia? Herpes? Nongonococcal urethritis [in men]? Epididymitis or infection of the testicles [in men]? Pelvic inflammatory disease or infection of the fallopian tubes or uterus [in women]? Proctitis (infection of the rectum)?"

Because many patients do not know the medical names of the diseases for which they were treated, more information can be collected if the clinician asks about syndromes; for example: "Have you ever been treated for urethral discharge? Burning on urination? Vaginal discharge? Genital sores or ulcers? Testicular pain? Lower

Table 31–1. Key aspects of obtaining a useful sexual history.

Assure confidentiality and be nonjudgmental
Remind patients of why the information is clinically
   relevant
Be specific and use nonmedical terminology
Ask about sexually transmitted diseases as well as
   preventive and sexual risk behaviors, including type
   of sex, condom use, and number and types of
   partners
Make no assumptions based on patient characteristics
Explore situations that place individuals at increased
   risk (eg, alcohol or substance use) and, together,
   develop a concrete risk-reduction plan
Use direct questions such as, "Do you have sex with
   men, women or both?"; "How many partners have
   you had in the past 2 months, past 1 year"; and "How
   do you protect yourself from getting STDs?"

---

abdominal pain? Discharge from the rectum?" If any of these questions are answered in the affirmative the approximate date and treatment received for each episode should be documented.

Patients with a history of STDs are at increased risk for future STDs, and repeat infection with the same bacterial pathogen (eg, chlamydia, gonorrhea, syphilis) is common due to reinfection from untreated sex partners or reexposure from continued sexual activity within a high-risk sexual network. As a result, a relatively recent history of a prior STD increases the likelihood of a similar diagnosis in a patient with (or without) relevant symptoms. In addition, the natural history of viral STDs such as genital warts and genital herpes includes recurrences; thus, patients with a prior history are more likely to have a similar diagnosis at the current evaluation.

Genital herpes deserves further mention. Although most studies show that between 20% and 25% of sexually active adults have been infected with herpes simplex virus type 2 (HSV-2), as defined by the serologic presence of HSV-2 antibody, most (80%) of those infected report no history of illness. When further educated, however, about the broad range of signs and symptoms of genital herpes (eg, genital pain, burning, redness, or unusual recurrent lesions), many (75%) of those without a history of herpes identify past syndromes consistent with clinical disease. The remaining 20% of those infected may have truly asymptomatic disease.

After the STD history, the clinician should proceed to inquire about relevant immunizations for STDs such as hepatitis A and B. Although many patients do not know specific dates or the number of completed doses, their responses open the way for further communication and the possible need for the initiation or completion of

immunization or an assessment of hepatitis A or B antibody status. After the history of STDs and immunizations is collected, it is recommended that information on sexual behavior be collected next.

ASSESSMENT OF SEXUAL BEHAVIOR

The clinician should begin by asking if the patient is sexually active with men, women, or both. No assumptions should be made about the gender of patients' sex partners based on a patient's marital status, occupation, attire, or mannerisms. The clinician should next ask the patient how many sex partners of either gender he or she has had in the past year. Again, assumptions about monogamy should be avoided, and the clinician should not allow his or her facial expressions, tone of voice, or body language to convey surprise or judgment in anyway. The patient should be asked how many sex partners he or she has had in the past 2 months (the average maximum incubation period for gonorrhea and chlamydia), and the date of his or her most recent sexual encounter. Some experts recommend asking about the lifetime number of sex partners, and in low- to moderate-risk populations (those with fewer than 10 lifetime partners), that number may be more predictive of current risk for specific infections than in those with substantially greater number of partners (more than 100). An alternate approach for evaluation of persons with lower numbers of sexual partners is to ask when the patient had sex with a partner different from his or her most recent sex partner.

If the patient has more than one partner, the clinician should ask the patient about the frequency of sex with each partner and attempt to classify each partner as a steady or regular partner or casual partner. Both risk for STD and use of preventative measures such as condoms tend to vary with differences in partner type. Thus, the type and number of different sex partners can have important implications for counseling about risk reduction on how to avoid STDs, including HIV infection.

The clinician should reinforce that the same questions are asked of all patients. The importance of honest answers should be emphasized, by noting that they enable the clinician to provide better care. Because different STDs are more or less likely to be transmitted by different types of sexual activity, it is crucial to discuss the type of sex the patient is having. In a patient with vaginitis, for example, oral-vaginal sex is more likely to be associated with bacterial vaginosis, whereas penile-vaginal sex is more often associated with trichomoniasis.

When asking about sexual activity the clinician must be explicit. The patient should be asked if he or she has oral sex—defining for the patient what is meant by oral sex (eg, when the patient puts his or her mouth on the partner's genitals or when the partner puts his or her mouth on the patient's genitals); if he or she has vaginal sex—again defining what is meant by vaginal sex (eg, when the patient puts his penis in his partner's vagina or the patient's partner puts his penis in her vagina), and if he or she has anal sex (eg, when the patient puts his penis in the partner's anus, rectum, or butt or the partner put his penis in the patient's anus, rectum, or butt). Lay terms for anatomic parts should be used to assure the communication is clear and responses valid.

The clinician should inquire about the use of any sex toys or sexual devices that may be associated with genital trauma or genitourinary infection. A difficult-to-diagnose dermatitis on the scrotum may be a result of the use of a genital constricting device (eg, "cock ring") that the patient may not consider disclosing unless specifically asked. Similarly, foreign bodies in the vagina can result in pain and alterations in vaginal odor and discharge that might go undetected without a thorough history.

The patient should be asked about behaviors he or she may practice to provide protection from STDs. It is usually best to ask an open-ended question about what the patient does to protect himself or herself from STDs. Prompting is often necessary; for example, suggesting several protective behaviors such as a reduction in the number of sex partners, use of condoms, lower risk sexual activity (eg, oral sex), nonpenetrative sexual activity (eg, mutual masturbation), or regular screening for STDs. Because protective behaviors often vary by sex partner type in a patient with multiple sex partners, it is important to ask about protective behaviors by different types of sex partners (ie, steady, regular, or casual).

Finally, the clinician should ask about behaviors that may increase the patient's risk for acquiring an STD; in particular, the use of alcohol or illicit drugs. Alcohol or drug intoxication is known to disinhibit individuals, and often patients engage in riskier sexual activity (eg, lack of condom use, sexual intercourse with new partners, increased number of partners, anal sex or other sexual acts that patients may not have participated in if sober) while under the influence of these substances. If identified as a potential problem, treatment for alcohol and substance use can be an effective means to reduce a patient's risk for STDs, including HIV infection. Of interest, the cost of alcohol in some communities has been shown to be directly related to gonorrhea rates, and recent increases in HIV and other STDs among gay men in the United States have been strongly associated with increases in methamphetamine use.

ASSESSMENT OF SEXUAL SATISFACTION

A complete sexual history should also include assessment of a patient's satisfaction with sexual activity and the identification or any potential problems related to the inability to initiate or maintain an erection, premature ejaculation, pain with intercourse, or lack of orgasm. Further discussion of these areas is beyond the scope of this chapter, but readers are encouraged to review materials on sexual dysfunction by Dr Raymond Rosen (Center for Sexual and Marital Health, Robert Wood Johnson Medical School, Piscataway, NJ).

Other considerations

During the interview process, the clinician should acknowledge the honesty of the patient and reinforce the value of his or her sharing of personal information. The interview should conclude with an opportunity for the patient to share any additional information; for example: "Is there anything else you'd like to tell me about your sexual history or anything else I should know to help take of you in this regard?" The patient should be asked if he or she has any questions or would like further information and reminded that sexuality is an important area of health that the patient and clinician will revisit together in the future.

As with any clinical skill, regular practice will result in continued improvement in sexual history taking. Ultimately, the ability to obtain a useful and thorough sexual history will become a key characteristic of an outstanding medical provider.

Klausner JD. Patient-centered care: A model for managing sexually transmitted infections. In: *Johns Hopkins Advanced Studies in Medicine*, vol 6. Galen Publishing, 2006:89–90. (Practical discussion of patient-centered care in the evaluation of patients with an STD.)

Nusbaum MR, Hamilton CD. The proactive sexual health history. *Am Fam Physician* 2002 ;66:1705–1712. [PMID: 12449269] (Review of sexual history taking for the general practitioner, highlighting how to make that practice routine and nonjudgmental with the ultimate goal of enhanced well-being and longevity in the patient.)

Young F. How to take a sexual history. *J Fam Health Care* 2005;15:149–151. [PMID: 16315683] (Offers a structured approach to sexual history taking and describes the often sensitive core questions that the professional may need to ask to obtain an effective sexual history and determine the risks for a particular patient.)

 PRACTICE POINTS

- The interview should be in a private space with the patient in street clothes sitting at a level equal to or higher than the clinician.
- The body language of the clinician should suggest openness and acceptance, with hands and legs uncrossed.

Appendix: Centers for Disease Control and Prevention 2006 Treatment Guidelines for Sexually Transmitted Diseases

Jeffrey D. Klausner, MD, MPH

Table 1. CDC STD treatment guidelines for adults and adolescents, 2006.

Disease	Recommended Regimens	Dose/Route	Alternative Regimens
Bacterial Vaginosis			
Adults and adolescents	Metronidazole *or*	500 mg PO twice daily for 7 d	Clindamycin, 300 mg PO twice daily for 7 d *or*
	Metronidazole gel *or*	0.75%, one full applicator (5 g) intravaginally once daily for 5 d	Clindamycin ovules, 100 g intravaginally at bed time for 3 d
	Clindamycin cream[a]	2%, one full applicator (5 g) intravaginally at bedtime for 7 d	
Pregnant women	Metronidazole *or*	500 mg PO twice daily for 7 d	
	Metronidazole *or*	250 mg PO 3 times daily for 7 d	
	Clindamycin	300 mg PO twice daily for 7 d	
Cervicitis[b]			
	Azithromycin *or*	1 g PO	
	Doxycycline[c]	100 mg PO twice daily for 7 d	
Chancroid			
	Azithromycin *or*	1 g PO	
	Ceftriaxone *or*	250 mg IM	
	Ciprofloxacin[c] *or*	500 mg PO twice daily for 3 d	
	Erythromycin base	500 mg PO 3 times daily for 7 d	
Chlamydia			
Uncomplicated, infections adults and adolescents[d]	Azithromycin *or*	1 g PO	Erythromycin base, 500 mg PO 4 times daily for 7 d *or*
	Doxycycline[c]	100 mg PO twice daily for 7 d	Erythromycin ethylsuccinate, 800 mg PO 4 times daily for 7 d *or*
			Ofloxacin,[c] 300 mg PO twice daily for 7 d *or*
			Levofloxacin,[c] 500 mg PO once daily for 7 d

Condition / Drug	Dose	Alternative
Pregnant women[e] Azithromycin *or* Amoxicillin	1 g PO 500 mg PO 3 times daily for 7 d	Erythromycin base, 500 mg PO 4 times daily for 7 d *or* Erythromycin base, 250 mg PO 4 times daily for 14 d *or* Erythromycin ethylsuccinate, 800 mg PO 4 times daily for 7 d *or* Erythromycin ethylsuccinate, 400 mg PO 4 times daily for 14 d

Epididymitis[b]

Condition / Drug	Dose	Alternative
Likely due to gonorrhea or chlamydia Ceftriaxone *plus* Doxycycline	250 mg IM 100 mg PO twice daily for 10 d	
Likely due to enteric organisms Ofloxacin[f] *or* Levofloxacin[f]	300 mg PO twice daily for 10 d 500 mg PO once daily for 10 d	

Gonorrhea[g]

Condition / Drug	Dose	Alternative
	Fluoroquinolones are no longer recommended for treatment of gonococcal infections in men who have sex with men or in California or Hawaii because of increasing resistance to that class of drugs. If fluoroquinolones are the only drug available and must be used, "test-of-cure" after treatment is recommended.	
Uncomplicated infections, adults and adolescents Ceftriaxone *or* Cefixime[h,i] *plus* Treatment for chlamydia if chlamydial infection has not been ruled out	125 mg IM 400 mg PO	Spectinomycin, 2 g IM *or* Single-dose cephalosporin regimens; cefpodoxime, 400 mg PO, or cefuroxime axetil, 1 g PO, may be additional alternatives *or* Single-dose quinolone regimens (see note above) include ciprofloxacin, 500 mg PO (preferred); ofloxacin, 400 mg PO; levofloxacin, 250 mg PO; gatifloxacin, 400 mg PO; norfloxacin, 800 mg PO; or lomefloxacin, 400 mg PO
Pharyngeal infections Ceftriaxone *or* Ciprofloxacin *plus* Treatment for chlamydia, if chlamydial infection has not been ruled out	125 mg IM 500 mg PO	

(Continued)

235

Table 1. CDC STD treatment guidelines for adults and adolescents, 2006. (*Continued*)

Disease	Recommended Regimens	Dose/Route	Alternative Regimens
Pregnant women	Ceftriaxone *plus* Treatment for chlamydia, if chlamydial infection has not been ruled out	125 mg IM	Single-dose cephalosporin *or* Spectinomycin, 2 g IM
Herpes Simplex Virus[j]			
First clinical episode	Acyclovir *or* Acyclovir *or* Famciclovir *or* Valacyclovir	400 mg PO 3 times daily for 7–10 d 200 mg PO 5 times daily for 7–10 d 250 mg PO 3 times daily for 7–10 d 1 g PO twice daily for 7–10 d	
Episodic therapy for recurrent episodes	Acyclovir *or* Acyclovir *or* Acyclovir *or* Famciclovir *or* Famciclovir *or* Valacyclovir *or* Valacyclovir	400 mg PO 3 times daily for 5 d 800 mg PO twice daily for 5 d 800 mg PO 3 times daily for 2 d 125 mg PO twice daily for 5 d 1000 mg PO twice daily for 1 d 500 mg PO twice daily for 3 d 1 g PO once daily for 5 d	
Suppressive therapy	Acyclovir *or* Famciclovir *or* Valacyclovir *or* Valacyclovir	400 mg PO twice daily 250 mg PO twice daily 500 mg PO once daily 1 g PO once daily	
HIV co-infected[k]			
Episodic therapy for recurrent episodes	Acyclovir *or*	400 mg PO 3 times daily for 5–10 d	

	Famciclovir	500 mg PO twice daily for 5–10 d
	or	
	Valacyclovir	1 g PO twice daily for 5–10 d
Suppressive therapy	Acyclovir	400–800 mg PO 2–3 times daily
	or	
	Famciclovir	500 mg PO twice daily
	or	
	Valacyclovir	500 mg PO twice daily
Human Papillomavirus		
External genital warts	***Patient applied***	
	Podofilox[l] 0.5% solution or gel	Twice daily for 3 d, followed by 4 d with no therapy, for a total of 4 wk
	or	
	Imiquimod,[m] 5% cream	Once daily at bedtime, 3 times weekly for up to 16 wk
	Provider administered	
	Cryotherapy	Repeat 1–2 wk
	or	
	Podophyllin[l] resin 10—25% in tincture of benzoin	Apply, air dry, repeat weekly
	or	
	Trichloroacetic acid (TCA)	Apply, air dry, repeat weekly
	or	
	Bichloroacetic acid (BCA) 80–90%	Apply, air dry, repeat weekly
	or	
	Surgical removal	Tangential scissor excision, tangential shave excision, curettage, or electrosurgery
Mucosal genital warts	Cryotherapy	Vaginal, urethral, and anal
	or	
	TCA or BCA 80–90%	Vaginal and anal
	or	
	Podophyllin[l] resin 10–25% in tincture of benzoin	Urethral
	or	
	Surgical removal	Anal
Lymphogranuloma Venereum		
	Doxycycline[c]	100 mg PO twice daily for 21 d
		Erythromycin base, 500 mg PO 4 times daily for 21 d

The right-most column also lists:

Intralesional interferon
or
Laser surgery

237

(Continued)

Table 1. CDC STD treatment guidelines for adults and adolescents, 2006. (*Continued*)

Disease	Recommended Regimens	Dose/Route	Alternative Regimens
Nongonococcal Urethritis[b]			
	Azithromycin	1 g PO	Erythromycin base, 500 mg PO 4 times daily for 7 d
	or		*or*
	Doxycycline	100 mg PO twice daily for 7 d	Erythromycin ethylsuccinate, 800 mg PO 4 times daily for 7 d
			or
			Ofloxacin, 300 mg PO twice daily for 7 d
			or
			Levofloxacin, 500 mg PO once daily for 7 d
Pelvic Inflammatory Disease[b]			
	Parenteral[n]		***Parenteral***[n]
	Either cefotetan	2 g IV q 12 h	*Either* ofloxacin,[c,f] 400 mg IV q 12 h
	or		with or without
	Cefoxitin	2 g IV q 6 h	Metronidazole, 500 mg IV q 8 h
	plus		*or*
	Doxycycline[c]	100 mg PO or IV q 12 h	Levofloxacin,[c,f] 500 mg IV once daily
	or		with or without
	Clindamycin	900 mg IV q 8 h	Metronidazole, 500 mg IV q 8 h
	plus		*or*
	Gentamicin	2 mg/kg IV or IM followed by 1.5 mg/kg IV or IM q 8 h	Ampicillin/sulbactam, 3 g IV q 6 h
			plus
			Doxycycline,[c] 100 mg PO or IV q 12 h
	Oral/IM		***Oral***
	• Levofloxacin[c,f]	500 mg PO once daily for 14 d	Either ofloxacin,[c,f] 400 mg PO twice daily for 14 d
	or		*or*
	Ofloxacin[c,f]	400 mg PO twice daily for 14 d	Levofloxacin,[c,f] 500 mg PO once daily for 14 d
	with or without		*plus*
	Metronidazole	500 mg PO twice daily for 14 d	Metronidazole, 500 mg PO twice daily for 14 d
	• Either ceftriaxone or	250 mg IM	
	Cefoxitin	2 g IM	
	with		
	Probenecid	1 g PO	
	plus		
	Doxycycline[c]	100 mg PO twice daily for 14 d	
	with or without		
	Metronidazole	500 mg PO twice daily for 14 d	

Syphilis[o]

Primary, secondary, and early latent	Benzathine penicillin G	2.4 million units IM as a single dose	Doxycycline, 100 mg PO twice daily for 14 d *or* Tetracycline, 500 mg PO 4 times daily for 14 d *or* Ceftriaxone, 1 g IM or IV once daily for 8–10 d *or* Azithromycin, 2-g single oral dose (All of the above should be used with caution and close follow-up)
Late latent and unknown duration	Benzathine penicillin G	7.2 million units, administered as 3 doses of 2.4 million units IM, at 1-wk intervals	Doxycycline, 100 mg PO twice daily for 28 d *or* Tetracycline 500 mg PO 4 times daily for 28 d (All of the above should be used with caution and close follow-up)
Neurosyphilis[p]	Aqueous crystalline penicillin G	18–24 million units daily, administered as 3–4 million units IV q 4 h for 10–14 d	Procaine penicillin G, 2.4 million units IM once daily for 10–14 d *plus* Probenecid, 500 mg PO 4 times daily for 10–14 d

Pregnant women[q]

Primary, secondary, and early latent	Benzathine penicillin G	2.4 million units IM as a single dose	None
Late latent and unknown duration	Benzathine penicillin G	7.2 million units, administered as 3 doses of 2.4 million units IM, at 1-wk intervals	None
Neurosyphilis[p]	Aqueous crystalline penicillin G	18–24 million units daily, administered as 3–4 million units IV q 4 h for 10–14 d	Procaine penicillin G, 2.4 million units IM once daily for 10–14 d *plus* Probenecid, 500 mg PO 4 times daily for 10–14 d

HIV co-infected

Primary, secondary and early latent	Benzathine penicillin G	2.4 million units IM	Doxycycline, 100 mg PO twice daily for 14 d *or* Tetracycline, 500 mg PO 4 times daily for 14 d *or* Ceftriaxone, 1 g IM or IV once daily for 8–10 d *or* Azithromycin, 2-g single oral dose (All of the above should be used with caution and close follow-up)

(Continued)

Table 1. CDC STD treatment guidelines for adults and adolescents, 2006. (*Continued*)

Disease	Recommended Regimens	Dose/Route	Alternative Regimens
Late latent, and unknown duration[q] with normal CSF examination	Benzathine penicillin G	7.2 million units, administered as 3 doses of 2.4 million units IM, at 1-wk intervals	None
Neurosyphilis[p,q]	Aqueous crystalline penicillin G	18—24 million units daily, administered as 3—4 million units IV q 4 h for 10—14 d	Procaine penicillin G, 2.4 million units IM once daily for 10—14 d *plus* Probenecid, 500 mg PO 4 times daily for 10—14 d
Trichomoniasis[r]	Metronidazole Tinidazole	2 g PO 2 g PO	Metronidazole, 500 mg PO twice daily for 7 d

[a]Might weaken latex condoms and diaphragms because oil based; not recommended in pregnancy.

[b]Testing for gonorrhea and chlamydia is recommended because a specific diagnosis may improve compliance and partner management. These infections are reportable in all states.

[c]Contraindicated for pregnant and nursing women.

[d]Annual screening for women aged 25 years or younger. Nucleic acid amplification tests (NAATs) are recommended. Women with chlamydia should be rescreened 3–4 mo after treatment.

[e]"Test-of-cure" follow-up is recommended in pregnancy.

[f]If gonorrhea is documented, change to a medication regimen that does not include a fluoroquinolone. "Test-of-cure" follow-up is recommended to ensure patient does not have untreated, resistant gonorrhea infection.

[g]Co-treatment for Chlamydia trachomatis infection is indicated unless chlamydia has been ruled out using sensitive technology or 2-g azithromycin dose is used.

[h]Cefixime is available in liquid formulation only.

[i]For patients with significant anaphylaxis-type (IgE-mediated) allergies to penicillin, in whom the use of cephalosporins is a concern, or patients with allergies to cephalosporins, spectinomycin (2 g IM) or azithromycin (2 g PO) may be used.

[j]Counseling about natural history, asymptomatic shedding, and sexual transmission is an essential component of herpes management.

[k]If lesions persist or recur while receiving antiviral treatment, antiviral resistance should be suspected and a viral isolate should be obtained for sensitivity testing.

[l]Contraindicated during pregnancy.

[m]Safety in pregnancy has not been well established.

[n]Discontinue 24 h after patient improves clinically and continue with oral therapy for a total of 14 d.

[o]Benzathine penicillin G (the generic name) is the recommended treatment for syphilis not involving the central nervous system and is available in multiple formulations. Bicillin L-A (or long acting; the trade name) contains only benzathine penicillin G. Other combination products, such as Bicillin C-R, should not be used to treat syphilis.

[p]Some specialists recommend 2.4 million units of benzathine penicillin G weekly for 1–3 wk after completion of neurosyphilis treatment. Although doxycycline may be used to treat late latent syphilis in penicillin-allergic patients, this drug is not recommended for the treatment of neurosyphilis.

[q]Patients allergic to penicillin should be treated with penicillin after desensitization.

[r]If reinfection is ruled out and persistence of trichomoniasis is documented, evaluate for metronidazole-resistant Trichomonas vaginalis. Consultation and T vaginalis suscepti-bility testing is available from the CDC at 770-488-4115.

CDC, Centers for Disease Control and Prevention; CSF, cerebrospinal fluid; STD, sexually transmitted disease.

Based on Centers for Disease Control and Prevention; Workowski KA, Berman SM. Sexually transmitted diseases treatment guidelines, 2006. MMWR Recomm Rep 2006;55(RR-11):1–94.

Table 2. Highlights from the CDC STD treatment guidelines, 2006.

Topic	CDC Comment	Note
Diagnosis of cervicitis	*Criteria:* 1. Purulent or mucopurulent endocervical exudate visible in endocervical canal or on an endocervical swab specimen, and 2. Sustained cervical bleeding easily induced by gentle passage of a cotton swab through the cervical os	Assess for pelvic inflammatory disease and test for *Chlamydia trachomatis, Neisseria gonorrhoeae*, bacterial vaginosis, and trichomoniasis
Diagnosis of trichomoniasis	Diagnostic tests include microscopy, Osom *Trichomonas* Rapid Test, immunochromatographic capillary flow dipstick, Affirm VPIII, and culture	Commercially available assays may be more costly; culture remains the "gold standard"
Treatment of trichomoniasis	*Additional treatment regimen:* tinidazole 2-g PO single dose	Avoid alcohol during and up to 72 h after treatment with tinidazole
Treatment of chlamydia in pregnancy	Clinical experience and studies suggest that azithromycin (1 g PO as a single dose) is safe and effective	Pregnant women with chlamydial infection should undergo "test-of-cure" >3 wk after treatment
Role of *Mycoplasma genitalium* in urethritis	*Ureaplasma urealyticum* and *M genitalium* have been implicated as etiologic agents of nongonococcal urethritis in some studies; however, detection of these organisms is frequently difficult	Nucleic acid amplification tests (NAATs) may be available for *M genitalium* diagnosis
Role of *M genitalium* in cervicitis	Limited data indicate that infection with *M genitalium* and bacterial vaginosis as well as frequent douching may cause cervicitis	
Treatment of *M genitalium*	Infections with *M genitalium* may respond better to azithromycin than to tetracyclines	
Management of lymphogranuloma venereum proctocolitis in men who have sex with men	*Recommended treatment regimen:* doxycycline, 100 mg PO twice daily for 21 d Sex partners within 60 d should be examined, tested, and treated with standard chlamydia regimen	
CSF examination in evaluation of neurosyphilis	Patients who have syphilis and who demonstrate any of the following criteria should undergo prompt CSF examination: · Neurologic or ophthalmic signs or symptoms · Evidence of active tertiary syphilis (eg, aortitis and gumma) · Treatment failure, or · HIV infection with late latent syphilis or syphilis of unknown duration	
Emergence of azithromycin-resistant *Treponema pallidum*	Several cases of azithromycin treatment failure have been reported, and resistance to azithromycin has been documented in several geographic areas	Azithromycin is not recommended in the treatment of syphilis

(Continued)

Table 2. Highlights from the CDC STD treatment guidelines, 2006. (Continued)

Topic	CDC Comment	Note
Increase in fluoroquinolone-resistant N gonorrhoeae in men who have sex with men	In 2004, quinolone-resistant N gonorrhoeae was more common among men who have sex with men than among heterosexual men (23.9% vs 2.9%)	Quinolones should not be used in the treatment of gonorrhea among men who have sex with men
Sexual transmission of hepatitis C	Findings indicate that sexual transmission of hepatitis C virus is possible but inefficient	
Use of postexposure prophylaxis after sexual assault	*Recommended:* • Postexposure hepatitis B vaccination • Empiric antimicrobial regimen for chlamydia, gonorrhea, trichomoniasis, and bacterial vaginosis (see next column) • Emergency contraception, if pregnancy is possible • Postexposure prophylaxis for HIV infection, depending on characteristics of the assailant and the assault	*Suggested antimicrobial regimen after sexual assault:* Ceftriaxone, 125 mg IM as a single dose *plus* Metronidazole, 2 g PO as a single dose *plus* Azithromycin, 1 g PO as a single dose *or* Doxycycline, 100 mg PO twice daily for 7 d
STD prevention approaches	*Recommended:* • Abstinence and reduction in number of sex partners • Preexposure vaccination • Male condoms • Female condoms Emergency contraception is effective; providers should counsel women concerning the option for emergency contraception, if indicated, and provide emergency contraception in a timely fashion	*Not recommended:* • Vaginal spermicide and diaphragms • Condoms and N-9 vaginal spermicides • Rectal use of N-9 spermicides • Non—barrier contraception, surgical sterilization, and hysterectomy (offer no protection against STDs)
Partner management	When medical evaluation, counseling, and treatment of a partner cannot be done because of the particular circumstances of a patient or partner or because of resource limitations, other partner management options can be considered; one option is patient-delivered therapy Patient-delivered therapy can prevent reinfection of the index case and has been associated with a higher likelihood of partner notification, compared with unassisted patient referral of partners	Patient-delivered therapy is a partner management option in which partners of infected patients are treated without previous medical evaluation or prevention counseling

CDC, Centers for Disease Control and Prevention; CSF, cerebrospinal fluid; N-9, nonoxynol-9; STD, sexually transmitted disease.

Index

Note: Page numbers followed by "*f*" denote figures; those followed by "*t*" denote tables